P9-CPY-511

ACSM's Introduction to
Exercise Science

Jeffrey A. Potteiger, PhD, FACSM
Director, Center for Health Enhancement
Professor, Department of Kinesiology and Health
Miami University
Oxford, Ohio

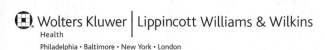
Wolters Kluwer | Lippincott Williams & Wilkins
Health
Philadelphia • Baltimore • New York • London
Buenos Aires • Hong Kong • Sydney • Tokyo

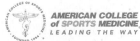
AMERICAN COLLEGE
of SPORTS MEDICINE
LEADING THE WAY

Acquisitions Editor: Emily Lupash
Product Manager: Andrea M. Klingler
Marketing Manager: Christen Murphy
Designer: Doug Smock
ACSM's Publications Committee Chair: Jeffrey L. Roitman, Ed. D., FACSM
ACSM's Group Publisher: Kerry O'Rourke
Compositor: SPi Technologies

First Edition

Copyright © 2011 Lippincott Williams & Wilkins, a Wolters Kluwer business

351 West Camden Street
Baltimore, MD 21201

530 Walnut Street
Philadelphia, PA 19106

Printed in China

All rights reserved. This book is protected by copyright. No part of this book may be reproduced or transmitted in any form or by any means, including as photocopies or scanned-in or other electronic copies, or utilized by any information storage and retrieval system without written permission from the copyright owner, except for brief quotations embodied in critical articles and reviews. Materials appearing in this book prepared by individuals as part of their official duties as U.S. government employees are not covered by the above-mentioned copyright. To request permission, please contact Lippincott Williams & Wilkins at 530 Walnut Street, Philadelphia, PA 19106, via email at permissions@lww.com, or via website at lww.com (products and services).

Library of Congress Cataloging-in-Publication Data
Potteiger, Jeffrey Aaron, 1958–
   ACSM's introduction to exercise science / Jeffrey A. Potteiger.—1st ed.
      p. ; cm.
   Includes bibliographical references and index.
   ISBN 978-0-7817-7811-4 (alk. paper)
 1. Exercise—Physiological aspects. 2. Sports medicine. 3. Human mechanics. I. American College of Sports Medicine.
II. Title. III. Title: Introduction to exercise science.
   [DNLM: 1. Sports Medicine. 2. Exercise. 3. Physical Fitness. QT 261 P865a 2011]
   QP301.P637   2011
   612'.044—dc22

                                                                                                2009043245

DISCLAIMER
Care has been taken to confirm the accuracy of the information present and to describe generally accepted practices. However, the authors, editors, and publisher are not responsible for errors or omissions or for any consequences from application of the information in this book and make no warranty, expressed or implied, with respect to the currency, completeness, or accuracy of the contents of the publication. Application of this information in a particular situation remains the professional responsibility of the practitioner; the clinical treatments described and recommended may not be considered absolute and universal recommendations.

The authors, editors, and publisher have exerted every effort to ensure that drug selection and dosage set forth in this text are in accordance with the current recommendations and practice at the time of publication. However, in view of ongoing research, changes in government regulations, and the constant flow of information relating to drug therapy and drug reactions, the reader is urged to check the package insert for each drug for any change in indications and dosage and for added warnings and precautions. This is particularly important when the recommended agent is a new or infrequently employed drug.

Some drugs and medical devices presented in this publication have Food and Drug Administration (FDA) clearance for limited use in restricted research settings. It is the responsibility of the health care provider to ascertain the FDA status of each drug or device planned for use in their clinical practice.

To purchase additional copies of this book, call our customer service department at **(800) 638-3030** or fax orders to **(301) 223-2320**. International customers should call **(301) 223-2300**.

Visit Lippincott Williams & Wilkins on the Internet: **http://www.lww.com**. Lippincott Williams & Wilkins customer service representatives are available from 8:30 am to 6:00 pm, EST.

9 8 7 6 5 4 3 2 1

*To Ellen, Tate, and Caroline for their limitless love
and never-ending support*

Preface

Exercise science is an umbrella term used to describe the study of numerous aspects of physical activity, exercise, sport, and athletic performance that have the common characteristic of movement and the adaptations that occur as a result of physical activity and regular exercise. Exercise science broadly includes the physiological, psychological, nutritional, motor, and functional adaptations and responses to physical activity, exercise, sport, and athletic competition. Physical activity and exercise play very important roles in promoting overall health, healthy living, and reducing the risk for numerous lifestyle diseases. Proper regular exercise and physical training are crucial for maximizing individual and team performance in sports and athletic competitions and for reducing the risk of injury. Exercise science students must therefore be well prepared for understanding how human movement assists individuals in their pursuit of good health and successful sport performance.

ACSM's Introduction to Exercise Science provides an overview of the components important to developing a solid understanding and appreciation of all aspects of exercise science. This book is designed for first year students in exercise science or any of the related areas, including athletic training and sports medicine, clinical and sport biomechanics, clinical exercise physiology, exercise and sport nutrition, exercise physiology, exercise and sport psychology, and motor control and learning. The 12 chapter topics and content were chosen to represent both the foundational and the broad-based professional areas and issues of exercise science.

FEATURES

Learning Objectives at the beginning of each chapter highlight concepts of importance. Boxes throughout the chapters also highlight important **terms and their definitions**, helping students to identify immediately terminology that may be new or unfamiliar. **Interviews** with prominent exercise science professionals are featured within the chapters; these individuals provide helpful insight into proper preparation for developing a successful professional career. **Critical Thinking Questions** are placed throughout the chapters as well to help facilitate discussion and deeper application of concepts. **Review Questions** at the end of each chapter provide a brief review of the material covered.

SUPPLEMENTAL MATERIALS

Supplemental materials for both students and instructors are available at http://thepoint.lww.com/ACSMIntroExSci.

Available for instructors are

- PowerPoint Lecture Outlines
- Image Bank, including all figures and tables from the text

- Brownstone Test Generator
- Full Text Online

For students, Full Text Online, flashcards of key terms in the text, and answers to the in-text review questions are available.

This book is designed to provide beginning students with an overview of the foundational content within the areas of exercise science as well as options available for professional career opportunities, career development, and employment. A look into the future focuses on several key paths that exercise science may possibly take in the 21st century. We hope that this book provides the students with valuable insight as they explore the wonderful world of exercise science.

Jeffrey A. Potteiger

Acknowledgments

I wish to extend a heartfelt thank you to all my professional colleagues who shared their thoughts and insights with me about the content and direction of this textbook. I would like to specifically acknowledge Jeffrey L. Roitman and D. Mark Robertson, for their support and belief in me to complete this project, and Ellen E. Adams, for her critical review of the material. Finally, a special thank you is extended to Randal P. Claytor for his thoughtfulness and unending ability to listen.

Reviewers

Rudy Aguilar, MEd, CSCS, ATC
Head Athletic Trainer
Kinesiology, Health & Athletics
Pasadena City College
Pasadena, CA

Scott R. Collier, PhD
Assistant Professor
Appalachian State University
Boone, NC

Shawn H. Dolan, PhD, RD, CSSD
Assistant Professor
Department of Kinesiology
California State University
Long Beach, CA

Craig A. Harms, PhD
Associate Professor
Department of Kinesiology
Kansas State University
Manhattan, KS

Susan Keith
Associate Professor
Department of Kinesiology
Angelo State University
San Angelo, TX

Mark Knoblauch, MS ATC, LAT, CSCS
Department of Health and Human Performance
University of Houston
Houston, TX

Contents

1

Introduction to Exercise Science

After completing this chapter you will be able to:

1. Explain the importance of exercise science as it relates to enhancing our understanding of physical activity, exercise, sport, and athletic performance.
2. Identify the different disciplines, subdisciplines, and specialty areas of exercise science, and describe how they relate to exercise science.
3. Describe the key highlights in the historic development of exercise science.
4. Identify the key influential accomplishments of the American College of Sports Medicine for promoting exercise science.
5. Name the general and advanced undergraduate coursework necessary for a career in exercise science or a related healthcare profession.
6. Define the different types of research conducted by exercise science professionals.

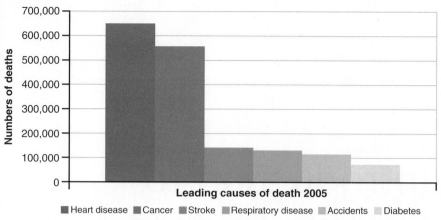

FIGURE 1.1 ▼ Common causes of mortality in the United States for the year 2005 (24).

Physical activity, exercise, sport, and athletic performance are integral parts of so many societies and cultures around the world that it is hard to imagine a time when people were not physically active and participating in competitive games and sport. Our earliest recordings of history mention the importance of what we have come to know as health and physical activity. For example, many of the Greek philosopher Aristotle's teachings mentioned of the importance of physical health to a good life (9). Indeed, current research and knowledge support the role of being physically active and participating in regular exercise for promoting good health and decreasing the risk of **morbidity** and **mortality** (2,5,10,32). Despite this information, the morbidity and mortality rates from lifestyle-related diseases are at an all-time high (19,28). Figure 1.1 shows the most common causes of mortality in the United States for the year 2005 (26). For many of these diseases, there is a lifestyle component that can be significantly affected by regular participation in physical activity and exercise.

In developed countries of the world, the changing work and living environment has for many people resulted in a decrease in physical labor and activity, but at the same time an increase in the opportunity for participation in leisure time activities (12,14). Many individuals in the general population, however, do not exercise enough or are insufficiently physically active to promote good health and reduce disease risk (3). For example, Figure 1.2 shows the percentage of individuals by age group who were physically inactive during leisure time for the years 2002–04 (38). Partly as a result of the high levels of physical inactivity, the United States and other countries have experienced a dramatic increase in the number of individuals who are overweight or obese, prompting healthcare experts to declare an obesity epidemic (35). Figure 1.3 illustrates the age-adjusted

Morbidity The relative incidence of a particular disease.
Mortality The rate of death.

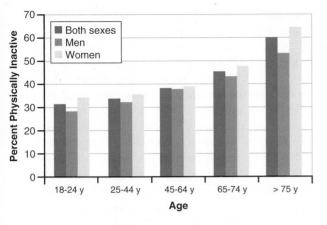

FIGURE 1.2 ▼ Percentage of individuals who are physically inactive during leisure time for 2002 to 04 (38).

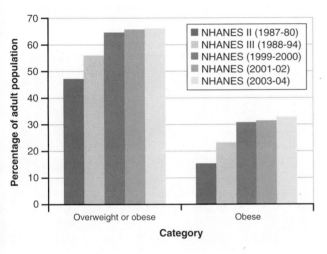

FIGURE 1.3 ▼ Age-adjusted prevalence of overweight and obesity among U.S. adults, aged 20 to 74 years as reported by the National Health and Nutrition Examination Surveys (18,31).

prevalence of overweight and obesity among the U.S. adults aged 20 to 74 years as reported by the National Health and Nutrition Examination Surveys (18,31). There has also been a rise in other diseases and health conditions linked to a lack of physical activity and exercise. It is also apparent that individuals who exhibit poor eating habits have an increased risk of cardiovascular disease and some forms of cancer (20). Exercise science professionals have an extremely important responsibility in helping individuals understand the importance of physical activity and exercise in promoting fitness and good health, the benefits of improved nutrition, the best practice for preventing and recovering from injury, and how to design and implement personal fitness and exercise programs.

Throughout history, physical prowess and the ability to succeed in sport and athletic competition have been highly valued by people and societies. The early Greeks held their successful athletes in high regard. The importance of athletic competition was so revered that regularly scheduled Olympic Games were held in Greece from 776 BC until 393 AD (33). Early sports and athletic competitions primarily involved individual events such as wrestling and running and often emerged from activities related to obtaining food or personal survival (e.g., javelin throwing and boxing) (17). As societies and cultures continued to develop, sports and games that often started from activities initiated in the rural working class became increasingly popular (17). In modern society, we have the Winter and Summer Olympic Games (Figure 1.4) alternating on a 2 year cycle, as well as regularly scheduled national and international competitions. Professional, college, and high school sporting events are an integral part of our social fabric binding communities, societies, and cultures together. There are more opportunities for individuals of all ages to participate in sporting events and athletic competitions than ever before. For example, the number of individuals participating in high school athletics has increased for 18 consecutive years with over 7.3 million students participating in high school sports and athletics in 2006–07 (Figure 1.5) (29). This trend has continued at the college and university level. According to the National Collegiate Athletic Association (NCAA), the number of students participating in intercollegiate sports increased by almost 150,000 participants from the 1982 to 2006 academic year (Figure 1.6) (11). Countless other individuals

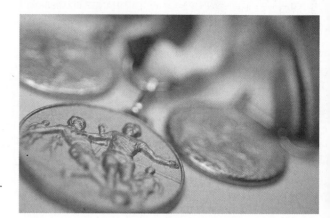

FIGURE 1.4 ▼ The Olympic Games are held every 2 years. (Photo from Medioimages/ Photodisc/GettyImages.)

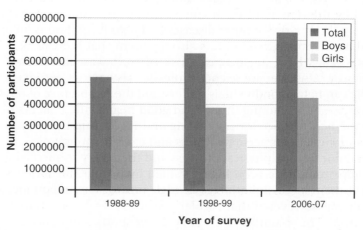

FIGURE 1.5 ▼ Participants in high school athletics (29).

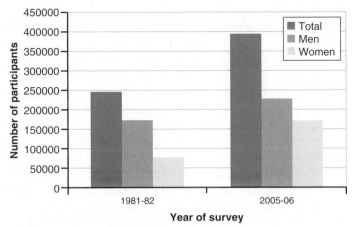

FIGURE 1.6 ▼ Individuals participating in NCAA-sponsored inter-collegiate athletics (11).

are participating in professional, amateur, and recreational sport and athletic competitions each year.

Athletes are continuously looking for exercise science professionals to assist them in developing an effective training program, the safest equipment, a sound nutrition program, and the best treatment for their acute and chronic injuries: all in an effort to improve their performance. Unfortunately, the desire and pressure to succeed has created a culture of win at all cost for some individuals leading to performance-enhancing drug use and other forms of cheating in competition. For example, recent research has indicated that as many as 5.4% of male and 2.9% of female adolescents have used androgenic anabolic steroids (25). Each year, athletes of all ages are disqualified from participation and competition in sports because of using performance-enhancing drugs.

The benefits derived from regular participation in physical activity and exercise and involvement in sport and athletic competition are important to us personally and as a society. Individuals can gain improvements in physical and mental health, and society gains from reduced levels of lifestyle diseases and illness. Exercise science professionals play an important role in promoting individual and population health, physical activity, and exercise, and contributing to successful performance in sport and athletic competition. The professionals who constitute exercise science include exercise and clinical exercise physiologists, athletic trainers, sports medicine physicians, exercise and sport nutritionists, clinical and sport biomechanists, exercise and sport psychologists, and motor behavior specialists. These professionals contribute to promoting good health, reducing disease risk, and assisting those individuals participating in sports in a wide variety of ways. To understand how exercise science and the associated professionals who came to be such an integral component of physical activity, exercise, sport, and athletic participation, it is important to provide a clear definition of exercise science.

WHAT IS EXERCISE SCIENCE?

Many scholars and professionals have a difficult time agreeing on a definition of exercise science. For the purpose of this textbook, **exercise science** will be used to describe the study of numerous aspects of physical activity, exercise, sport, and athletic performance that have the common characteristic of movement and the adaptations that occur as a result of physical activity and regular exercise. The term exercise science has evolved primarily from the disciplines of physical education and exercise physiology to be much more inclusive of related areas. Exercise science broadly includes the nutritional, physiologic, psychological, and functional adaptations to movement and sport. Over time we have seen exercise science become part of our educational and professional activities so that we now have Departments of Exercise Science in our colleges and universities, curricular programs of exercise science that can gain accreditation from national organizations, and students graduating with undergraduate and/or graduate degrees in exercise science. Kinesiology is another term commonly used to describe the study of movement. Kinesiology, however, is generally used to reflect a more broadly defined study of movement including the components of exercise science and the additional areas of physical education, sport history, and sport sociology. Kinesiology also often includes areas of study such as sport management, sport marketing, and sport journalism. Exercise science is more commonly used to reflect study, preparation, and professional practice in more basic science– and applied science– based areas that are specifically related to physical activity, exercise, sport, and athletic competition.

Areas of Study in Exercise Science

A discipline is defined as an organized formal body of knowledge (23). Generally, in most academic disciplines the body of knowledge is limited to a specific subject matter. For example, the traditional academic areas of biology, chemistry, and mathematics are defined as disciplines because they have specific bodies of knowledge. Each of these disciplines has developed subdisciplines or specialty areas such as plant biology, nutritional biochemistry, and biostatistics. As the traditional academic disciplines have evolved, there is continuing development of subdisciplines and specialty areas. Determining whether exercise science is a specific academic discipline such as chemistry or mathematics is beyond the scope

Exercise science An umbrella term used to describe the study of numerous aspects of physical activity, exercise, sport, and athletic performance that have the common characteristic of movement and the adaptations that occur as a result of physical activity and regular exercise

Physical activity Movement activities of daily living including work- and job-related activities, leisure time activities, and activities performed around the home.

Exercise A structured movement process that individuals consciously and voluntarily engage in and includes those activities that improve or maintain fitness and health.

Sport and athletic competition Movement in structured and organized activities that include a competitive aspect including all athletic events.

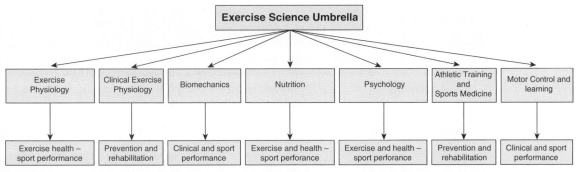

FIGURE 1.7 ▼ Relationships of the disciplines, subdisciplines, and specialty areas of exercise science.

of this book. It is clear that related areas in exercise science such as exercise physiology and exercise and sport psychology have been recognized as disciplines (36) because each contains a distinct body of knowledge that is organized in a formal course of learning. In this book, exercise science is used as an umbrella term to include exercise and clinical exercise physiology, athletic training and sports medicine, exercise and sport nutrition, biomechanics, exercise and sport psychology, and motor behavior. Figure 1.7 illustrates the disciplines, subdisciplines, and specialty areas covered under the exercise science umbrella. Many of the areas of study in exercise science draw on information developed by professionals in other areas making exercise science a truly interdisciplinary field of study. Table 1.1 provides some examples of areas of study by exercise science students and professionals.

As you read through the chapters of this textbook, you will realize that each area of study in exercise science has movement as a central theme or focus. Therefore, it is worthwhile at this point to operationally define these different types of movement. **Physical activity** is defined as those movement activities of daily living including work- and job-related activities, leisure time activities, and activities performed around the home. Sufficient levels of physical activity can result in improvements of fitness and health. **Exercise** is defined as a structured movement process that individuals consciously and voluntarily engage in. Exercise includes those activities that improve or maintain fitness and health and those activities that improve performance in a sport or athletic competition. **Sport and athletic competition** are defined as movement in structured and organized activities that consist of a competitive aspect including all individual and team athletic events. Combined, these types of movement activities underlie the study and professional practice of exercise science.

Exercise Science as a Field of Study

Historically, the study of physical activity, exercise, sport, and athletic performance originated from the academic discipline of physical education. Many of the early educational and professional leaders in physical education studied and promoted the role of exercise and sport in the development of the whole person. It is clear, however, that the areas of study in exercise science are moving farther

Table 1.1	Areas of Study by Students and Professionals in Exercise Science
AREAS OF EXERCISE SCIENCE	**AREAS OF STUDY**
Exercise physiology	Physiologic responses to physical activity, exercise, sport, and athletic competition.
Clinical exercise physiology	Using movement in the prevention and rehabilitation of acute and chronic diseases
Athletic training and sports medicine	Prevention, treatment, and rehabilitation of sport and athletic injuries
Exercise and sport nutrition	Nutritional aspects of disease prevention and improvement of sport and athletic performance
Exercise and sport psychology	Behavioral and mental aspects of exercise, sport, and athletic performance
Motor behavior	Control of body movement in healthy and diseased conditions and improvement of sport and athletic performance
Clinical and sport biomechanics	Mechanical aspects of movement in disease, injury, sport, and athletic performance

away from physical education as the base academic discipline. Many of the early pioneers and leaders in the disciplines and areas of study in exercise science were in fact physical educators. Numerous distinguished professionals and leaders of our professional organizations began their careers as physical education students and teachers, but would no longer refer to themselves as physical educators but as exercise scientists, athletic trainers, sport psychologists, or some other professional term that provides greater clarity and meaning to what they do. The areas of study in exercise science programs have moved curricular requirements further away from the coursework and content knowledge of current physical education teacher licensure programs. College and university programs of study may still require physical education students to enroll in coursework in exercise physiology, biomechanics, nutrition, and motor behavior. Students of exercise science, however, are rarely required to take coursework in many of the content areas of physical education. Over the last 50 years, professionals and leaders of the disciplines of exercise science and physical education have made concerted efforts to clearly define the parameters of each discipline. It is now more appropriate to define physical education as a discipline with a purpose to investigate how the teaching process can be used most effectively to acquire movement skill (15). As a discipline, physical education is primarily interested in how a body of knowledge can be developed to help individuals be better prepared as teachers, manage classroom environments, enhance student interaction and socialization, improve instruction, and enhance movement skill acquisition. Conversely, exercise science is primarily interested in the study of the nutritional, physiologic, psychological, and functional adaptations to physical activity, exercise, sport, and athletic performance (15). As the discipline of physical education continues to evolve to meet the expectations for the preparation of licensed teachers, there will be a further clarification of the body of knowledge required to be a successful physical education teacher. Similarly, as exercise science responds to the demands of preparing students for work in exercise and healthcare facilities or competitive sport and athletic environments so too will the disciplines, subdisciplines, and specialty areas of exercise science continue to evolve.

> ➤ *Thinking Critically*
> *Exercise science has expanded from its origins in physical education to the broad array of disciplines and subdisciplines that it encompasses today. Why do you think this has occurred? Is this a good change for promoting physical activity, exercise, sport, and athletic competition?*

HISTORIC DEVELOPMENT OF EXERCISE SCIENCE

Exploring the historic background of a specific academic discipline can provide considerable insight into the events that help shape current educational experiences and practice. This is especially true for exercise science. Answering the question "When did exercise science officially begin?" is very difficult however, because there is no clear and definable birth of exercise science owing to its structure as a collection of disciplines and areas of study. Although a complete historic account of the evolution of exercise science can be found elsewhere, there are significant periods and events that deserve mentioning to allow for an understanding of how exercise science shapes our current educational programs and professional activities. Noted American College of Sports Medicine Historian Jack W. Berryman presents an excellent historic account of the important events that laid the foundation for the development of exercise science (9) and students are encouraged to read this account and others (36).

Early Influences

Exercise science has evolved historically from several significant influences. Early history (~450 BC) has Greek scholars such as Hippocrates, Plato, Aristotle, and Socrates exploring physical activity in a scientific fashion (9). Early Greek and Roman artists portrayed humans performing various feats of athletic endeavors (9). For example, one of the most well-known artistic sculptures showing an athlete is the Diskobolos or more commonly known as Discus Thrower (Figure 1.8). From Greek and Roman times throughout the medieval period (ca. 400 AD to 1400 AD), there was a continued interest in physical activity, exercise, and sports, primarily through studies of anatomy, physiology, and medicine (9).

During the Renaissance period (ca. fourteenth to seventeenth century), artists and scientists such Leonardo da Vinci and Galileo Galilee had a strong analytic interest in human physical activity. Famous physicians such as Bombastus von Hohenheim and Thomas Linacre wrote in the areas of physiology and hygiene, respectively. In the seventeenth century pioneers from the disciplines of biology, physics, mathematics, and chemistry were doing significant work in the area of physiology. For example, William Harvey's discovery of the circulation of the

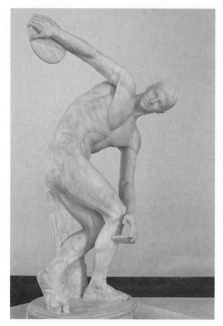

FIGURE 1.8 ▼ Diskobolos—more commonly known as Discus Thrower. (From the Esquiline Hill; former collection Massimo-Lancellotti.)

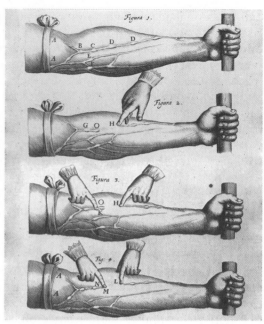

FIGURE 1.9 ▼ William Harvey's discovery of the circulation of the blood through arteries and veins. (Courtesy of the National Library of Medicine.)

blood through arteries and veins (Figure 1.9) was instrumental in developing new concepts in physiology and medicine. Harvey's most influential writings often included specific references to exercise. A significant development at this time was the use of mechanical principles to solve physiologic questions, leading to the construct of the human body as a machine. Questions about skeletal muscular contraction and pulmonary respiration interested physicians and scientists such as Robert Boyle and Robert Hooke in the 1600s. The famous English physician John Mayow wrote extensively on exercise and more specifically on muscle fibers, strength, and muscular contraction (9).

The era of Enlightenment (ca. eighteenth century) saw physicians and scientists publish major works summarizing the knowledge to date on exercise, health, and longevity. Sir John Floyer described the change in heart rate in response to moderate intensity walking, whereas London physician James Keill added to previous work on the muscular system by describing various aspects of muscle fiber size, structure, and contraction. Stephen Hales was the first to make accurate measurements of blood pressure (Figure 1.10), which ultimately contributed to Daniel Bernoulli, a Dutch mathematician making exact calculations of the amount of blood pumped by the heart (now known as cardiac output). During this time, John Desaguliers invented the first mechanical dynamometer that was used to assess muscular force and strength. Joseph-Clement Tissot was the first to describe the effects of time, location, intensity, and duration of exercise on the physiologic processes of the body. Work by the famous French chemist Antoine-Laurent

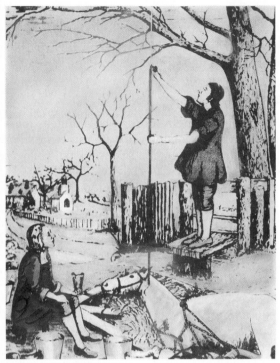

4E786.11   STEPHEN HALES (1677-1761).
Credit: The Granger Collection, New York

FIGURE 1.10 ▼ Stephen Hales making the first measurement of blood pressure. (From the Granger Collection, New York.)

Lavoisier and French mathematician Pierre de Laplace led to the understanding of the use of oxygen to burn carbon in the body and that during physical work (i.e., exercise) oxygen consumption was increased. Additional work by Lavoisier and Armand Seguin allowed for the development of the basic ideas of energy transformation and the source of heat, particularly that which occurred during exercise (9).

Nineteenth-Century Influences

In the early nineteenth century, the study of exercise received more attention from physicians because of its important role in the maintenance of good health and from scientists who were interested in how physical exertion and exercise affected the human body (9). During this period there was experimentation in respiratory physiology, metabolism, and nutrition with the first experiments conducted on how diet and exercise influence the urinary system (9). The term physical education was introduced as a way to promote the education of individuals about their bodies and as a result, physical exercise became more popular. The publication of several books on calisthenics and gymnastics forms of exercise promoted by Swedish and German physicians occurred in the late nineteenth century.

In the early nineteenth century, sport and athletic competition began to be popularized in private schools and colleges and through the formation of professional teams. As a result, there was an increased interest in training the human body to improve the chance of success in sports. Sir John Sinclair of Scotland was one of the first individuals to write extensively about the role of physical training for improving performance during sport and athletic competition (9).

Early Twentieth-Century Influences

Exercise science continued to develop in the twentieth century extending its roots from the discipline of physical education. Two factors played a prominent role in providing the foundation for the development of exercise science. First, colleges and universities developed specific health and physical activity–related courses in their academic curricula to promote the physical and emotional well-being of the whole person. The second prominent factor was the formation of specific programs of study in colleges and universities to prepare professional physical education teachers and athletic coaches (36). Early leaders in physical education, many of whom had their academic preparations in medicine, were proponents of scientifically based, systematic programs of study. Students enrolled in physical education and coaching programs were required to take coursework in anatomy, physiology, **anthropometry,** and physics. Throughout the early to mid-twentieth century, the primary focus in the field of physical education was the preparation of teachers and coaches for public schools, colleges, and universities (36). In the 1930s and 1940s, the writings of two prominent scholars, Jay Bryan Nash and Charles H. McCloy, began to set the stage for a separation of exercise science from the discipline of physical education. Specifically, Nash believed that children should be educated for lifelong leisure-time pursuits, whereas McCloy believed that physical education should be used to develop the human body (36).

Other principal twentieth century figures in the development of exercise science came from a variety of disciplines. One of the leading pioneers in the study of physical activity was Dudley Allen Sargent. Sargent received a medical degree from Yale University in 1879 and immediately became the director of the Hemenway Gymnasium at Harvard University. Sargent pioneered an all-inclusive system for individual exercise prescriptions using information from physical examinations, strength assessments, and anthropometric measurements. His work in measuring strength and power and for recording and evaluating anthropometric measurements of the human body was instrumental in the development of assessment measures of human performance (22). One might say that Sargent was the first personal trainer of the twentieth century.

Sargent's advances in the field strongly influenced George W. Fritz who graduated from Harvard University with a medical degree in 1891. Fritz was an enthusiastic proponent of developing theories and beliefs regarding exercise and its effect on the human organism using scientifically based physiologic research (13,37). Through this work, Fritz established the Physiologic Laboratory at Harvard University, which ultimately led to the establishment of the first college degree program

---

Anthropometry The study of the physical measurements and characteristics of humans and animals.

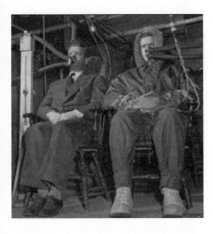

FIGURE 1.11 ▼ Experiments conducted in the Harvard Fatigue Laboratory (ca. 1945).

in physical education. Graduates of this program received a Bachelor of Science degree in anatomy, physiology, and physical training. Throughout his career, Fritz explored the relationships among physical training, anatomy, and physiology, and some consider Fritz the "father of exercise physiology" (34).

Without question, the faculty and scholars working in the Harvard Fatigue Laboratory (Figure 1.11) were the key leaders in the study of physical activity and exercise in the early twentieth century. In existence from 1927 to 1947, the laboratory was home to some of the most prominent researchers at the time, including Lawrence J. Henderson and David Bruce Dill. As the first and only director of the Harvard Fatigue Laboratory, Dill was instrumental in leading laboratory research activities. Although much of the experimental research focused on exercise and environmental physiology, many of the scientists who worked in the laboratory also conducted research in related areas such as clinical physiology, gerontology, nutrition, and physical fitness (13,22,37). The work conducted in this laboratory provided the foundation for many of the basic theories used in exercise science today.

Perhaps, the most significant accomplishment of the Harvard Fatigue Laboratory in the evolution of exercise science was its role in the development of other prominent laboratories for the study of exercise. For example, Steven M. Horvath a student of Dill started the Institute for Environmental Stress at the University of California Santa Barbara. Some of the most well-known exercise scientists were trained at the institute under Horvath including Jack H. Wilmore and Barbara L. Drinkwater, two influential exercise science leaders and researchers. The Laboratory for Physiologic Hygiene at the University of Minnesota, established by Ancel Keys, produced the renowned exercise scientists Ellsworth R. Buskirk and Henry Longstreet Taylor (37). These scientists significantly promoted our understanding of physical activity and exercise. Many other individuals had a profound influence on the expansion of exercise science across the United States during the early to mid-twentieth century. For example, in 1923 Author Stienhaus founded the second laboratory devoted to the study of physiology, physical activity, and exercise at the George Williams College in Chicago. Peter V. Karpovich of Springfield College is credited with introducing physiology to physical education in the United States and was instrumental in promoting the use of weightlifting for enhancing health and human performance. Another prominent exercise scientist, Thomas K. Cureton began his professional career at Springfield College and then later moved to the University of Illinois where he established the Physical Fitness Research Laboratory in 1941 and an adult fitness program in 1961 (37).

Late Twentieth-Century Influences

Several landmark events following World War II resulted in significant changes to the relationship between physical education and exercise science. In 1953, the poor performance of U.S. children compared to European children in the Kraus-Weber physical fitness tests stimulated an increased interest in fitness assessment and the promotion of physical fitness programs (Figure 1.12). The formation of the American College of Sports Medicine in the mid 1950s joined physical education–based researchers with scholars from the medical community to form an organization that continues to offer significant support and promotion of exercise science and sports medicine (36). In addition, other organizations, such as the National Athletic Trainers Association (1950), the International Society of Biomechanics (1973), and the Association for Applied Sport Psychology (1986), were created to provide support to students and professionals and to advance the mission of these professions. The decade of the 1960s brought about the beginning of the separation of exercise science from physical education (36) and the establishment of many of the areas of study in exercise science as a stand-alone body of knowledge.

During the last 25 years of the twentieth century, academic departments in colleges and universities developed programs of study and specializations in many of the areas that today constitute exercise science. Throughout the 1980s and 1990s, the debate continued as to the exact relationship between and among

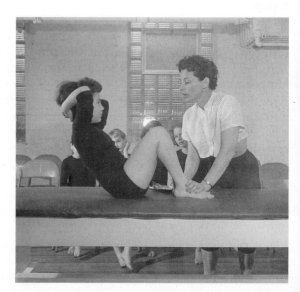

FIGURE 1.12 ▼ Administration of the Kraus-Weber physical fitness test (ca. 1954). (Photo by Orlando/Three Lions/Getty Images.)

the various disciplines, subdisciplines, and specialty areas that are contained under exercise science. As we move further into the twenty-first century, scholars and professionals will continue to clarify the roles and create the history that exercise sciences plays in the promotion of health, physical activity, exercise, sport, and athletic performance. In an effort to gain a greater understanding of how the areas of exercise science have evolved, each chapter of this textbook will further examine the historic development of these areas identified in Table 1.1.

> ### ▶ *Thinking Critically*
>
> *In what specific ways has exercise science contributed to a broader understanding of how physical activity and exercise influence physical fitness and health?*
>
> *In what specific ways has exercise science contributed to a broader understanding of how exercise and training influence sport and athletic performance?*

EXERCISE SCIENCE AND THE AMERICAN COLLEGE OF SPORTS MEDICINE

There is probably no organization that has been more effective in developing and promoting exercise science than the America College of Sports Medicine (ACSM). One only has to attend a national conference of the ACSM and observe the broad array of exercise science and sports medicine topics presented by professionals from around the world to truly appreciate the vast influence of the ACSM. Although many of the disciplines, subdisciplines, and specialty areas under the exercise science umbrella have their own professional organizations, none is so broad reaching in exercise science as the ACSM. Several significant events are worth discussing so that students of exercise science may have an understanding of how physical activity, exercise, sport, and athletic performance have been shaped by the ACSM over the past 60 years. For a more detailed study of the history and influence of the ACSM, students are directed to an additional reading (8).

Early Development of the ACSM

The first meeting of the organization that eventually became the ACSM occurred in 1954 as part of the afternoon program of the American Association for Health, Physical Education, and Recreation national meeting. The initial name chosen by the founding members "Federation of Sports Medicine" was changed to the ACSM in 1955 when the organization was officially incorporated. There were 11 professionals from the disciplines of physical education, physiology, and medicine who were instrumental in the establishment of the ACSM (8).

The ACSM developed as a result of increased interest in health and exercise (8). Two other factors also played a prominent role in the evolution of ACSM: the interest by the U.S. military in physical fitness, physical training, and rehabilitation of soldiers in the post–World War II period and the growth of sports medicine in the international arena prompted by the Federation Internationale Medico Sportive (FIMS). At the time, FIMS was a world leader in the areas of sport and athletics. College and university team physicians and athletic trainers also contributed significantly to the formal development of the ACSM. The influence of the above factors catalyzed the founding members of the ACSM to define sports medicine as a "unique blend of physical education, medicine, and physiology" (8).

From its establishment, the ACSM and its members provided significant public outreach and worked to shape public policy. For example, in 1955, members of the ACSM provided professional guidance to U.S. President Dwight D. Eisenhower's National Conference on Physical Fitness. This commitment to public involvement has continued throughout ACSM's history and currently includes programs such as ACSM's annual Health and Fitness Summit and the Team Physician Program, which provide opportunities for practicing professionals to receive the most current information in all areas of exercise science and sports medicine. Publications, such as the *ACSM's Health and Fitness Journal* and the *Fit Society Page*, allow ACSM professionals to provide meaningful health and fitness information to the general public.

The membership of the ACSM has always been actively involved in performing scholarly research. ACSM members have provided valuable insight into the prevention of lifestyle-related diseases such as coronary artery disease, hypertension, diabetes, and cancer, and the rehabilitation of stroke patients and injured athletes. Much of this information is broadly available in the **peer-reviewed** journal *Medicine and Science in Sports and Exercise*, published by ACSM since 1969. Early in its development as an organization, the ACSM maintained an emphasis on and commitment to science and research. This commitment remains strong as the ACSM funds promising young scholars with support from the ACSM Foundation (8).

ACSM has been considered the world's leader in exercise science and sports medicine since 1974, when it published its first position stand "Prevention of thermal injuries during distance running" (1). Throughout its history, ACSM has continued to publish position stands and opinion papers that have helped shape health, physical activity, exercise, sport, and athletic performance in the United States and around the world. Table 1.2 provides a list of the current positions stands published by the ACSM (8). Copies of these position stands can be found on the ACSM Web page at www.acsm.org.

The initial edition of the highly acclaimed book *Guidelines for Graded Exercise Testing and Exercise Prescription* first became available in 1974. This book continues to be a valuable source of information for exercise science and sports medicine professionals. During the 1970s, the ACSM first awarded certification to individuals who completed training as exercise program directors and exercise specialists. The ACSM continues to furnish practical information through continuing education activities, periodical and nonperiodical publications, certification opportunities, and annual meetings (8).

Recent Role of the ACSM

During the early 1980s, interest in exercise and sports medicine in the United States greatly increased and ACSM responded strongly to this interest. In 1983, a little less than 30 years after its founding, the ACSM membership was well over 10,000 professional and student members. During the 1980s, the professional certification program in the ACSM continued to grow and included two categories: rehabilitation and prevention. Individuals who demonstrated competencies in

Peer-reviewed The evaluation of a professional colleague's work.

Table 1.2	Positions Stands from the American College of Sports Medicine	
POSITION STAND		**YEAR PUBLISHED**
Automated external defibrillators in health/fitness facilities		2002
Appropriate intervention strategies for weight loss and prevention of weight regain for adults		2009
Exercise and acute cardiovascular events: placing the risks into perspective		2007
Exercise and fluid replacement		2007
Exertional heat illness during training and competition		2007
Exercise and hypertension		2004
Exercise and physical activity for older adults		2009
Exercise and type II diabetes		2002
Exercise for patients with coronary artery disease		1994
Female athlete triad		1997
Nutrition and athletic performance		2009
Physical activity and bone health		2004
Prevention of cold injuries during exercise		2006
Progression models in resistance training for healthy adults		2009
Recommended quantity and quality of exercise for developing and maintaining cardiorespiratory fitness and muscular fitness, and flexibility in healthy adults		1990
The use of alcohol in sports		1982
The use of anabolic-androgenic steroids in sports		1984
The use of blood doping as an ergogenic aid		1996
Weight loss in wrestlers		1996

the rehabilitation category could become certified as program directors, exercise specialists, and exercise test technologists. By demonstrating competences in the prevention category, members became certified as a health/fitness director, health/fitness instructor, and exercise leader/aerobics (8). These programs continue today with opportunities for certification in health and fitness (ACSM Certified Personal Trainer and ACSM Health Fitness Instructor) and clinical (ACSM Exercise Specialist and ACSM Registered Clinical Exercise Physiologist) tracks. During the late 1980s, the ACSM established formal relationships with the President's Council on Physical Fitness and Sports and the Office of Disease Prevention and Health Promotion within the Department of Health and Human Services (8).

Throughout the 1990s, ACSM continued to promote its research and outreach activities by making *Medicine and Science in Sports and Exercise* a monthly publication, offering the Team Physician Course, and disseminating exercise science and sports medicine position stands to ACSM members and the general public (8). These position stands continue to shape policy and practice in the areas of health, physical activity, exercise, sport, and athletic competition. In 1994, ACSM provided consultation to the U.S. Centers for Disease Control and Prevention (CDC) and the President's Council on Physical Fitness as new recommendations for physical activity were being developed. The resulting report from the U.S. Surgeon General provided guidelines for the amount of physical activity required to obtain significant health benefits and reduce the risk of developing chronic diseases such as heart disease, hypertension, diabetes, and osteoporosis (39). Furthering its commitment to physical activity, the ACSM joined with several other professional organizations and government agencies in 1995 to form the National Coalition for Promoting Physical Activity (NCPPA) (8). The mission of the NCPPA is to unite the strengths of public, private, and industry efforts into collaborative partnerships that inspire and empower all Americans to lead more physically active lifestyles (http://www.ncppa.org). A current listing of prominent ACSM publications is shown in Table 1.3.

ACSM has partnered with other professional organizations to promote improved safety and care for competitive athletes. In 1994 the ACSM, working with

Table 1.3	Key Exercise Science–Related Publications from the American College of Sports Medicine
ACSM Fitness Book, Third Edition	
ACSM's Advanced Exercise Physiology	
ACSM's Certification Review, Third Edition	
ACSM's Exercise is Medicine™: A Clinician's Guide to Exercise Prescription	
ACSM's Exercise Management for Persons with Chronic Diseases and Disabilities, Third Edition	
ACSM's Guidelines for Exercise Testing and Prescription, Eighth Edition	
ACSM's Health/Fitness Facility Standards and Guidelines, Third Edition	
ACSM's Health-Related Physical Fitness Assessment Manual, Third Edition	
ACSM's Metabolic Calculations Handbook	
ACSM's Primary Care Sports Medicine, Second Edition	
ACSM's Resources for the Personal Trainer, Third Edition	
ACSM's Resource Manual for Guidelines for Exercise Testing and Prescription, Sixth Edition	
ACSM's Resources for Clinical Exercise Physiology: Musculoskeletal, Neuromuscular, Neoplastic, Immunologic and Hematologic Conditions, Second Edition	
ACSM's Worksite Health Handbook: A Guide to Building Healthy and Productive Companies, Second Edition	
Preparticipation Physical Evaluation, Fourth Edition	

the American College of Cardiology, developed recommendations for determining eligibility for competition in athletes with cardiovascular abnormalities (27). In 1996, the ACSM partnered with the American Medical Society for Sports Medicine (AMSSM) and the American Orthopaedic Society for Sports Medicine (AOSSM) to present the first Advanced Team Physician Course. ACSM remains committed to educating team physicians through publications such as *ACSM's Handbook for Team Physicians*, *ACSM's Essentials of Sports Medicine*, and *ACSM's Sports Medicine Review*. The Team Physician Consensus statement, a collective effort by members of ACSM, AOSSM, AMSSM, and the American Academy of Orthopaedic Surgeons was first published in 2000. This statement provided physicians, school administrators, team owners, the general public, and individuals who are responsible for making decisions regarding the medical care of athletes and teams with guidelines for choosing a qualified team physician and an outline of the duties expected of a team physician (4).

More than 50 years after its inception, the ACSM continues to expand by working to shape public policy, supporting research, expanding educational opportunities for exercise science and sports medicine professionals, and disseminating knowledge to the general public. The ACSM has made commitments to influence world health through its roles with the Active Aging Partnership/National Blueprint, Musculoskeletal Partnership, and Exercise is Medicine[Rx] initiative. At the 52nd Annual Meeting in 2005, the ACSM and the President's Council on Physical Fitness and Sports announced a collaboration to benefit public health by jointly promoting physical activity, fitness, and sports. In 2006, the Federation of American Societies for Experimental Biology accepted ACSM into the Federation, further solidifying ACSM as a leader in the study of health, physical activity, exercise, sport, and athletic performance.

The ACSM (www.acsm.org) continues to build upon its rich history established and fostered by its world leaders in exercise science and sports medicine as it adheres to its mission:

> To promote and integrate scientific research, education, and practical applications of sports medicine and exercise science to maintain and enhance physical performance, fitness, health, and quality of life guides the activities of the organization.

The fulfillment of this mission will allow the ACSM to remain instrumental in helping exercise science professionals to disseminate valuable information and shape policy affecting health, physical activity, exercise, sport, and athletic performance.

> ➤ *Thinking Critically*
> *In what significant ways has the American College of Sports Medicine contributed to the development of exercise science and the related fields of study?*

ACADEMIC PREPARATION IN EXERCISE SCIENCE

As presented in this chapter and others throughout the book, you will see that exercise science professionals come from a variety of educational backgrounds and disciplines. Appropriate academic preparation is critical to developing and preparing for a successful career as an exercise science or sports medicine professional. Students entering into a program of study in exercise science must pay particular attention to meeting certain requirements, especially in a program or

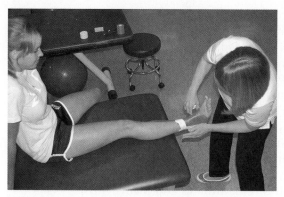

FIGURE 1.13 ▼ Athletic trainers work with individuals injured during exercise, sport, or athletic competitions.

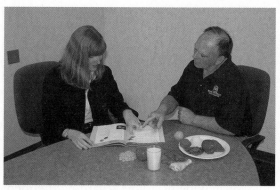

FIGURE 1.14 ▼ Registered dietician counseling a patient.

major that requires the successful completion of a licensure or certification examination upon graduation with an undergraduate degree. For example, exercise science students interested in becoming certified athletic trainers (Figure 1.13) or registered dieticians (Figure 1.14) must complete the program requirements and graduate from an accredited program in athletic training or dietetics. Exercise science can also be a valuable and effective program of study for those who want to enter into postbaccalaureate study in the medical or **allied healthcare** fields or for completing further graduate education.

Undergraduate Coursework

Undergraduate exercise science programs and the associated majors are typically broad based and include general studies in biology, chemistry, biochemistry, anatomy, physiology, human development, psychology, physics, mathematics, and statistics. Coursework in these fields provides a solid foundation for understanding how and why humans move. Advanced coursework provides enhanced knowledge in particular areas of study. For example, depending on the major area of study students can expect coursework in exercise physiology, fitness programming in health and disease, motor development, control, and behavior, nutrition, structural and functional biomechanics, exercise testing and prescription, exercise and sport psychology, evaluation and assessment of athletic injuries, and rehabilitation modalities. The foundational and advanced coursework is designed to provide basic and applied knowledge to prepare exercise science students for the next phase of their professional career including employment, certification or licensure examinations, graduate study, and professional schools. Students interested in careers in medicine or another allied health field must also meet the major requirements for entry into that chosen field.

Allied healthcare The professional field that works to deliver patient care services for the identification, prevention, and treatment of diseases, disabilities, and disorders.

Table 1.4	Foundation Recommendations for Continued Professional Development	
CONTINUED PROFESSIONAL DEVELOPMENT	**RECOMMENDATION**	
Graduate study	Complete the degree requirements for the intended graduate program of study	
Professional schools	Meet the prerequisites for the professional program of study	
Certification/licensure	Meet the eligibility requirements established by the professional certifying or licensing agency	
Employment	Gain internship or field experience in the potential field of employment	

As you begin your course of study, it is very important that you understand the requirements of the career path you wish to take after graduation. Chapter 11 provides valuable information about professional employment and career opportunities. It is important to make sure your coursework at the undergraduate level provides you with the knowledge, skills, and abilities necessary for your chosen career path. Although the information contained in the following section provides a general overview of the requirements for continued preparation, it is essential that you speak with a career advisor in your academic department at your college or university. He or she will guide you to the most appropriate coursework and experiences for achieving your career goals. Table 1.4 provides key foundational recommendations for educational and professional development.

Preparation for Careers in Healthcare

It is becoming increasingly common for students to major in an exercise science program as an undergraduate student and then complete postbaccalaureate work in a healthcare field (Figure 1.15). An undergraduate degree in exercise science allows the flexibility of course programming to fulfill the requirements necessary for entry into medical, chiropractic, or dental school, a physician assistant program, and physical or occupation therapy programs. Obtaining a degree in exercise science will provide additional benefits in preparation for advanced healthcare education. Coursework in physical activity and exercise prescription for healthy and diseased populations, exercise testing and evaluation, nutrition for health and athletic performance, and exercise and sport psychology can be valuable supplements for advanced study in healthcare. The following sections serve as a general overview for those students intending to pursue postbaccalaureate study in a healthcare field or graduate school. If you have decided to pursue a career in medicine or allied healthcare, you are strongly encouraged to obtain information from those schools you may consider attending so that you have all necessary information regarding the schools' specific entrance requirements. You are strongly encouraged to contact your college or university chief premedical or healthcare advisor to assist you in developing your undergraduate coursework and program of study in exercise science.

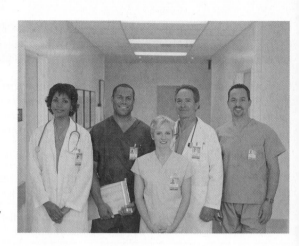

FIGURE 1.15 ▼ Allied healthcare professionals. (Photo from Lifesize/ Ryan McVay/Getty Images.)

Preparation for Medical School

There are approximately 140 allopathic (MD) and 20 osteopathic (DO) medical schools in the United States and Canada. Generally, the minimum academic requirements for acceptance into these schools include one academic year of coursework in English, biology, general chemistry, organic chemistry, and physics. Additional coursework in cell biology, mammalian physiology, and biochemistry provides valuable preparation for medical school. Some medical schools also require a year of college mathematics, including coursework in statistics. Becoming proficient in a foreign language may also be helpful.

To enter medical school following graduation from college, you must complete all premedical requirements at least one year prior to your expected matriculation into medical school. You should take the Medical College Aptitude Test (MCAT) at least 3 to 6 months before submitting your application. Medical school admissions committees evaluate candidates largely, although not completely, on objective criteria. Therefore, a high overall grade point average, a high science course grade point average, and competitive MCAT scores are important. Other factors considered by admissions committees include well-developed interpersonal skills, evidence of leadership potential, supportive letters of recommendation, prior work or volunteer experience in a healthcare facility, and performance in a personal interview. Additional information for preparing for a career in medicine may be obtained from the following organizations: Association of American Medical Colleges (www.aamc.org) and American Association of Colleges of Osteopathic Medicine (www.aacom.org).

Preparation for Dental School

There are currently 66 schools or programs of dentistry in the United States, Canada, and Puerto Rico. Preparation for entry into dentistry should include knowledge of the basic physical and biological sciences and proficiency in communication skills. Minimum academic course requirements for acceptance into a dental program generally include one academic year of English, inorganic chemistry, organic chemistry, physics, mathematics, and introductory biology (with each of the science courses having a laboratory component). Additional coursework in comparative anatomy, developmental biology, genetics, microbiology, human physiology, histology, biochemistry, and cell biology may also provide valuable preparation for entering a program in dentistry. Owing to the visual, mechanical, and personal nature of the activities you will participate in as a dentist, it may be advantageous to also consider taking courses in art, psychology, personal communication, and business.

The Dental Admissions Test (DAT) is required by all dental schools and programs and should be taken in the spring or the summer before you apply to dental schools. Your application materials should be completed and submitted approximately 1 year prior to your anticipated starting date. Dentistry programs consider a variety of factors in selecting students including a high grade point average, good DAT scores, strong letters of recommendation (including those from a practicing dentist), and at least 20 hours of observation with a practicing dentist. Other important factors considered by admissions committees include a strong interest in dentistry, awareness of the terminology used in dentistry, demonstrated good manual dexterity, and performance during a personal interview. Additional information for preparing for a career in dentistry may be obtained from the following associations: American Dental Association (www.ada.org) and the American Academy of Pediatric Dentistry (www.aapd.org).

Preparation for Chiropractic School

There are presently 17 fully accredited colleges of chiropractic medicine in the United States. All individuals practicing chiropractic medicine must pass the State Board of Health Examination. Although all states sanction the practice of chiropractic medicine, most of the state boards of health also require that an applicant for a licensing examination be a graduate of an accredited college program. The primary focus of Chiropractic medicine is spine manipulation, for which X-rays may be used as a diagnostic tool. Doctors of Chiropractic medicine also use nutrition and patient counseling as part of the complete practice. Neither drug treatment nor surgery may be performed by a Doctor of Chiropractic medicine. Most chiropractic programs require 4 years of study, although some colleges may offer a 3-year program.

Schools of chiropractic medicine vary in the number of credit hours and specific courses required for admission. Students interested in applying to a program of study in chiropractic medicine should check on the exact entrance requirements. In general, a minimum of 2 years of college coursework must be completed prior to entering a chiropractic school and several states require chiropractic physicians to have a baccalaureate degree in addition to the chiropractic degree to be licensed to practice chiropractic medicine.

The following list of minimal entrance requirements should serve as a general guide, although specific entrance requirements may vary slightly at each school. Students are encouraged to check the Association of Chiropractic Colleges directory or individual school admissions requirements. Students are required to have 1 year of the following courses: biological sciences, general chemistry, organic chemistry, and physics (with a laboratory component for each). Students should also have 1 year of English or communication, one semester of psychology, and coursework in the humanities or social sciences. Generally, three letters of recommendation are required with at least one from a practicing chiropractic physician. Applicants are generally evaluated on the basis of their undergraduate grade point average and coursework, the MCAT (if required by the school), clinical exposure and experience, personal attributes, involvement in extracurricular activities, service to others, and a personal interview with the admissions committee. Additional information for preparing for a career in chiropractic medicine may be obtained from the following associations: The Association of Chiropractic Colleges www.chirocolleges.org and the Association for Chiropractic Medicine www.chiromed.org.

Preparation for Physician Assistant Programs

There are presently 136 fully accredited physician assistant programs in the United States. The typical physician assistant program is 24 to 32 months in duration and requires at least 4 years of college and some healthcare experience prior to admission. Applicants to physician assistant programs must complete approximately 2 years of college courses in basic science and behavioral science as prerequisites to physician assistant training. This is similar to the premedical requirements for medical students. Students interested in physician assistant programs should take coursework in the basic sciences, including anatomy, physiology, biochemistry, pharmacology, physical diagnosis, pathophysiology, microbiology, clinical laboratory sciences, behavioral sciences, and medical ethics. Additional coursework in communication and psychology is encouraged. Preference in admission is usually given to candidates who have prior experience in a healthcare setting. The hallmark of physician assistant education is the clinical training in a variety of inpatient and outpatient settings including family medicine, internal medicine, obstetrics and gynecology, pediatrics, general surgery, emergency medicine, and psychiatry (Figure 1.16).

The independent Accreditation Review Commission on Education for the Physician Assistant accredits all physician assistant programs. Only graduates of accredited programs are eligible to sit for the Physician Assistant National Certifying

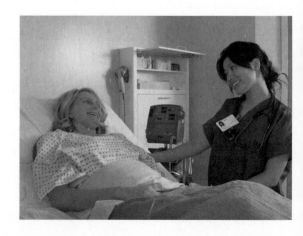

FIGURE 1.16 ▼ Physician assistant. (Photo from Rubberball Productions/ Getty Images.)

Exam administered by the independent National Commission on Certification of Physician Assistants and developed by the National Board of Medical Examiners. All 50 states and the District of Columbia have enacted laws or regulations authorizing physician assistant practice and authorize physician assistants to prescribe controlled medicines. Once a physician assistant is certified, she or he must be recertified every 6 years to keep her/his certification current. Additional information for preparing for a career as a physician assistant may be obtained from the following associations: the American Academy of Physician Assistants www.aapa.org and Physician Assistant Education Association at www.paeaonline.org.

Preparation for Physical and Occupational Therapy

There are presently 210 fully accredited physical therapy and 153 fully accredited occupational therapy programs in the United States. Undergraduate degree programs in exercise science provide excellent preparation for graduate study in physical and occupational therapy because many exercise science programs offer the required coursework for direct entry into a physical or occupational therapy program (Figure 1.17). The American Physical Therapy Association (APTA) has mandated that all physical therapy programs offer a master's degree (MS) or a doctoral degree in physical therapy (DPT) to earn or retain certification. Therefore, students interested in physical therapy must earn a baccalaureate degree before entering into an MS or DPT program. Each school has its own prerequisite courses for admission into a program and therefore it is strongly recommended that you contact the programs you may wish to attend and obtain a list of requirements for admission. In general, most programs require the following courses for admission: one academic year of biology, chemistry, and physics (with a laboratory component for each). Additionally, most programs require at least one course in each of the following: human anatomy, human physiology, statistics, biomechanics, exercise physiology, English composition, general psychology, and developmental psychology. Additional coursework in organic chemistry, biochemistry, philosophy or medical ethics, and speech composition may also be valuable.

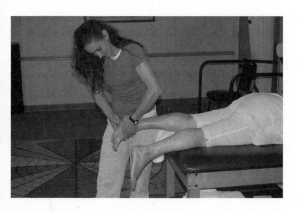

FIGURE 1.17 ▼ Physical therapy professional at work.

The majority of schools offering MS and DPT programs require the Graduate Record Examination as part of the admission materials, whereas other schools require the Allied Health Professions Aptitude Test. Physical and occupational therapy programs require that candidates have volunteered in physical therapy or occupational therapy clinics. Many physical therapy and occupational therapy admissions committees look for evidence of exposure to the types of patients with whom you will eventually be working and for experience in a variety of clinical settings. The number of required volunteer hours varies by school and program and must be certified by a healthcare professional. A general recommendation is that you complete at least 100 hours of volunteer service. Other important factors considered by admissions committees include well-developed interpersonal skills and performance during a personal interview. Additional information for preparing for a career in physical or occupational therapy may be obtained from the following associations: APTA (www.APTA.org) and the American Occupational Therapy Association, Inc. (www.aota.org).

Preparation for Graduate School

Obtaining an undergraduate degree in exercise science provides excellent preparation for continuing education in graduate school. Each of the areas of study in exercise science may be offered as graduate programs in many colleges and universities. Furthermore, an exercise science degree can provide solid preparation for graduate work in areas such as public health, epidemiology, physiology, biochemistry, psychology, and engineering. Most graduate programs require 1 to 2 years of study for a master's degree and 3 to 5 years of study for a doctoral degree. Graduate programs have specific requirements for entry into the program and completion of the degree that are often unique to the particular college or university. Obtaining a master's or doctoral degree will generally result in a higher salary and greater job responsibility. In addition, some professional employment opportunities require an advanced degree beyond a bachelor's degree. Additional information about specific graduate programs can be obtained by visiting the homepage of the college or university of which you are interested in attending.

> ➤ *Thinking Critically*
>
> *How does your choice of undergraduate coursework in exercise science best prepare you for a career in the professional fields of medicine and allied health?*

RESEARCH IN EXERCISE SCIENCE

Research and the dissemination of the knowledge gained from the research are key activities of many exercise science professionals. Much of what we know about health, physical activity, exercise, sport, and athletic performance is derived from

Basic research Research directed toward the increase of knowledge, the primary aim being a greater knowledge or understanding of the subject under study.

research and experiments conducted by exercise science professionals. Researchers work to gain or accumulate knowledge for a discipline, subdiscipline, or specialty area. The scientific method is the most commonly used way to generate knowledge in exercise science. As you begin your program of study in exercise science, you will quickly learn that exercise science is founded in well-designed and well-conducted research. It is therefore important to provide a general overview of research in exercise science so that you may have a greater appreciation and understanding for the research work performed in the areas comprising exercise science.

Research procedures

Exercise science professionals may conduct research using human and animal models, tissue and cell cultures, computer modeling, and advanced statistical procedures. Many of the different types of equipment and procedures used in exercise science research are discussed in Chapter 10. The specific processes and methods used in research are employed to assure that the conclusions reached at the end of an experiment or study are factual and stand up to rigorous analysis. These methods include the formulation of hypotheses and alternative hypotheses to test the objectivity of the experiment and experimenter (30). Researchers and scholars publish results in peer-reviewed journals to allow others to review and often replicate the work that was conducted (30). Investigators and researchers use the scientific method to solve interesting problems and answer specific questions. Individuals conducting high quality scientific research acquire specific personal and intellectual characteristics that enable them to think and act in a scientific manner. Some examples of these attitudes and characteristics are provided in Table 1.5 (6).

Types of Research

Investigative work performed by researchers and scientists is typically characterized as either basic or applied research. **Basic research** is sometimes referred to as pure or fundamental research and aims to expand the knowledge base by formulating, evaluating, or expanding a theory (7). Research in certain areas of exercise science can be categorized as basic research if there is, for example, a biochemical or biological approach. In general, basic research aims to discover new and unknown

Table 1.5	Attitudes and Characteristics of Scientists (6)
Scientists are essentially doubters, who maintain a highly skeptical attitude toward the data derived from science	
Scientists are objective and impartial, and they do not have any personal bias toward the observations they make	
Scientists deal with facts and make conclusions based on the data, and they do not make personal decisions about what is good or what is bad	
Scientists are not satisfied with isolated facts but seek to put things known into an orderly system	

knowledge often without concern for the practical application of the information that has been gained. The practical application of the information that has been generated is considered at a later time, often years in the future. To some students of exercise science this type of research often seems of limited value, but many of the advances seen in physical activity, exercise, sport, and athletic performance have arisen from practical applications of discoveries made in basic research (7).

Applied research attempts to solve practical problems, although it uses the same methods as basic research. In applied research, theoretical concepts are tested in real world situations. Applied research acquires solutions to an immediate practical problem. However, applied research is often used to make inferences beyond the specific group or situation being studied. The results of applied research are intended to be generalized and to extend to the target population setting. Applied research is not conducted in controlled laboratories, but rather in classrooms, hospitals, clinics, and field settings. Much of the research in exercise science is applied because it is concerned with testing the processes of movement and behavior in a real life condition. Basic or applied research conducted by exercise scientists must depend on each other for the proper research process to take place and for theories to be developed and evaluated (7). Table 1.6 provides some examples of basic research and applied research conducted in physical activity, exercise, sport, and athletic performance.

Research in exercise science can also be classified as quantitative or qualitative (7). **Quantitative research** uses a scientific approach designed for the collection and analysis of numerical data typically obtained from subjects through direct testing or questionnaires. Quantitative approaches are used to illustrate existing conditions or phenomena, investigate the relationships between two or more variables, and explore cause and effect relationships between phenomena. The methods used in quantitative research are based on a paradigm adopted from the natural sciences that believes in the assumption that reality is relatively stable, uniform, measurable, and governed by rational laws that enable generalizations to a larger population be made (7). The quantitative research approach involves the following characteristics:

1. clearly stated research questions,
2. rationally conceived hypotheses and alternative hypotheses,
3. fully developed and valid research procedures,
4. controlling, as much as possible, those extraneous factors that might interfere with the data collected,
5. using sufficiently large enough samples of participants to provide meaningful data, and
6. employing data analysis techniques based upon statistical procedures (16,21).

Applied research Research directed toward finding solutions to an immediate practical problem.

Quantitative research Research that uses a scientific approach designed for the collection and analysis of numerical data typically obtained from subjects through direct testing or questionnaires.

Qualitative research Research that uses extensive observations and interviews to provide nonnumeric data obtained in natural environments.

Table 1.6	Examples of Basic and Applied Research in Areas of Exercise Science	
AREAS OF EXERCISE SCIENCE	**BASIC RESEARCH**	**APPLIED RESEARCH**
Exercise physiology	The effect of muscle pH levels on lactic acid movement out of the muscle fibers	Does alteration of whole body pH levels through the use of an ergogenic aid improve distance running performance?
Clinical exercise physiology	The effect of different drugs on cardiac muscle fiber contractile strength	Do different drug therapies combined with exercise decrease the recovery time after a myocardial infarction?
Athletic training and sports medicine	The effect of different durations of cold application on the change in intramuscular temperature	Does the duration of cold application improve the healing process of an injured muscle?
Exercise and sport nutrition	The effect of different meal composition on muscle glycogen resynthesis	Do enhanced muscle glycogen levels improve endurance exercise performance?
Exercise and sport psychology	The effect of different types of music on psychological arousal	Does listening to music before an athletic competition improve performance during the competition?
Motor control and learning	The role of different levels of neurotransmitters in the control of movement	Does the administration of the neurotransmitter dopamine improve the quality of life in patients with Parkinson's disease?
Clinical and sport biomechanics	The role of different stride lengths during ambulation on balance	Does a mechanical knee brace improve the ability to freely ambulate in patients recovering from injury?

Qualitative research uses extensive observations and interviews that provide nonnumeric data obtained in natural environments. Qualitative research seeks to interpret phenomena and discover meaning of situations. Qualitative research, sometimes called naturalistic research, is frequently conducted in natural settings and does not attempt to control the context or conditions surrounding the research setting (7,30). Unlike quantitative research, qualitative research does not subscribe to the viewpoint that the world is stable and uniform and can be explained by laws that govern phenomena. Instead, qualitative researchers use the constructionist perspective. This perspective suggests that meaning and reality are situation specific, and allow for many different interpretations, none of which is necessarily more valid than another. In qualitative research, there is usually not an attempt to generalize the results to the entire population being studied because the context of the study is situational specific. Specific research methods are not established prior to the beginning of the study and tend to evolve as the research is performed. In the qualitative research approach, the analysis and interpretation of the collected data is mainly interpretive and descriptive in nature. This results in a categorization of the data into trends and patterns. Qualitative research rarely uses statistical procedures (7,30).

The use of quantitative and qualitative research methods should be based on the type of research question that is being posed. Each research method has advantages and disadvantages. Many researchers in exercise science are also beginning to use mixed method approaches to investigate interesting research questions related to physical activity, exercise, sport, and athletic performance.

Additional Research Descriptions

A description of the different types of quantitative research and qualitative research is beneficial for understanding the strengths and weaknesses of each type (7,30). Often research is categorized as either descriptive or experimental.

1. **Descriptive research**
   - describes the current state of the problem
   - does not require the manipulation of the experimental variables
   - provides no conclusions about why an effect occurs
   - offers no explanation of what happens
2. **Experimental research**
   - manipulates a variable or variables to investigate the effect on some outcome
   - provides conclusions about why an effect occurs

There are also three primary forms of experimental research: longitudinal, cross-sectional, and sequential (7,30).

1. The **longitudinal research** method is the study of change over time:
   - probably the most reliable of the three types of experimental research, because societal and technological factors usually do not have a large effect on the results
   - learning or familiarization is often a problem because repeated testing may affect the data because individuals learn how to take the test
2. The **cross-sectional research** method requires the collection of data on individuals of different characteristics who represent different attributes being investigated (e.g., age, gender, race, fitness levels):
   - allows all the data to be collected at once

Descriptive research A type of research that describes specific characteristics about a question or problem.

Experimental research A type of research that requires the manipulation of at least one variable to answer a question or problem.

Longitudinal research A type of research that involves the study of change over time.

Cross-sectional research A type of research that requires the collection of data on individuals of different characteristics who represent different attributes being investigated.

Sequential research A type of research that combines both cross-sectional and longitudinal research.

- performance might be affected for reasons other than the variables being measured (e.g., societal or technological factors)
3. The **sequential research** method combines the longitudinal and cross-sectional methods:
   - involves studying several different samples (cross-sectional) over several years (longitudinal)
- allows individuals differing in some characteristic (e.g., age or fitness level), to be compared at the same time to identify current differences

> ➤ **Thinking Critically**
> *How does basic and applied research contribute to our improved understanding of health, physical activity, exercise, sport, and athletic performance?*

I N T E R V I E W

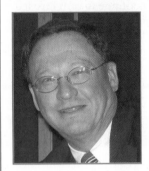

Jack W. Berryman, PhD, FACSM, Professor of Medical
History at the University of Washington School of Medicine, Seattle, Washington. Jack currently serves as the ACSM Historian.

Brief Introduction

I began my college education as a health and physical education major at Lock Haven University in Pennsylvania. In the early 1970s, I completed two master's degrees at the University of Massachusetts, Amherst: one in exercise science and the other in history. During this time, I became involved in the early stages of the exercise science and sport studies movement. I completed a PhD at the University of Maryland in physical education and history, and I joined the University of Washington faculty in 1975. In 1992, I was voted a fellow in the American Academy of Kinesiology and Physical Education and in 1994, was named ACSM's official historian. Two of my books of special interest are *Sport and Exercise Science: Essays in the History of Sports Medicine* (1992) and *Out of Many, One: A History of the American College of Sports Medicine* (1995). I have been honored as ACSM's D. B. Dill Historical Lecturer an unprecedented two times, in 1994 and 2004.

➤ **What is ACSM's importance in the development of exercise science?**

Because of ACSM's unique multidisciplinary membership that included physicians, physical educators, exercise scientists, and many other professions directly related to the health benefits of exercise, the organization became a leader in the field by the late 1950s. ACSM's annual meetings, along with its significant journals and books, as well as position stands and scientific roundtables, put ACSM in the forefront of health promotion and exercise science very quickly. With a strong scientific and clinical base, the ACSM has continued to be the most respected authority in the field of exercise science. The ACSM has

played a leadership role in the National Coalition for Promoting Physical Activity (1995) and in the writing of *Physical Activity and Health: A Report of the Surgeon General* (1996). The College has been a dominant force in the institutionalization of exercise in the prevention, diagnosis, and treatment of cardiac and other degenerative diseases such as diabetes, osteoporosis, and obesity.

➤ **What is ACSM's importance in the development of sport and athletic performance?**

Although ACSM's early emphasis was on health and fitness, the ACSM began to move more in the direction of clinical sports medicine and athletic

(Continued)

training in the 1970s. Through annual meetings and publications, those with sports medicine expertise were gradually attracted to the ACSM. By the 1980s, ACSM had as professional members some of the leading sport team physicians and athletic trainers in the world. Research and publications began to focus on the prevention and treatment of sports injuries, peak athletic performance, the role of the team physician, and other important aspects of athleticism, such as the female athlete triad. The ACSM also offers a series of team physician courses, which are important in disseminating information to practicing physicians.

➤ **How will ACSM contribute as a world leader in exercise science into the twenty-first century?**

ACSM has in its membership the leaders in exercise science and sports medicine worldwide.

This highly scientific international membership continues to position the ACSM at the forefront of any major development in the field. The ACSM also has a very proactive and highly talented professional staff at its headquarters in Indianapolis who work tirelessly to further ACSM's goals. Publications, annual meetings, special symposia, certifications, and position stands, among numerous other projects, have a constant impact on the field. Because of its stature, the ACSM has had a significant impact on policy decisions and continues to be the most dynamic force to view exercise deficiency as a serious health problem. The ACSM believes that exercise is in fact good medicine and will continue to convince federal, state, and local officials that physical activity is the key to good health and the prevention of disease.

I N T E R V I E W

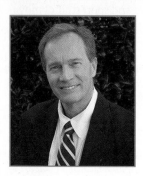

Scott K. Powers, EdD, PhD, FACSM, Professor of Exercise Physiology, Department of Applied Physiology and Kinesiology at the University of Florida. Scott is a past-president of the ACSM.

Brief Introduction

I earned my BS degree in physical education from Carson Newman College in Tennessee. After completing a master's degree at the University of Georgia, I then earned a doctoral degree in exercise science (with an emphasis in exercise physiology) from the University of Tennessee. I desired additional training in basic science and cell biology, and subsequently completed a PhD in physiology and cell biology from Louisiana State University.

➤ **What are your most significant career experiences?**

I began my professional career as a faculty member in the Department of Kinesiology at Louisiana State University, and I am currently a professor within the Department of Applied Physiology and Kinesiology at the University of Florida. Citing my research and teaching accomplishments, the University of Florida honored me with an endowed professorship in 2004 followed by the title of "distinguished professor" in 2005.

Throughout my career, I have been active in both the American Physiologic Society and the American College Sports Medicine having served both organizations via committee memberships and as an elected officer.

➤ **Why did you choose to become an exercise science professional?**

My personal interest in exercise physiology began during my undergraduate studies at Carson Newman College. As a distance runner on our

(Continued)

collegiate track team, I became fascinated with the physiology of human performance and began to read all of the exercise physiology texts available at the time. I quickly realized that knowledge in exercise physiology was limited in many areas and hence, a need for additional research existed. Fueled by natural curiosity, I decided to pursue a graduate degree in exercise physiology to learn more about this exciting topic. My experience in graduate school served to motivate me further to expand my knowledge about exercise physiology and to dedicate my career to research and teaching in exercise physiology.

➤ Which individuals or experiences were the most influential in your career development?

Two individuals played major roles in my early career development. First, my mother, who was a public school teacher and a high school guidance counselor, played a major role in motivating me toward academic endeavors. Second, Dr Edward T. Howley, professor in exercise physiology at the University of Tennessee, had a major positive influence on my professional development. Specifically, Professor Howley was my doctoral mentor at the University of Tennessee and served as an ideal role model during my graduate studies in exercise physiology. Indeed, Dr Howley was both a master teacher and accomplished scholar and he passed along his enthusiasm for learning to all of the graduate students that he mentored during his highly successful career.

➤ What are your top two or three professional accomplishments?

From a research perspective, my primary achievements have come in three different areas of inquiry. First, during the 1980s, my laboratory investigated the factors that control breathing and regulate pulmonary gas exchange during exercise. An important finding related to this work was that pulmonary gas exchange limits maximal oxygen uptake in many elite endurance athletes. This novel observation revealed that the lung and not the cardiovascular system limits maximal oxygen uptake in this population of elite athletes. In 1990, my research focus shifted toward two new areas of investigation: (a) exercise-induced

cardioprotection; and (b) disuse muscle atrophy. By studying how exercise changes the heart, my research group has made significant contributions to our understanding of how and why regular bouts of endurance exercise protects the heart during a heart attack. This form of cardiac safeguard is termed exercise-induced cardioprotection and provides direct evidence about the importance of exercise. In this regard, our work demonstrates that as few as 3 to 5 days of aerobic exercise can produce cardioprotection. However, this exercise-induced protection is lost quickly (i.e., within 18 days) after the cessation of exercise. Moreover, our research has revealed some of the key cellular mechanisms that are responsible for exercise-induced cardioprotection. Finally, my laboratory has also made some important discoveries regarding the mechanisms responsible for disuse muscle atrophy (i.e., muscle loss owing to inactivity resulting from prolonged bed rest, limb immobilization, etc.). By investigating the mechanisms responsible for this type of muscle wasting, our research team hopes to develop countermeasures to prevent this type of muscle atrophy and prevent or retard this cause of muscle atrophy.

➤ What advice would you have for a student exploring a career in exercise science?

Successful individuals in any profession share many of the same traits. A key trait of all successful people is that they are passionate about what they do. So, my best advice for students exploring career options is to find your passion in life. In short, what career would make you happy so that you enjoy going to work each morning? Is it possible to enjoy going to work? YES! A job is only work if you do not like it. So, find your passion and you will never work a day in your life! Although locating your passion in life is the first important step in developing your career, it is also very important to receive the best possible education to assist you in achieving your professional goals. Therefore, before choosing a major or professional career track, do your homework and research the best courses and experiences and faculty mentors can then provide you with the cutting edge training that will allow you to begin your career on the right track.

SUMMARY

- Exercise science refers to the application of science to the phenomenon of movement in physical activity, exercise, sport, and athletic performance.
- Exercise science has evolved from the work of scholars and professionals from a variety of disciplines, subdisciplines, and specialty areas.
- Much of the educational coursework provided in a curriculum of study is valuable preparation for professional employment or continued study in graduate or professional school.
- Teachers, coaches, exercise specialists, healthcare providers, scholars, and researchers use the knowledge gained from exercise science in both basic and applied contexts.
- Exercise science is truly interdisciplinary with individuals from a wide array of backgrounds working together to provide the most relevant information and answer important questions related to individual health, exercise, medicine, public health, sport, and athletic competition.

FOR REVIEW

1. What is the difference between morbidity and mortality?

2. What disciplines, subdisciplines, and specialty areas constitute exercise science?

3. Describe the characteristics of an academic discipline?

4. What are the unique differences between physical activity, exercise, sport, and athletic competition?

5. What major factors have contributed to the separation of exercise science from the discipline of physical education?

6. In what significant ways did the Harvard Fatigue Laboratory contribute to the development of exercise science?

7. What are the primary ways the American College of Sports Medicine disseminates information to the professional membership and general population?

8. Why must exercise science students pay close attention to required coursework if planning on obtaining certification or licensure after graduation?

9. What are the primary requirements for entry into a professional career in a healthcare field after graduation?

10. What is the difference between basic and applied research?

11. What is the difference between quantitative and qualitative research?

REFERENCES

1. American College of Sports Medicine. Prevention of thermal injuries during distance running. *Med Sci Sports Exerc.* 1974;19:529.

2. American College of Sports Medicine. Position stand: Exercise and physical activity for older adults. *Med Sci Sports Exerc.* 1998;30:992–1008.

3. American College of Sports Medicine. The recommended quantity and quality of exercise for developing and maintaining cardiorespiratory and muscular fitness, and flexibility in health adults. *Med Sci Sports Exerc.* 1998;30:975–91.

4. American College of Sports Medicine. Team physician consensus statement. *Med Sci Sports Exerc.* 2000;32:877–8.

5. American College of Sports Medicine. Physical activity and bone health. *Med Sci Sports Exerc.* 2004;36:1985–96.

6. Ary D, Jacobs L, Razevieh A. *Introduction to Research in Education.* New York (NY): Holt, Rinehart, and Winston; 1985.

7. Baumgartner TA, Hensley LD. *Conducting and Reading Research in Health and Human Performance.* New York (NY): McGraw-Hill Publishers; 2006.

8. Berryman JW. *Out of Many, One: A History of the American College of Sports Medicine.* Champaign (IL): Human Kinetics; 1995.

9. Berryman JW. Ancient and early influences. In: Tipton CM, editor. *Exercise Physiology: People and Ideas.* New York (NY): Oxford University Press; 2003. p. 1–38.

10. Bish CL, Blanck HM, Serdula MK, Marcus M, Kohl HW, Khan LK. Diet and physical activity behaviors among americans trying to lose weight: 2000 behavioral risk factor surveillance system. *Obes Res.* 2005;13:596–607.

11. Bracken, N. *NCAA® Sports Sponsorship and Participation Rates Report.* Indianapolis (IN): National Collegiate Athletic Association; 2008. p. 1–233. Available at www.ncaapublications.com

12. Burton NW. Occupation, hours worked, and leisure-time physical activity. *Prev Med.* 2000;31:673–81.

13. Buskirk ER, Tipton CM. Exercise physiology. In: Massengale JD, Swanson RA, editor. *The History of Exercise and Sport Science.* Champaign (IL): Human Kinetics; 2003. p. 367–438.

14. Centers for Disease Control and Prevention. Prevalence of no leisure-time physical activity – 35 States and the District of Columbia, 1988–2002. *Morb Mortal.* 2004;53:82–6.

15. DeVries HA. History of exercise science. In: Housh TJ, Housh DJ, Johnson GO, editor. *Introduction to Exercise Science.* San Francisco (CA): Benjamin Cummings; 2008. p. 17–40.

16. Drew CJ, Hardman ML, Hart AW. *Designing and Conducting Research: Inquiry into Education and Social Sciences.* Needham Heights (MA): Allyn & Bacon; 1996.

17. Durant J. *Highlights of the Olympics: From Ancient Times to the Present.* New York (NY): Hastings House Publishers; 1973.

18. Flegal KM, Carroll MD, Kuczmarski RJ, Johnson CL. Overweight and obesity in the United States: Prevalence and trends, 1960–1994. *Int J Obes.* 1998;22:39–47.

19. Flegal KM, Williamson DF, Pamuk ER, Rosenberg HM. Estimating deaths attributable to obesity in the United States. *Am J Public Health.* 2004;94:1486–9.

20. Friedenreich CM. Physical activity and cancer: Lessons learned in nutrition epidemiology. *Nutr Rev.* 2001;59:349–57.

21. Gay LR, Airasian P. *Educational Research: Competencies for Analysis and Application.* Upper Saddle River (NJ): Prentice-Hall; 2000.

22. Gerber EW. *Innovators and Institutions in Physical Education.* Philadelphia (PA): Lea and Febiger; 1971.

23. Henry FM. Physical education: An academic discipline. *J Health Phys Educ Recreation.* 1964;35:32–3,69.

24. Hivert MF, Sullivan LM, Fox CS, et al. Associations of adiponectin, resistin, and tumor necrosis factor-{alpha} with insulin resistance. *J Clin Endocrinol Metab.* 2008;93:3165–72.

25. Irving LM, Wall M, Nuemark-Sztainer D, Story M. Steroid use among adolescents: Findings from Project EAT. *J Adolesc Health.* 2008;30:243–52.

26. Kung HC, Hoyert DL, Xu J, Murphy SL. Deaths: Final data for 2005. Centers for Disease Control and Prevention. National Vital Statistics Report. 2008;56(10):1–121.

27. Maron BJ, Isner JM, McKenna WJ. 26th Bethesda conference: Recommendations for determining eligibility for competition in athletes with cardiovascular abnormalities. Task Force 3: Hypertrophic cardiomyopathy, myocarditis and other myopericardial diseases and mitral valve prolapse. *J Am Coll Cardiol.* 1994;24:880–5.

28. Minino AM, Heron MP, Murphy SL, Kochanek KD. Deaths: Final Data for 2004. U.S. Department of Health and Human Services. National Vital Statistics Report. 2007;55(19): 1–120.

29. National Federation of State High School Associations. National Federation of State High School Associations 2006–07 Athletics Participation Summary. 2008. Available from: http://www.nfhs.org/.

30. Neutens JJ, Rubinson L. *Research Techniques for the Health Sciences.* San Francisco (CA): Benjamin Cummings; 2002.

31. Ogden CL, Carroll MD, Curtin LR, McDowell MA, Tabak CJ, Flegal KM. Prevalence of overweight and obesity in the United States, 1999–2004. *JAMA.* 2006;295:1549–55.

32. Pate RR, Pratt M, Blair SN, et al. A recommendation from the Centers for Disease Control and Prevention and the American College of Sports Medicine. *JAMA.* 1995;273:402–7.

33. Senn AE. *Power, Politics, and the Olympic Games.* Champaign (IL): Human Kinetics; 1999.

34. Sidentop D. *Introduction to Physical Education, Fitness, and Sport.* Mountain View (CA): Mayfield Publishing Company; 1994.

35. Slyper AH. The pediatric obesity epidemic: Causes and controversies. *J Clin Endocrinol Metab.* 2004;89:2540–7.

36. Swanson RA, Massengale JD. Exercise and sport science in 20th-century America. In: Massengale JD, Swanson RA, editors. *The History of Exercise and Sport Science*. Champaign (IL): Human Kinetics; 1997. p. 1–14.

37. Tipton CM. Exercise physiology, part II: A contemporary historical perspective. In: Massengale JD, Swanson RA, editors. *The History of Exercise and Sport Science*. Champaign (IL): Human Kinetics; 1997. p. 396–438.

38. U.S. Department of Health and Human Services. Health behaviors of adults: United States, 2002–04. 2006. p. 10–230, 1–156.

39. U.S. Department of Health and Human Services, Centers for Disease Control and Prevention, National Center for Chronic Disease Prevention and Health Promotion, and The President's Council on Physical Fitness and Sports. Physical Activity and Health: A Report of the Surgeon General. 1995.

2

Exercise Science: A Systems Approach

At the completion of this chapter you will be able to do the following:

1. Describe the meaning and context of a systems approach to the study of exercise science.
2. Understand the primary functions of each system of the body.
3. Provide examples of how each system of the body can influence physical activity and exercise.
4. Provide examples of how each system of the body can influence sport and athletic performance.

As identified in Chapter 1, several interrelated disciplines, subdisciplines, and specialty areas constitute exercise science. Collectively, the study of each component of exercise science is based on a core understanding of the structure (anatomy) and function (physiology) of the human body. It is expected that beginning exercise science students enroll in courses in human anatomy and physiology, often in the first year of study in college. The knowledge acquired in these courses provides the necessary foundation for advanced study in exercise science at both the undergraduate and graduate levels.

A systems approach to the study of exercise science allows students to understand how the various systems of the body respond to acute and chronic stimuli and conditions. Each system has specific functions that cannot be performed in the expected manner in isolation and without interaction with other systems of the body. This system integration provides for the coordinated control of the body environment and allows the body to respond to the challenges encountered every day. Appropriate responses to challenges such as physical activity, regular exercise, stress, changes in nutritional intake, and extreme environmental conditions allow us to be healthy and perform at optimal levels during sport and athletic competition.

This chapter presents a systems approach to the study of exercise science. To maintain a current and accurate knowledge base with today's rapid generation of information, exercise science students must be able to draw on their conceptual understanding of how systems work together instead of merely recalling isolated facts. Athletic trainers, clinical exercise physiologists, sport biomechanists, and other exercise science professionals are better prepared to perform their job by having a solid understanding of how the various structures and systems of the body interrelate and function together. For example, a clinical exercise physiologist designing a rehabilitation program for an individual recovering from a heart attack must understand how the cardiovascular, pulmonary, and muscular systems work together to create movement and respond to physical activity and exercise. Only with a sound understanding of the structure and functioning of the body's integrated systems can the clinical exercise physiologist design a rehabilitation program that is safe and effective in preparing the individual to return to activities of daily living and occupational activities without an elevated level of risk for an adverse medical event. Figure 2.1 illustrates the various systems of the body. This chapter will provide a short description of the systems of the body and examples of how each system is affected by or responds to (a) physical activity and exercise and (b) sport and athletic performance. This information should provide a foundation for which exercise science students begin to understand the integrated systems approach to the study of exercise science.

NERVOUS SYSTEM

The nervous system is one of the two primary control systems of the body (the other primary control system is the endocrine system). The nervous system controls the voluntary and involuntary actions and functions of the body and works with other systems to regulate and respond to challenges such as exercise or disease conditions. For ease of study, we generally divide the nervous system into the central and peripheral components, but in reality the two components function

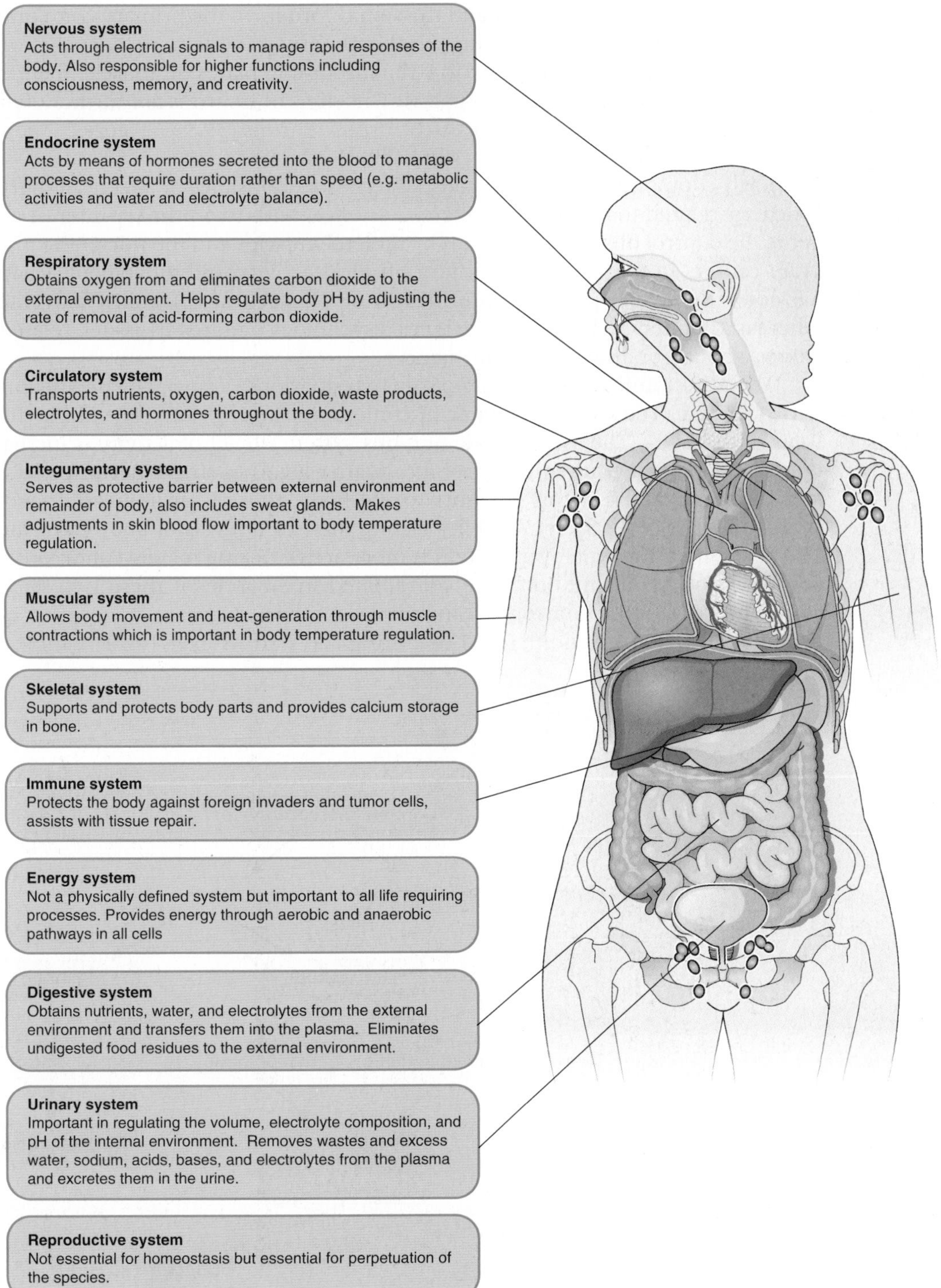

Nervous system
Acts through electrical signals to manage rapid responses of the body. Also responsible for higher functions including consciousness, memory, and creativity.

Endocrine system
Acts by means of hormones secreted into the blood to manage processes that require duration rather than speed (e.g. metabolic activities and water and electrolyte balance).

Respiratory system
Obtains oxygen from and eliminates carbon dioxide to the external environment. Helps regulate body pH by adjusting the rate of removal of acid-forming carbon dioxide.

Circulatory system
Transports nutrients, oxygen, carbon dioxide, waste products, electrolytes, and hormones throughout the body.

Integumentary system
Serves as protective barrier between external environment and remainder of body, also includes sweat glands. Makes adjustments in skin blood flow important to body temperature regulation.

Muscular system
Allows body movement and heat-generation through muscle contractions which is important in body temperature regulation.

Skeletal system
Supports and protects body parts and provides calcium storage in bone.

Immune system
Protects the body against foreign invaders and tumor cells, assists with tissue repair.

Energy system
Not a physically defined system but important to all life requiring processes. Provides energy through aerobic and anaerobic pathways in all cells

Digestive system
Obtains nutrients, water, and electrolytes from the external environment and transfers them into the plasma. Eliminates undigested food residues to the external environment.

Urinary system
Important in regulating the volume, electrolyte composition, and pH of the internal environment. Removes wastes and excess water, sodium, acids, bases, and electrolytes from the plasma and excretes them in the urine.

Reproductive system
Not essential for homeostasis but essential for perpetuation of the species.

FIGURE 2.1 ▼ Systems of the body. (Adapted from Sherwood L. *Fundamentals of Physiology: A Human Perspective.* Belmont (CA): Thompson Publishing; 2006.)

together very closely. The brain and the spinal cord form the primary components of the central nervous system. The peripheral nervous system includes the **afferent neurons** and **efferent neurons**, the motor end plates on muscle fibers, and the sensory receptors on sensory organs. The efferent neurons are further divided into the **somatic** neurons and the **autonomic** neurons (39,99). Figure 2.2 depicts the organization of the nervous system (99).

Each component of the nervous system is responsible for several important functions related to the study of exercise science, with two primary interest areas being the control of body movement by skeletal muscles and the role of the higher brain centers in performing voluntary physical activity and movement. Chapter 8 (Motor Behavior) provides information on the neural control of movement, whereas Chapter 7 (Exercise and Sport Psychology) addresses issues related to exercise behavior and sport performance.

The autonomic nervous system has two divisions: **sympathetic** and **parasympathetic**. These systems work in conjunction to regulate the various functions of the body. The sympathetic nervous system's level of activity is increased when the body is required to respond to higher levels of stress. Because physical activity and exercise act as stressors to the body, there is an increased level of sympathetic nervous system activity during increased levels of body movement. The parasympathetic nervous system is more active during resting conditions and following food consumption. The coordinated interaction of these two systems allows for both subtle and significant changes in body function to occur. A good example of this interaction would be during the start of exercise. The increased

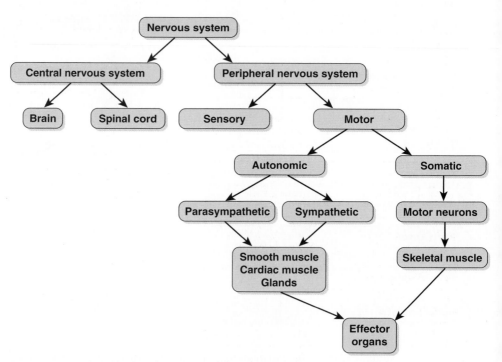

FIGURE 2.2 ▼ Organizational structure of the nervous system.

sympathetic activity and the decreased parasympathetic activity results in an increase in heart rate, strength of cardiac contraction, and blood pressure, as well as a redistribution of blood flow from inactive tissues (e.g., stomach and kidneys) to active tissues (e.g., heart and skeletal muscle). These changes allow the body to coordinate an appropriate response to meet the demands of exercise.

Nervous System and Exercise Science

Although many neurologic disorders can affect the body's response to physical activity and exercise, many affected individuals can achieve significant health benefits with participation in regular physical activity and exercise programs. For example, the disease condition cerebral palsy interferes with the normal development of areas of the brain that control muscle tone and spinal reflexes. This results in limited ability to move and maintain balance and posture (63). The location and extent of the injury within the brain will influence the resulting changes in muscle tone and spinal reflex sequelae that occurs (63). Medical doctors classify individuals based on functional ability, which can be beneficial for helping to identify an appropriate exercise program (63). Individuals with cerebral palsy can benefit from participation in an exercise program focusing on the development of muscular strength, flexibility, and cardiovascular fitness (74,86,87). Owing to the nature of the disorder resistance exercise may be a more suitable type of exercise for individuals with cerebral palsy to perform. Exercise science professionals can play a valuable role in helping individuals affected with many neurologic disorders. Table 2.1 lists the various neurologic disorders that can have improved health and fitness outcomes as a result of well-planned and appropriate physical activity and exercise program (5). For additional information about the role of exercise in treatment programs for neurologic disorders, the reader is directed to *ACSM's Exercise Management for Persons with Chronic Disease and Disability* (5).

Various components of the nervous system can play an important role in sport and athletic performance. For example, it is believed that as an aerobic endurance athlete becomes better trained there are changes to the autonomic nervous system that could lead to improvements in performance (23,36,37). Following training, increases in parasympathetic nervous activity allow for a reduced heart rate leading to a longer filling time of the heart during the period of diastole. The increased filling results in a greater **stroke volume** during each contraction of the heart, which

---

Afferent neurons Nerves that carry electric impulses toward the brain and spinal cord.

Efferent neurons Nerves that carry electric impulses away from the brain and spinal cord.

Somatic Part of the nervous system that controls voluntary action.

Autonomic Part of the nervous system that regulates involuntary action.

Sympathetic Part of the autonomic nervous system that tends to act in opposition to the parasympathetic nervous system especially under conditions of stress.

Parasympathetic Part of the autonomic nervous system that tends to act in opposition to the sympathetic nervous system.

Stroke volume The volume of blood pumped from the heart with each contraction.

Table 2.1	Neurologic Disorders and the Potential Benefits of Exercise (5)
NEUROLOGIC DISORDER	**BENEFITS OF EXERCISE**
Alzheimer disease	Increased fitness, physical function, cognitive function, and positive behavior
Amyotrophic lateral sclerosis	Maintain strength in healthy muscle fibers and range of motion in joints
Cerebral palsy	Improved fitness, work capacity, and sense of wellness
Deaf and hard of hearing	Improved fitness, balance, self-image, and confidence, with enhanced socialization skills
Epilepsy	Improved fitness
Mental illness	Improved fitness, mood, self-concept, and work behavior with decreased depression and anxiety
Mental retardation	Improved functional capacity and strength
Multiple sclerosis	Improved fitness and functional performance
Muscular dystrophy	Slow down or possibly reverse the deterioration in muscle function
Parkinson disease	Enhanced functionality and movement
Polio and postpolio syndrome	Improved fitness and lower leg strength
Spinal cord injury	Improved fitness and sense of well-being
Stroke and head injury	Improved fitness and muscular strength
Visual impairment	Improved fitness, balance, self-image, and confidence, with enhanced socialization skills

in turn causes a higher **cardiac output,** and hence more blood being pumped to working tissues. The changes in autonomic nervous system activity also allow for an increased blood flow to active tissues (i.e., skeletal muscle) during exercise (14). The higher cardiac output and enhanced blood flow to working tissues would result in a greater oxygen delivery to skeletal muscle and most likely an improvement in aerobic endurance performance (14). Table 2.2 provides a summary of the major functions of the nervous system and some examples of how those functions relate to physical activity, exercise, sport, and athletic performance.

MUSCULAR SYSTEM

The muscular system works in conjunction with both the nervous system and the skeletal system to create movement of the human body. In response to nervous system input, the various muscles of the body can contract and generate force.

Table 2.2	Functions of the Nervous System and their Relationship to Physical Activity, Exercise, Sport, and Athletic Performance (99)
FUNCTION	**RELATIONSHIP TO PHYSICAL ACTIVITY, EXERCISE, SPORT, AND ATHLETIC PERFORMANCE**
Afferent neurons provide central nervous system (CNS) with sensory and visceral information	Allows for a rapid and coordinated control of body systems in response to movement
Control centers for cardiovascular, respiratory, and digestive systems	Allows for a rapid and coordinated response to movement
Controls activity of smooth muscle, cardiac muscle, and glands through the autonomic nervous system	Allows for a rapid and coordinated response of body systems to movement
Efferent neurons control movement of skeletal muscle through somatic nervous system	Allows for the body to contract skeletal muscle and create movement
Maintenance of balance	Allows for correct positioning of the body during movement
Regulation of temperature control, thirst, urine output, and food intake	Allows for the body to regulate the internal environment, remove waste products, and supply energy to the tissues in response to movement
Voluntary control of movement, thinking, memory, decision making, creativity, self-consciousness, role in motor control	Allows for control of the body during participation in any type of movement

The contraction of skeletal muscle causes the bones to which they are attached to move, creating movement of the body parts. Skeletal muscle, because of its ability to generate energy and heat, also helps maintain an appropriate body temperature. Contraction of smooth muscle, found in the walls of the hollow organs and tubes in the body, regulates the movement of blood through the blood vessels, food through the digestive tract, air through the respiratory airways, and urine through the urinary tract. Contraction of cardiac muscle, found in the walls of the heart, generates the force by which the heart delivers blood to the tissues of the body (39,99).

The primary components of the muscular system are the individual muscle fibers (i.e., muscle cells). Muscle fibers can generate force through the interaction of various contractile and regulatory proteins. This force allows the different types of muscle to perform their specific functions in very unique ways. Muscle fibers have distinct characteristics depending on the type of muscle (skeletal, smooth, and cardiac). Skeletal muscle fibers are typically named based on certain contractile or

Cardiac output The volume of blood pumped by the heart per unit of time, usually 1 minute.

Table 2.3	**Nomenclature, and Specific Contractile, and Metabolic Characteristics of Skeletal Muscle Fibers (38,58)**		
	TYPE OF FIBER		
CHARACTERISTIC	**TYPE I—SLOW OXIDATIVE**	**TYPE IIA—FAST OXIDATIVE**	**TYPE IIB—FAST GLYCOLYTIC**
Speed of contraction	Slow	Fast	Fast
Resistance to fatigue	High	Intermediate	Low
Myosin ATPase activity	Low	High	High
Oxidative energy capacity	High	High	Low
Nonoxidative energy capacity	Low	Intermediate	High
Color of fiber	Red	Red	White

metabolic characteristics. Table 2.3 illustrates the different nomenclature, along with the specific contractile and metabolic characteristics of skeletal muscle (38,58).

Smooth muscle and cardiac muscle share some basic properties with skeletal muscle, yet each type also displays unique characteristics regarding the force and speed of contraction. In general, the contraction process in all three types of muscle is the same. For example, the initiation of contraction in muscle occurs through a calcium-dependent process and the generation of force occurs via the sliding protein filament theory. There are some other significant differences among the three muscle types. For example, skeletal muscle is under voluntary control, whereas smooth and cardiac muscles are controlled by the autonomic nervous system. Furthermore, the force of smooth and cardiac muscle contraction can be influenced directly by various hormones from the endocrine system, whereas skeletal muscle cannot (39,99).

Muscular System and Exercise Science

Previously sedentary individuals who begin an exercise program for improving their health and fitness are likely to experience delayed onset muscle soreness in the active muscles. This muscle soreness generally appears 24 to 48 hours after strenuous exercise and can last for up to 72 to 96 hours. Delayed onset muscle soreness is believed to result from tissue injury caused by excessive mechanical force exerted upon the muscle fibers and connective tissue (12,30,31,92,101). Delayed onset muscle soreness occurs most frequently following unaccustomed exercise that is of high intensity (92). It is thought that delayed onset muscle soreness is a result of cellular damage that breaks down cellular proteins in the muscle. This causes the immune system to create an inflammatory response in the muscle that leads to the formation of swelling. Afferent nerves then become stimulated, and pain is felt in the muscle. **Eccentric muscle actions** appear to cause greater damage to the tissues and more substantial soreness and pain in the affected muscle (16). The phenomenon of delayed onset muscle soreness has been studied by exercise science and allied healthcare professionals for decades in an effort to understand how this soreness develops and to determine if there are any preventive measures that might eliminate or at least reduce the amount of muscular soreness experienced. Gradually beginning an exercise program, while simultaneously avoiding strenuous eccentric muscle actions, appears to be the best way to avoid delayed onset muscle soreness. Other preventive and treatment measures such as hyperbaric oxygen therapy and prostaglandin-inhibiting drugs seem to provide little protection or relief from delayed onset muscle soreness (42,61,79).

High-intensity resistance exercise training results in significant gains in muscle size and strength that can result in an improvement in sport and athletic performance. The increase in muscle size can occur as a result of either increases in the size of the individual muscle fibers (called **muscle fiber hypertrophy**) or increases in the individual muscle fibers (called **muscle fiber hyperplasia**). Muscle fiber hypertrophy has been demonstrated to occur in response to resistance exercise training, however, there is still some question as to whether muscle fiber hyperplasia occurs (66). Growth-promoting agents from the endocrine system help stimulate muscle hypertrophy. Athletes who have engaged in high intensity and high volume resistance exercise training for many years appear to have more muscle fibers per motor unit than the average person (62). Additionally, the use of anabolic steroids and other human and synthetic growth-promoting agents may result in an increase in the number of individual fibers within a muscle (54). If hyperplasia does occur, it could result from one of two proposed mechanisms (2,54,57). Fiber number could increase, if the existing fibers hypertrophied to the extent that the individual fiber became so large that it split into more than one fiber. A second mechanism for increasing muscle fiber number could occur if existing **undifferentiated satellite cells** in the muscle are stimulated to grow into fully developed muscle fibers. Regardless of the mechanism involved in muscle fiber hyperplasia, the increase in number appears to be small and dependent on a variety of factors including genetic profile, training history, nutritional intake, and the use of growth-promoting substances (54,57). Figure 2.3 shows a resistance-trained athlete who has experienced muscle hypertrophy. Table 2.4 provides the functions of the muscular system and examples of how those functions relate to physical activity, exercise, sport, and athletic performance (99).

> ➤ **Thinking Critically**
>
> *In what ways has a systems approach to exercise science contributed to a broader understanding of the muscular and skeletal factors that influence successful sport and athletic performance?*

Eccentric muscle actions When the muscle fibers lengthen when generating force.
Muscle fiber hypertrophy An increase in the muscle fiber cross-sectional size.
Muscle fiber hyperplasia An increase in the number of muscle fibers in a muscle.
Undifferentiated satellite cells An undeveloped cell that has the potential to convert to a developed cell.

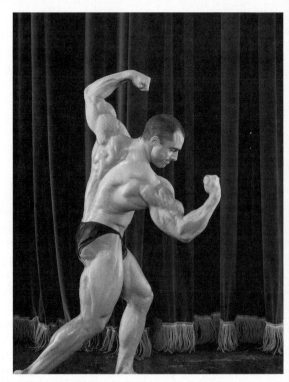

FIGURE 2.3 ▼ A resistance-trained athlete who has experienced muscle hypertrophy. (Photo from Blend Images/John Lund/Sam Diephuis/ Getty Images.)

SKELETAL SYSTEM

The skeletal system serves as a structural framework of the body, protecting underlying organs and tissues of the body, providing a lever system for movement, and serving as a storage area of minerals important to the body's function. The skeletal system is also involved in blood cell formation. During body movement, the skeletal system works with the muscular system to create movement or respond to nervous system stimulus. This close interaction of the muscular and skeletal systems often leads to the two systems being discussed together as the musculoskeletal system (81,99).

The minerals calcium and phosphorus and the different cells that constitute the bone marrow are the primary components of the skeletal system. The bones provide structural support, which transfers the weight of the body to the ground through the lower extremities. The bones also provide a site to which muscles can attach, subsequently acting as a lever system for the movement of body parts. Bone tissue is a rigid mass and therefore offers protection to underlying structures such as the brain, spinal cord, heart, and lungs. The skeletal system serves as a reservoir for calcium, so when calcium levels are insufficient to meet the body's needs calcium can be taken from bone and then replaced when calcium levels are returned to normal. Several bones of the body contain red bone marrow, which produces all types of blood cells (red, white, platelets) in a process called **hematopoiesis** (81,99).

Table 2.4	Functions of the Muscular System and their Relationship to Physical Activity, Exercise, Sport, and Athletic Performance	
FUNCTION	**RELATION TO PHYSICAL ACTIVITY, EXERCISE, SPORT, AND ATHLETIC PERFORMANCE**	
Cardiac muscle contraction propels blood through the circulatory system	Delivers nutrients and oxygen to the working tissues of the body and removes waste products	
Skeletal muscle generates movement, which increases energy expenditure and heat production	Allows for body movement, responsible for the majority of daily energy expenditure	
Smooth muscle contraction and dilation regulates diameter of passageways in the cardiovascular and respiratory systems	Allows for coordinated flow of blood to working tissues and air to the lungs for gas exchange	

Skeletal System and Exercise Science

The interaction of physical activity, exercise, nutrition, and aging has significant implications for the health of the skeletal system. Without appropriate levels of physical activity and adequate calcium intake in the diet, the risk for developing osteoporosis can increase in any individual regardless of age. Osteoporosis is a disease condition characterized by low bone mineral density. Figure 2.4 illustrates the differences in bone mineral density between normal bone and osteoporotic bone. An individual is clinically defined as having osteoporosis when the bone mineral density is less than the bone mineral density of the lowest 2.5% of the population of gender-matched young adults (56). The two primary strategies for decreasing the risk of developing osteoporosis are (a) maintaining peak bone mass by age 30 years and (b) slowing the rate of bone loss over the remaining years of life (6). Maximizing peak bone mass can be best accomplished by performing moderately intense exercise that requires some structural support such as walking or jogging (6,33,68). Consuming at least a minimal daily level of calcium also maximizes bone mass. Although the optimal level of calcium intake for all individuals has yet to be determined, clearly consuming an inadequate amount of calcium when young will prohibit an individual from maximizing bone mineral density (6,44,45). Exercise science professionals are instrumental in developing effective nutrition and physical activity and exercise programs for reducing the risk of osteoporosis in men and women of all ages.

Hematopoiesis   The formation and development of red blood cells.

Osteoporosis   A disorder in which the bones become increasingly porous, brittle, and subject to fracture, owing to loss of calcium and other mineral components.

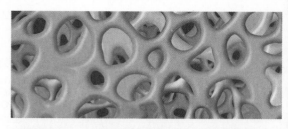

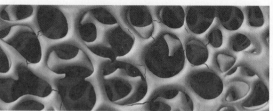

FIGURE 2.4 ▽ The differences in bone mineral density between normal bone (**top panel**) and osteoporotic bone (**bottom panel**).

The skeletal system also plays an important role in determining success in sport and athletic performance. One of the many important factors in determining success in aerobic endurance events is the ability to deliver oxygen to the working tissues of the body. Almost all of the oxygen delivery in the body occurs via red blood cells (39). The red marrow in bone generates red blood cells. The endocrine hormone **erythropoietin** controls this process (39). If the number of red blood cells can be increased in the body, oxygen delivery to the tissues increases as well and we usually see improvements in cardiovascular fitness and endurance exercise performance (14). Aerobic endurance athletes can benefit from an increase in red blood cell number. The development and production of **recombinant human erythropoietin** (rEPO) have been demonstrated to increase red blood cell formation and reduce the risk of anemia as part of the therapy for a wide variety of clinically ill patients (35). If rEPO can increase red blood cell formation in athletes, there exists the potential for improving performance through an increased delivery of oxygen to the working tissues. In fact, rEPO has been demonstrated to improve cycling performance (10) and there have been numerous implications of illegal rEPO use by aerobic endurance athletes. Sports-governing associations have routinely expelled athletes from competition because the athletes test positive for rEPO during drug testing (9). Altitude training may be a legal way to induce bone marrow to produce more red blood cells (64). Living at high altitudes where there is less oxygen and training at lower altitudes may be a legal and ethical way to stimulate bone to increase the red blood cell level, enhance oxygen delivery by the cardiovascular system, and improve aerobic endurance exercise performance (64). In response to the potential for improving aerobic endurance performance with this type of living and training environment, commercial companies have developed altitude tents that allow individuals to rest and sleep at "high altitudes" and train at low altitudes regardless of an individual's physical living location. Table 2.5 provides the functions of the skeletal system and examples of how those functions relate to physical activity, exercise, sport, and athletic performance.

Table 2.5	Functions of the Skeletal System and their Relationship to Physical Activity, Exercise, Sport, and Athletic Performance	
FUNCTION	**RELATION TO PHYSICAL ACTIVITY, EXERCISE, SPORT, AND ATHLETIC PERFORMANCE**	
Formation of red blood cells	Carries oxygen to the tissues of the body; a key step in aerobic energy production	
Lever system provides movement to the body	Allows for the contraction of the muscles to move body parts	
Provides a structural framework to the body	Allows for body position and movement	
Storage of minerals such as calcium and phosphorus	Appropriate levels are critical for normal physiologic function and strong bone health	

CARDIOVASCULAR SYSTEM

The cardiovascular system transports blood containing oxygen, nutrients, and other substances (e.g., hormones, electrolytes, and drugs) to the tissues of the body, whereas at the same time facilitating the removal of carbon dioxide and other waste products from the body. The cardiovascular system also assists in body temperature regulation. Owing to the unique interaction of the cardiovascular and respiratory systems, these two systems are often referred to as one system; the cardio-respiratory or the cardio-pulmonary system. Although the two systems do work in conjunction with each other, they each have other functions that allow them to be integrated with other systems of the body as well (39,99).

The primary components of the cardiovascular system include the heart, arteries, capillaries, veins, and blood. The heart is comprised of cardiac muscle and nervous tissue that generates the force that propels the blood through the body. The arteries and some of the veins are comprised of smooth muscle that helps distribute blood through the various tissues of the body. The capillaries are tubes, one cell thick, which facilitate the transfer of gases, nutrients, and waste products to and from the cells of the body. The blood is comprised of red and white blood cells and a watery fluid that carries the various gases, nutrients, and waste products to the body tissues (99). Figure 2.5 illustrates the various components of the cardiovascular system. Both cardiac muscle and smooth muscle respond to input from the nervous and endocrine systems. All of these systems function together to provide a coordinated response to the challenges of physical activity and exercise.

Erythropoietin A hormone that stimulates the production of red blood cells and hemoglobin.
Recombinant human erythropoietin The laboratory production of human erythropoietin.

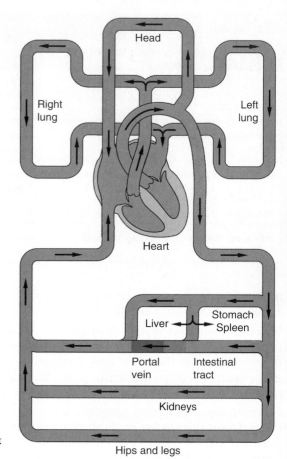

FIGURE 2.5 ▼ Components of the cardiovascular system. (LifeART image
copyright © 2010 Lippincott, Williams &
Wilkins. All rights reserved.)

Cardiovascular System and Exercise Science

A disease free cardiovascular system with strength sufficient to respond to the
demands of daily living, physical activity, and exercise is critical to good health.
Cardiovascular disease is one of the leading causes of death in the United States
(80). Years of research by public health experts and exercise science professionals have provided great insight into factors that lead to the development
of cardiovascular disease (11,20,75,76). Coronary artery disease (CAD) is the
primary cardiovascular disease in most Americans (20). **Atherosclerosis**, a disease process whereby cholesterol and blood lipids build up in the arteries sup-
plying blood to the heart, results in a reduction of blood flow to cardiac muscle
(39). If blood flow to the heart is reduced to a critical level, a heart attack can
result. Figure 2.6 shows how the buildup of plaque can cause a decrease in the
lumen of the artery. Increased levels of physical activity and regular exercise
are associated with a reduced risk of morbidity and mortality from cardiovascular disease (11,94,97). Physical activity and exercise enhance cardiac muscle
function and improve blood flow to the heart and other tissues of the body.

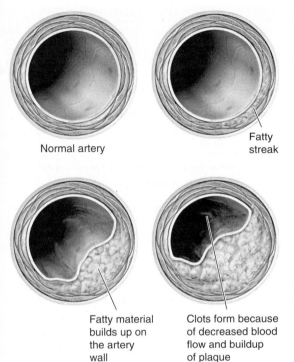

Normal artery

Fatty streak

Fatty material builds up on the artery wall

Clots form because of decreased blood flow and buildup of plaque

FIGURE 2.6 ▼ How the buildup of plaque can cause a decrease in the lumen of the artery is shown. (Asset provided by Anatomical Chart Co.)

When an individual has a heart attack, that person is often referred to a cardiac rehabilitation program. In these programs, exercise science professionals work to increase levels of physical fitness, improve nutritional intake, reduce stress, and change unhealthy behaviors. Cardiac rehabilitation programs use regular exercise as an integral component for helping individuals recover from a cardiac event. For more information on cardiac rehabilitation programs, please see Chapter 4 (Clinical Exercise Physiology).

The cardiovascular system also plays an important role in the successful performance of various types of sport and athletic events. The delivery of oxygen and nutrients to working muscles and the removal of metabolic waste products are key in determining success during aerobic endurance events (14). The cardiovascular system works in conjunction with the nervous, pulmonary, and endocrine systems to accomplish this. Athletic events that last longer than approximately 3 to 5 minutes rely heavily on the adequate delivery of oxygen to tissues. **Maximal oxygen consumption** (VO_{2max}) is defined as the maximal amount of oxygen consumed by the body during maximal effort exercise. Much

---

Atherosclerosis A disease process whereby cholesterol and blood lipids build up in the arteries causing a narrowing of the vessel opening.

Maximal oxygen consumption The maximum amount of oxygen the body can use during maximal effort exercise.

Table 2.6	Functions of the Cardiovascular System and their Relationship to Physical Activity, Exercise, Sport, and Athletic Performance
FUNCTION	**RELATION TO PHYSICAL ACTIVITY, EXERCISE, SPORT, AND ATHLETIC PERFORMANCE**
Assists with temperature regulation	Controls body temperature during periods of increased movement
Removes carbon dioxide and waste products	Allows for elimination of metabolic waste products of metabolism
Transports nutrients and other substances to the tissues of the body	Allows for delivery of macronutrients and substances to working tissues

of the available research indicates that the delivery of blood and oxygen to the working tissues by the cardiovascular system is the limiting factor in determining an individual's VO_{2max}. Because successful performance in most aerobic endurance events is determined in part by an individual's VO_{2max}, this makes the contribution of the cardiovascular system critical to endurance performance success (14,27,40). Exercise science professionals are frequently involved in developing new training programs, improving biomechanical movement, enhancing nutritional intake, and improving psychological factors in an effort to enhance oxygen delivery to the tissues and improving sport and athletic performance. Table 2.6 provides a summary of the functions of the cardiovascular system and examples of how those functions relate to physical activity, exercise, sport, and athletic performance.

> ➤ *Thinking Critically*
> *In what ways has a systems approach to exercise science contributed to a better understanding of the role of the cardiovascular system in promoting good health by reducing the risk for heart disease and enhancing aerobic endurance performance?*

PULMONARY SYSTEM

The pulmonary system brings air into the lungs, allows for oxygen to be removed from the air, and facilitates the elimination of carbon dioxide into the external environment. By regulating the carbon dioxide levels in the blood, the pulmonary system also helps maintain the acid–base balance of the body. The lungs and associated structures create a large surface area between the blood and the external environment that allows for the fast and efficient exchange of oxygen and carbon dioxide in a healthy individual. The pulmonary system works in close conjunction with the cardiovascular system and two systems are often referred to as the cardio-respiratory or cardio-pulmonary system (39,99).

The primary components of the pulmonary system are the respiratory muscles, the respiratory airways, and the respiratory unit. The respiratory muscles (internal and external intercostals, diaphragm, and abdominals) create a pressure gradient in the chest and lungs that allow for airflow into and out of the lungs. The respiratory airways, some of which contain smooth muscle, begin with the mouth and nose, continue with the trachea, right and left bronchus, bronchiole, and end with the terminal bronchiole. Those respiratory airways, which contain smooth muscle are able to dilate and constrict, in response to internal and external stimuli. The bronchodilation and bronchoconstriction of the air passageways allow for increased or decreased airflow into the lungs, respectively. The respiratory unit consists of individual alveoli (where gas exchange occurs) and the pulmonary capillaries, which surround the alveoli. The majority of the exchange of oxygen and carbon dioxide occurs in the respiratory unit (39,99). Figure 2.7 illustrates the primary components of the pulmonary system.

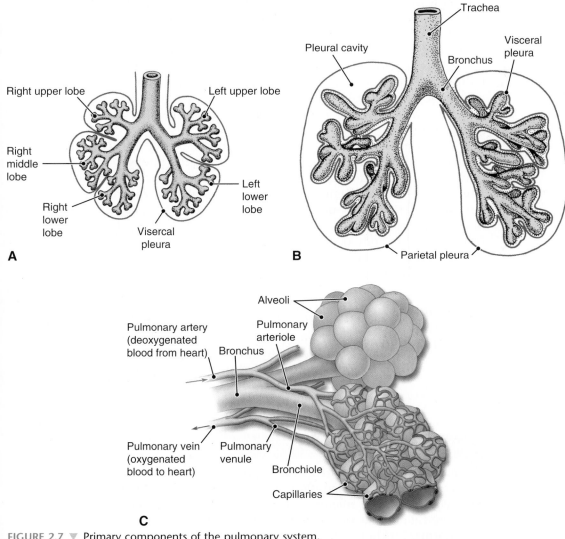

FIGURE 2.7 ▼ Primary components of the pulmonary system.

Pulmonary System and Exercise Science

Disease conditions of the pulmonary system play a significant role in the performance of physical activity and exercise by individuals. For example, chronic obstructive pulmonary disease (COPD) is a health condition that includes chronic bronchitis and emphysema and often results in a reduced ability to perform physical activity and exercise. Often the medical management team for an individual with COPD will include physical and respiratory therapists, pulmonologists, and clinical exercise physiologists. These individuals work together to improve the functional performance of the pulmonary system and increase the quality of the individual's life. Physical activity and exercise can also affect the pulmonary system and result in an asthmatic event triggered by an immune system response (103). This asthmatic event is typically referred to as **exercise-induced asthma**. Exercise-induced asthma can result in airway constriction, shortness of breath, and wheezing similar to those experienced with asthma, but in exercise-induced asthma symptoms occur on a transient basis (59). The type, intensity, and duration of exercise can all act to trigger an asthmatic event in susceptible individuals. Other environmental factors such as tobacco smoke, molds, dust, and cold temperatures may also play a role in triggering an exercise-induced asthma episode. An attack can result in difficult and labored exercise and reduce exercise compliance (51). The key to minimizing the occurrence of exercise-induced asthma is to avoid any predetermined factors that may trigger an episode (59).

The pulmonary system also plays an important role in successful sport and athletic performance. During very high to maximal intensity exercise, skeletal muscle breaks down carbohydrate and increases the production of lactic acid. The accumulation of lactic acid can cause the pH (a measure of the hydrogen ion concentration) in tissues of the body to decrease and become more acidic. To maintain pH of the body's fluids and tissues within an acceptable range, chemical reactions in the body occur and these reactions result in an increased production of carbon dioxide (39). The primary reaction that results in the formation of carbon dioxide as a result of an increase in hydrogen ion concentration is $H^+ + HCO_3^- \rightarrow H_2CO_3 \rightarrow H_2O + CO_2$. The increased carbon dioxide is ventilated outside of the body by the lungs and this helps keep the tissues of the body from becoming too acidic as it lowers the concentration of hydrogen ions (39). Table 2.7 provides a summary of the functions of the pulmonary system and examples of how those functions relate to physical activity, exercise, sport, and athletic performance.

> ➤ *Thinking Critically*
> *How would participation in a regular program of physical activity and exercise improve the functional ability of the pulmonary system to a disease condition of the lungs?*

URINARY SYSTEM

The urinary system eliminates waste products from the body and regulates the volume, electrolyte composition, and pH of the body fluids. All tissues of the body depend on the maintenance of a stable environment of the body fluids and removal of the toxic metabolic wastes produced by the cells as they perform their normal functions. Of special importance is the body's ability to regulate the

Table 2.7	Functions of the Pulmonary System and their Relationship to Physical Activity, Exercise, Sport, and Athletic Performance
FUNCTION	**RELATION TO PHYSICAL ACTIVITY AND EXERCISE AND SPORT AND ATHLETIC PERFORMANCE**
Brings oxygen into the body	Allows for energy production during movement through aerobic metabolism
Eliminates carbon dioxide from the body	Allows for the removal of carbon dioxide, a waste product of macronutrient metabolism
Helps regulate acid–base balance	Controls pH levels in the body during periods of high-intensity movement

volume and **osmolarity** (i.e., concentration) of the internal fluid environment by controlling sodium and water balance (39,99).

The primary components of the urinary system are the kidneys, renal artery and vein, ureter, urinary bladder, and urethra. The kidneys regulate the concentration of many of the plasma constituents, especially the electrolytes and water, and eliminate all the metabolic waste products (except for carbon dioxide). Plasma which is the watery portion of the blood progresses through the renal artery into the kidney where substances important to the body are retained, and the undesirable or excess materials are filtered into the urine for excretion from the body. The plasma then moves back to the central circulation through the renal vein. The ureter is responsible for transporting the fluid and waste products (now called urine) to the urinary bladder for storage until the urine is eliminated from the body through the urethra (39,99). Figure 2.8 illustrates the primary components of the urinary system.

Urinary System and Exercise Science

The urinary system regulates the total fluid volume and electrolyte concentration of the body and this function can have important implications for reducing the risk for certain diseases. Hypertension affects approximately 50 million individuals in the United States and can contribute to serious health effects (70). Individuals with this condition have an increased risk of developing cardiovascular disease (especially CAD and stroke) and kidney disease (20) Furthermore, all-cause mortality increases progressively with higher levels of both systolic blood pressure and diastolic blood pressure (20). The primary treatment of individuals with hypertension involves preventing morbidity and mortality associated with the high blood

Exercise-induced asthma A medical condition characterized by shortness of breath induced by sustained aerobic exercise.
Osmolarity A measure of the concentration of a solution.

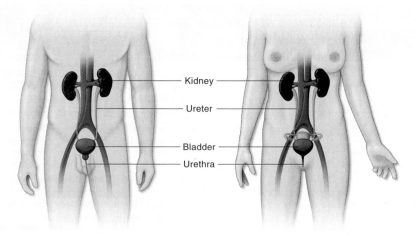

A **Anterior view**

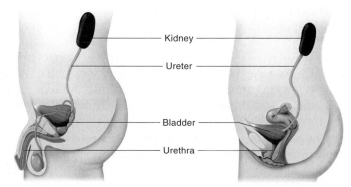

B **Lateral view**

FIGURE 2.8 ▼ Primary components of the urinary system. (From Premkumar K. *The Massage Connection Anatomy and Physiology*. Baltimore (MD): Lippincott, Williams & Wilkins; 2004.)

pressure and controlling blood pressure by the least invasive means possible (52). Individuals with a resting blood pressure of 140/90 mm Hg are treated for hypertension (52). Changes in physical activity and exercise habits and modification of nutritional intake are at the center of effective treatment programs for hypertension. The urinary system can play an important role in helping to manage blood pressure in hypertensive individuals by regulating fluid volume in the body.

Macronutrients The foodstuffs need in large quantities including carbohydrates, fats, and proteins that are used for numerous processes in the body.

Micronutrients The foodstuffs need in smaller quantities including vitamins and minerals that are used for numerous processes in the body.

Electrolytes The anions and cations that are distributed in the fluid compartments of the body.

Table 2.8	Functions of the Urinary System and their Relationship to Physical Activity, Exercise, Sport, and Athletic Performance	
FUNCTION	**RELATION TO PHYSICAL ACTIVITY, EXERCISE, SPORT, AND ATHLETIC PERFORMANCE**	
Eliminate waste products from the body	Removes waste products from increased levels of metabolism experienced during movement	
Long-term regulation of acid–base balance	Helps control body pH levels that may be affected by alterations in metabolism	
Regulate fluid volume and electrolyte concentrations	Controls levels of body fluids and electrolyte concentrations that are critical for efficient functioning of the body during movement	

Diuretics are a group of drugs that increase the excretion of sodium and water by the kidneys (60). Diuretics block the absorption of sodium from urine by the kidney and this in turn increases the volume of fluid excreted as urine. The reduction of sodium concentration in the blood results in a reduction of total blood volume and decreases the resistance by the blood vessels of the body. Both of these actions have the effect of reducing blood pressure (39).

The urinary system plays an important role in sport and athletic performance in many ways. Athletes who train and play sports in hot and/or humid conditions regulate body temperature primarily by sweating. As a result of sweating, the total body fluid volume decreases. In response to this decrease, the urinary system reabsorbs sodium and water from the urine in an effort to maintain an acceptable level of body water. The process of sodium and water reabsorption by the kidneys decreases the urine volume and makes the urine more concentrated. Exercise science professionals including sport nutritionists, athletic trainers, and sports medicine professionals encourage athletes to carefully examine the color of their urine as a way to monitor hydration status. When the urine is a dark concentrated color this usually indicates that the athlete is dehydrated and should consume more fluids (93). Athletes in sports using weight classes for competition may illegally use diuretics to increase the urine volume excreted from the body. This assists those athletes attempting to lose body weight to participate in a lower weight class. Athletes have also used diuretics to decrease the concentration of a drug in the urine by increasing the volume of urine excreted from the body. Increasing the volume of urine excreted will assist in lowering the concentration of the drug or its metabolites in the urine (39) and may help the athlete avoid the detection of illegal drug use. Table 2.8 provides a summary of the functions of the urinary system and examples of how those functions relate to physical activity, exercise, sport, and athletic performance.

DIGESTIVE SYSTEM

The digestive system works to transfer **macronutrients**, **micronutrients**, **electrolytes**, and water from the food we consume into the body so that normal functions can be performed and proper health can be maintained.

The macronutrients are carbohydrates, fats, proteins, and the micronutrients are vitamins and minerals. These macro- and micronutrients contained in the food we consume represent essential sources of compounds that form the basic structures of the body and regulate the various processes of cells and tissues. Without a consistent supply of nutrients, the ability to maintain good health, perform physical activity and exercise, and train at levels required for sport and athletic competition becomes severely compromised (39,99).

The primary components of the digestive system are the mouth, pharynx, esophagus, stomach, pancreas, liver, and small intestine and large intestine. The mouth and pharynx and the esophagus are responsible for chewing and swallowing food, respectively. The stomach mixes and promotes further digestion by using digestive juices that come from the pancreas and liver. The small intestine absorbs nutrients and most of the electrolytes and water. The large intestine is primarily responsible for absorbing salt and water and converting the remaining contents into fecal matter (39,99). Figure 2.9 illustrates the primary components of the digestive system.

Digestive System and Exercise Science

Increasing physical activity and exercise and altering nutritional habits may play a role in decreasing the risk of developing certain forms of cancer, one of the leading causes of death in the United States (80). Several lines of research have suggested that increasing dietary fiber intake may reduce the risk of developing colorectal cancer. A protective effect of increased fiber intake may occur as a result of the dilution of fecal **carcinogens** and **procarcinogens**, reduction in the time fecal matter moves through the bowel, production of short chain fatty acids (which promote **anticarcinogenic** action), and the binding of bile acids that are carcinogenic (65). However, the results of numerous large population studies examining the role of increased fiber intake in reducing cancer risk have been inconsistent (88). Environmental and case-controlled studies have found an inverse association between the dietary fiber intake and the incidence of colorectal cancer (53). Conversely, most prospective group studies have found little or no association between the dietary fiber intake and the risk of colorectal cancer (34,69,77,95,104) or adenomas (90), and randomized clinical trials of dietary fiber supplementation have failed to show any decrease in the recurrence of colorectal adenomas (4,67,78,96). One of the biggest contributors to the colorectal cancer–causing process is dietary fat. The consumption of a meal high in fat increases the amount of bile acids that are released into the digestive tract. Bile acids help break down the fats we consume, but when the large amounts of bile acids get into the colon, they may be converted to secondary bile acids, which

Carcinogens A cancer-causing substance or agent.
Procarcinogens Compounds or substances that can lead to the formation of cancer cells.
Anticarcinogenic Tending to inhibit or prevent the activity of a carcinogen or the development of carcinoma.

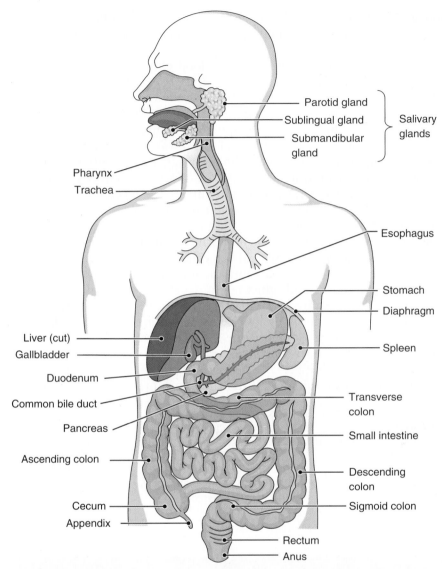

Parotid gland
Sublingual gland
Submandibular gland
Salivary glands
Pharynx
Trachea
Esophagus
Stomach
Diaphragm
Liver (cut)
Gallbladder
Duodenum
Common bile duct
Pancreas
Ascending colon
Cecum
Appendix
Spleen
Transverse colon
Small intestine
Descending colon
Sigmoid colon
Rectum
Anus

FIGURE 2.9 ▼ Primary components of the digestive system. Reprinted with permission from Cohen BJ, Wood DL. *Memmler's The Human Body in Health and Disease.* 9th Ed. Philadelphia, PA: Lippincott Williams & Wilkins, 2000.

could promote cancerous tumor growth. This is especially true of the cells that line the area of the colon (65).

The digestive system also plays an important role in sport and athletic performance. Carbohydrates are the preferred fuel of skeletal muscle for most high-intensity sports competitions and athletic events. An inadequate supply of dietary carbohydrate consumed prior to and during competition can lead to poor performance. Carbohydrate ingestion during exercise increases blood glucose availability and maintains the ability of the working tissues to use carbohydrate as an energy source during high-intensity exercise. The ingestion of carbohydrate during prolonged, high-intensity aerobic endurance exercise enhances performance (17,18) and can also increase performance during high-intensity short duration exercise (43).

There is a limit to the peak rate of blood glucose utilization during prolonged exercise when carbohydrates are ingested orally (17,19). The gastrointestinal system plays a key role in the delivery of carbohydrate to the body during exercise. The gastrointestinal tract has several potential sites for limiting carbohydrate use including gastric emptying and intestinal absorption (41). An examination of how the gastrointestinal, cardiovascular, and muscular systems interact can help demonstrate these limitations. Gastric emptying rates and the intestinal absorption of glucose from a 6% glucose electrolyte solution have been measured at 1.2 and 1.3 g per minute under resting conditions (25). As the concentration of glucose in the beverage rises, the rate at which ingested glucose is supplied to the blood is lower than the rate of carbohydrate used in the muscle. This suggests either a gastrointestinal limitation to using the ingested carbohydrate as a fuel or a failure of the cardiovascular system to deliver glucose from the gastrointestinal tract into the main blood supply (73). The simultaneous consumption of both glucose and fructose, which are absorbed from the gastrointestinal tract by different mechanisms, results in the greater use of the carbohydrates for energy by muscle than the ingestion of similar amounts of glucose or fructose consumed alone (3). Furthermore, if glucose is infused into the blood, rather than consumed orally, the glucose can be used to supply energy at a faster rate (21). Collectively, this information suggests that the delivery of ingested carbohydrate from the gastrointestinal tract to the cardiovascular system might be a limiting factor in the use of ingested carbohydrate as an energy source for contracting muscle during exercise (41). Table 2.9 provides a summary of the functions of the digestive system and examples of how those functions relate to physical activity, exercise, sport, and athletic performance.

➤ *Thinking Critically*
In what ways could consumption of a carbohydrate beverage improve performance during a competitive marathon or triathlon?

Table 2.9	Functions of the Digestive System and their Relationship to Physical Activity, Exercise, Sport, and Athletic Performance
FUNCTION	**RELATION TO PHYSICAL ACTIVITY AND EXERCISE AND SPORT AND ATHLETIC PERFORMANCE**
Delivery of macronutrients to the body	Carbohydrates, fats, and proteins are essential for the optimal function of the body during and after movement
Delivery of micronutrients to the body	Vitamins and minerals are essential for the optimal function of the body during and after movement

ENDOCRINE SYSTEM

The endocrine system is the other primary control system (along with the nervous system) of the body. It helps to regulate physiologic function and influence the function of other systems of the body. The endocrine system accomplishes these functions through the use of hormones secreted by the various endocrine glands of the body. Even though the endocrine glands are not connected anatomically, they function as a system in a practical sense. Many of these hormones are important for influencing both the acute responses and the chronic adaptations of the systems of the body to physical activity and exercise (39,99).

The primary components of the endocrine system are the glands of the body and the hormones that each gland secretes. Some endocrine glands only specialize in hormonal secretion, (e.g., anterior pituitary and thyroid), whereas other components of the endocrine system consist of organs that perform other functions in addition to secreting hormones (e.g., testes secrete testosterone and also produce sperm). The endocrine system, by means of the bloodborne hormones it secretes, generally regulates activities and functions at a much slower pace than the other primary control mechanism of the body, the nervous system. Most of the activities under the control of hormones are directed toward maintaining **homeostasis** (normal conditions of functioning) of the body (39,99). Table 2.10 illustrates various endocrine glands of the body of interest to exercise science and the primary hormones each secretes.

Endocrine System and Exercise Science

Hormones affect the systematic responses of the body in various ways and often work with other systems of the body to regulate normal functions during physical activity and exercise. For example, epinephrine and norepinephrine (also called adrenaline and noradrenaline) have been shown to increase heart rate and blood pressure in response to stress including physical activity and exercise (14). Insulin maintains blood glucose concentrations by increasing glucose uptake and utilization as an energy source in tissues of the body. The interaction of epinephrine, norepinephrine, and insulin has been associated with the development of hypertension in a disease condition called metabolic syndrome (110). Metabolic syndrome describes the clustering of several conditions of the body including obesity, hyperinsulinemia, elevated triglyceride levels, hypertension, and type 2 diabetes. Figure 2.10 shows the relationship among the clustering of metabolic syndrome risk factors. Central to the understanding of metabolic syndrome is the role insulin resistance plays in the development of some of the associated disease conditions. A diet high in fat and refined sugar (7) contributes significantly to the development of insulin resistance. A decreased ability of cells to absorb glucose at a given insulin concentration characterizes the condition of insulin resistance. In response to increasing insulin resistance by the tissues of the body, the pancreas secretes

Homeostasis   The maintenance of relatively stable internal physiologic conditions.

Table 2.10	Endocrine Glands and Selected Secreted Hormones (99)
ENDOCRINE GLAND	**HORMONES**
Hypothalamus	Releasing and inhibiting hormones
Posterior pituitary	Vasopressin
Anterior pituitary	Thyroid stimulating hormone, adrenocortico- tropic hormone, and growth hormone
Thyroid gland	Thyroxin, triiodothyronine, and calcitonin
Adrenal cortex	Aldosterone, cortisol, and androgens
Adrenal medulla	Epinephrine and norepinephrine
Pancreas	Insulin and glucagon
Parathyroid gland	Parathyroid hormone
Ovaries	Estrogen and progesterone
Testes	Testosterone
Kidneys	Renin and erythropoietin
Stomach	Gastrin
Liver	Somatomedins
Skin	Vitamin D
Heart	Atrial natriuretic peptide
Adipose tissue	Leptin and adiponectin

more insulin in an effort to promote blood glucose uptake into cells and return the blood glucose concentration to normal. If the pancreas cannot secrete sufficient amounts of insulin, the blood glucose concentration remains elevated and type 2 diabetes results (39). When the pancreas is forced to secrete additional insulin to address the insulin resistance, the plasma insulin level becomes elevated (called hyperinsulinemia). This condition can elevate blood pressure and contribute to the development of hypertension. Sympathetic nervous system activity increases in response to elevated insulin levels. This response can lead to an elevation of the hormones epinephrine and norepinephrine, which can lead to an increase in heart rate, stroke volume, and blood pressure. The elevated levels of epinephrine and norepinephrine can also interfere with insulin release from the pancreas and glucose uptake at the tissue, causing an aggravation of the problem. In this case, insulin resistance contributes significantly to the hypertension. Alternatively, given the complex interaction of the events hypertension may in fact cause the insulin resistance. Physical activity and regular exercise can benefit individuals with insulin resistance and hypertension by improving the body's sensitivity to the hormones insulin, epinephrine, and norepinephrine (47,71,92).

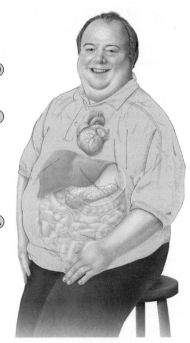

Elevated blood pressure: (D)
Equal to or greater than
130/85 mm Hg

Elevated fasting glucose: (E)
Equal to or greater than
100 mg/dL

(B) Elevated triglycerides:
Equal to or greater than
150 mg/dL

Elevated waist circumference: (A)
Men – Equal to or greater than
40 inches (102 cm)
Women – Equal to or greater
than 35 inches (88 cm)

(C) Reduced HDL ("good") cholestero
Men – Less than 40 mg/dL
Women – Less than 50 mg/dL

FIGURE 2.10 ▽ The relationship among the clustering of metabolic syndrome risk factors. (Asset provided by Anatomical Chart Co.)

Coaches and athletes have long been interested in the use of **exogenous** hormone supplementation to improve assorted types of sports and athletic performance. For example, the use of anabolic steroids (e.g., synthetic testosterone) and human growth hormone for improving athletic performance is common among certain groups of athletes (15,26,82,108). Anabolic steroids have both **androgenic effects** and **anabolic effects** (109). The anabolic actions cause the body to retain nitrogen, which can then lead to increased protein synthesis in skeletal muscles and other tissues. The increased protein synthesis results in increased muscle size and strength as well as increased body weight (39). For those sports that rely on body size or the generation of power and force by the muscle, the increase in mass and strength often result in improvements in sport and athletic performance. When used in high dosages, as often the case with athletes, there are potentially serious side effects that may be irreversible and cause serious health problems (109). Although the use of these types of substances and others like them is illegal and unethical, there is a considerable interest in understanding how these substances work and how the illegal use of these substances can be detected (109). Identifying

Exogenous Coming from outside the body.
Androgenic effects The development and maintenance of masculine characteristics.
Anabolic effects The development and maintenance of tissue, particularly skeletal muscle.

Table 2.11	Primary Hormones of the Endocrine System and how their Functions Relate to Physical Activity, Exercise, Sport, and Athletic Performance	
HORMONE	**FUNCTION**	**RELATION TO PHYSICAL ACTIVITY, EXERCISE, SPORT, AND ATHLETIC PERFORMANCE**
Adiponectin	Regulates glucose and fatty acid metabolism	Plays a role in the suppression of metabolic abnormalities
Aldosterone	Increases sodium reabsorption and potassium excretion in the kidneys	Helps regulated fluid balance to prevent dehydration
Calcitonin	Decreases plasma calcium concentration	Increases calcium deposition in bone
Cortisol	Increases blood glucose concentration; contributes to stress adaptation	Helps increase blood glucose concentration to avoid hypoglycemia
Epinephrine and norepinephrine	Reinforces sympathetic nervous system activity	Assists the body when responding to the stress of movement
Erythropoietin	Stimulates red blood cell production in bone marrow	Increases oxygen delivery to working tissues
Estrogen	Responsible for development of secondary sexual characteristics	Helps regulate lean mass and skeletal mass in the body
Glucagon	Promotes maintenance of nutrient levels in blood, especially glucose	Helps regulate blood glucose levels during exercise
Growth hormone	Essential for the growth of bones and soft tissue; protein anabolism; fat mobilization	Promotes the growth of lean and skeletal tissue
Insulin	Promotes uptake of absorbed nutrients, especially insulin	Helps regulate blood glucose levels after food consumption
Leptin	Assists the brain in regulating appetite and metabolism	Helps assist the body in the regulation of an appropriate body weight
Testosterone	Responsible for development of secondary sexual characteristics	Helps regulate lean mass in the body
Vitamin D	Increases absorption of ingested calcium and phosphate in the GI tract	Helps regulate levels of calcium in the body, especially bone

the mechanism by which these hormones work is important for determining how these substances can be detected in saliva, blood, and urine (55) for compliance with athletic-governing association rules. Issues surrounding effective drug testing include using equipment that is sensitive enough to detect drug metabolites in the blood or urine, identifying the various metabolites that are associated with synthetic anabolic steroids, and ensuring that effective drug testing is a deterrent to anabolic steroid and other anabolic substance use by athletes (55). Table 2.11 provides the primary hormones of the endocrine system and some examples of how those functions relate to physical activity, exercise, sport, and athletic performance.

IMMUNE SYSTEM

Overall, the immune system regulates susceptibility to, severity of, and recovery from infection, abnormal tissue growth, and illness. The immune system works with other body systems through a complex system of structures, compounds, and cells. The various components of the immune system are not connected anatomically yet they do constitute a functional system in the body. The immune system allows the body to make a distinction between its normal components and any foreign elements, with the purpose of protecting itself against those substances foreign to the body (39,99).

The primary components of the immune system are the physical, mechanical, chemical, blood, and cellular factors of the body. The **innate** (i.e., natural) and **acquired** (i.e., adaptive) components of the immune system function together in a complex interaction to protect the body from outside elements. The innate components of the body offer an immediate and predetermined general protection against any type of foreign challenge to the body. Conversely, the adaptive components of the immune system are extremely specific in the response to a given foreign invader (98). Table 2.12 illustrates the components of innate immunity and acquired immunity.

Immune System and Exercise Science

Since the 1980s, there has been steady growth in the study of physical activity, exercise, and immune function and how they all interact to positively and negatively affect health. Exercise may play a role in the prevention and treatment of certain illnesses such as cancer and acquired immune deficiency syndrome (AIDS) (48). Evidence from **epidemiologic** studies indicates an association between regular physical activity and lower rates of certain cancers (28). Animal studies also indicate that exercise training enhances resistance to

---

Innate Immunity existing from within the body at birth.
Acquired Immunity that is derived after birth.
Epidemiologic The branch of medicine dealing with the incidence and prevalence of disease in large populations.

Table 2.12	Components of Innate and Acquired Immunity (98)
INNATE IMMUNITY	**ACQUIRED IMMUNITY**
Skin	Antibodies
Epithelium	Immunologic memory
Mucus	T helper cells
Cilia	T suppressor cells
Turbulent airflow	Cytotoxic cells
Compliment factors	B cells
Lysozyme factors	Plasma cells
Acute phase proteins	
pH	
Various trace minerals	
Monocytes and macrophages	
Granulocytes	
Natural killer cells	

experimentally induced tumor growth (49). Furthermore, exercise may have a positive effect in stimulating the immune system during times of illness or reduced responsiveness (such as aging or AIDS). Recent studies over extended periods of 10 to 20 years have reported reduced incidence of cancer in physically active groups (24,49). There is also evidence that occupational physical activity is associated with a reduced risk of colorectal cancer (100) and that physical inactivity is associated with an increased risk of colorectal cancer (49). Increased levels of physical activity may also reduce the risk of cancer at other sites such as the breast and reproductive system in women (24,28). Exercise may positively affect autoimmune diseases such as rheumatoid arthritis, Graves disease, and systemic lupus erythematosus (29). In older adults, increased levels of physical activity and regular exercise may also enhance immune system function (22,72).

Some competitive athletes may appear to suffer high rates of certain illnesses such as mononucleosis and upper respiratory illness. The relationship between exercise and upper respiratory illness may be modeled in the form of a "J" curve as shown in Figure 2.11 (83). This model suggests that although the risk of upper respiratory illness may decrease below that of a sedentary individual when one engages in moderate exercise training, the risk may rise

Overtraining syndrome A condition whereby too much training results in the maladaptations of body responses.

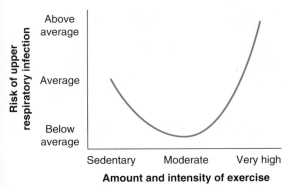

FIGURE 2.11 ▼ Relationship between exercise and upper respiratory illness may be modeled in the form of a "J" curve (83).

above average during periods of excessive amounts of high-intensity training such as that performed by some athletes (98). Frequent illness has also been observed in athletes experiencing a condition called **overtraining syndrome** (32,84). Although much of the evidence is anecdotal the few attempts to quantify rates of illness tend to support a higher incidence of illness among certain groups of athletes (85). In runners, the incidence of infectious illness increases with training volume and after major competitions. It is likely that training volume and competition exert a combined effect on the susceptibility to illness. Moderate-intensity exercise has been demonstrated to induce a much smaller change in the cellular components of the immune system. Short bouts of high-intensity exercise can cause temporary impairment of the immune response and repeated heavy training and the stress of top level competition can have a more serious effect on immune function. Research supports the concept that heavy exertion increases an athlete's risk of upper respiratory illness because of the changes in immune function and the elevation of the hormones epinephrine and cortisol (89). Table 2.13 provides the functions of the immune system and examples of how those functions relate to physical activity, exercise, sport, and athletic performance.

> ➤ *Thinking Critically*
> *How does exercise training for improving health and fitness differ from exercise training for enhancing performance during sport and athletic competitions as they relate to alterations in immune system function?*

Table 2.13	Functions of the Immune System and how Those Functions Relate to Physical Activity, Exercise, Sport, and Athletic Performance
FUNCTION	**RELATION TO PHYSICAL ACTIVITY, EXERCISE, SPORT, AND ATHLETIC PERFORMANCE**
Regulate susceptibility to, severity of, and recovery from infection, abnormal tissue growth, and illness	Provides protective effect from internal and external illness–causing agents

ENERGY SYSTEMS

The ability to produce energy is critical for ensuring normal function in all living cells and tissues of the body. The production of energy to support the functions of the body is tightly controlled and regulated so that energy production closely matches energy utilization. Energy exchange in humans occurs when the foods (carbohydrates, fats, proteins) we eat are broken down into a useable form of energy by the body. Although energy exchange in humans is not a system in a structural sense, the various processes by which the body produces energy do constitute a system in the functional sense (39,99).

The main components of the energy system are the chemical compounds contained in the energy pathways of the cells and the macronutrients carbohydrate, fat, and protein. When the cells of the body need energy, they break down a chemical compound call adenosine triphosphate (ATP). Immediately the body begins to resynthesize the ATP from the energy contained in the chemical bonds that hold together the macronutrients. Energy to resynthesize ATP comes from one of the three energy pathways: (a) immediate sources which use stored energy in the form of **creatine phosphate** (often called the ATP–CP energy system); (b) **glycolysis** and **glycogenolysis,** which use blood glucose and stored muscle glycogen, respectively, (often called the anaerobic energy system); and (c) **oxidative metabolism,** which use products of carbohydrate, fat, and protein metabolism (often called the aerobic energy system). The immediate stores rapidly resynthesize ATP in the muscle during the initiation of movement and during very high-intensity exercise. Because the immediate energy system is limited in capacity, the body quickly begins to provide energy through other pathways. The processes of glycolysis (using glucose) and glycogenolysis (using glycogen) involve the breakdown of carbohydrates into compounds called pyruvic acid and lactic acid. As the carbohydrate is broken down, energy is formed for use by the body. The need for energy by the body often determines the end product of carbohydrate metabolism. If energy requirements are high, then lactic acid is formed. If the energy requirements are lower, then pyruvic acid is formed, which is then used to produce energy in oxidative metabolism. Pyruvic acid, fats, and proteins can all be used to produce energy. Oxidative metabolism occurs in the mitochondria of cells and is an energy system that is powerful with a large capacity for producing energy (14). Energy production must match utilization during exercise or the exercise intensity must be reduced or exercise must be stopped. The energy pathway that

---

Creatine phosphate An organic compound found in muscle and cardiac tissue and capable of storing and providing energy for muscular contraction.

Glycolysis The breakdown of glucose to produce energy.

Glycogenolysis The breakdown of glycogen to produce energy.

Oxidative metabolism The use of oxygen to breakdown carbohydrates, fats, and proteins to produce energy.

Ergogenic aids Any substance or device that improves physiologic or psychological performance.

Body composition The amount of fat and nonfat tissue in the body.

Table 2.14	Energy Production Systems in the Body	
ENERGY SYSTEM	**SUBSTRATE USED**
Immediate Sources	ATP and creatine phosphate
Glycolysis and glycogenolysis	Blood glucose and muscle glycogen
Oxidative metabolism	By-products of carbohydrate, fat, and protein metabolism

predominates during physical activity or exercise will depend on the intensity and duration of the activity. Whether carbohydrates, fats, or proteins are used to produce energy will depend on the pathway being used, but can also be influenced by factors such as food consumption, training status, and the use of **ergogenic aids**. Table 2.14 illustrates the pathways for energy production in the body.

Energy Systems and Exercise Science

Identifying the appropriate physical activity and exercise intensity to promote the utilization of fat as an energy source is an important issue in the regulation of body weight and body composition. At the beginning of exercise, increases in energy utilization of the body are matched by increases in energy production from the immediate energy sources and the breakdown of glucose and glycogen. As the exercise duration continues, energy production shifts so that under certain circumstances more energy is produced from the breakdown of fats. Several factors influence which energy pathway is used to provide energy, including the nutritional status and training level of the individual, the exercise intensity and duration, and various hormonal concentrations in the body. Of those factors, exercise intensity and duration most often have the greatest influence on fat and carbohydrate utilization as energy sources (Figure 2.12). During physical activity and exercise, the percent contribution of carbohydrate and fat to energy production can be estimated by using the respiratory exchange ratio (RER). The RER is calculated as the ratio of the amount of carbon dioxide produced to the amount of oxygen consumed (14). When using the RER to estimate fuel utilization during rest or exercise, the role that protein contributes to energy production is usually ignored because protein generally contributes very little to energy production during physical activity (14). The RER can be used to estimate fuel utilization because carbohydrates and fat differ in the amount of oxygen consumed and carbon dioxide produced; fat requires more oxygen than carbohydrate when used for energy production (14).

The understanding of how body weight and **body composition** affects fat utilization is of great interest for understanding the mechanisms behind the obesity epidemic (50). Increases in body weight and body fat, as well as changes in fat utilization as an energy source have significant implications for the development of several chronic disease conditions such as insulin resistance, type 2 diabetes, and metabolic syndrome (106). Exercise science professionals are interested in determining the optimal intensity for utilizing fat during physical activity and

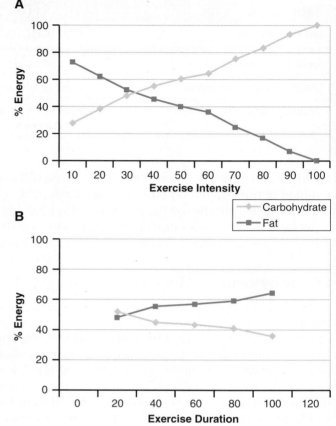

FIGURE 2.12 ▼ The relationship between exercise intensity **(A)** and duration **(B)** and the use of fat and carbohydrates as energy sources.

exercise to better assist those individuals seeking to decrease body fat and lose weight. Recent evidence would indicate that the exercise intensity at which there is maximal fat utilization is approximately 65% of an individual's VO_{2max} (1).

Determining the optimal exercise intensity during endurance events that are longer than 10 km is critical for maximizing sport and athletic performance. Success in endurance events can be determined by examining several factors. For example, one of the strongest predictors of successful performance in distance running is the running velocity at the **maximal lactate steady state** (105). During moderate- to high-intensity exercise, the majority of energy produced to power muscular contraction comes from the breakdown of carbohydrates. During the metabolism of glucose and glycogen, there is lactic acid formation that can contribute to fatigue unless it is removed from the contracting muscle (107). The removal of lactic acid occurs through several processes

Maximal lactate steady state The exercise intensity where maximal lactic acid production is matched by maximal lactic acid removal.

Table 2.15	Components of the Energy System and how Those Components Relate to Physical Activity, Exercise, Sport, and Athletic Performance	
ENERGY SYSTEM	**RELATION TO PHYSICAL ACTIVITY, EXERCISE, SPORT, AND ATHLETIC PERFORMANCE**
Immediate Sources: ATP and creatine phosphate	Provides energy during the initiation of movement and during high intensity exercise
Glycolysis and glycogenolysis	Provides energy during moderately high-intensity exercise
Oxidative metabolism	Provides energy during resting and low- to moderately high–intensity physical activity and exercise

in the body (8,13). There is an exercise intensity whereby the maximal formation of lactic acid in the muscle fiber is matched by the maximal clearance of lactic acid from the muscle fiber. This is called the maximal lactate steady state (46). Exercise above the maximal lactate steady state leads to a progressive increase in the lactic acid concentration in the muscle and ultimately a decrease in exercise performance or a cessation of exercise altogether (46). Endurance coaches and athletes develop and implement training programs with the intent on improving the exercise intensity at the maximal lactate steady state (14,91,102). Table 2.15 provides the components of the energy system and examples of how those components relate to physical activity, exercise, sport, and athletic performance.

> ➤ *Thinking Critically*
>
> *Why would an understanding of how the systems of the body interact contribute to a greater understanding of how physical activity and exercise influence health and how regular exercise training affects sport and athletic performance?*

SUMMARY

- The various systems of the body play important roles in regulating body functions prior to, during, and following physical activity, exercise, sport, and athletic performance.

- Proper control of the body functions require the systems to function together in a coordinated and controlled manner.

- Increased levels of physical activity and regular exercise training usually result in an improved function of the various systems whereas physical inactivity typically leads to a decrease in functional ability and often diseased conditions in the body.

- Successful performance in sport and athletic competition depends on optimal functioning of the systems of the body.

- Various subject and content areas of exercise science, as well as the professional careers graduates enter into, will rely heavily on a sound knowledge of the systems of the body.

FOR REVIEW

1. Why should the study of the systems of the body be examined from an integrated approach?

2. What are the primary functional components of the nervous system?

3. What are the three primary types of skeletal muscle fibers?

4. What are the principal functions of the skeletal system?

5. How does the cardiovascular system work to maintain challenges to homeostasis during exercise?

6. Discuss the role of the pulmonary system in maintaining normal acid–base balance.

7. What role does the urinary system play in the treatment of individuals with hypertension?

8. How does the gastrointestinal system influence the delivery of carbohydrate to working skeletal muscle?

9. Discuss how insulin resistance influences the development of metabolic syndrome.

10. What is the difference between innate immunity and acquired immunity?

11. Provide a list of the energy sources used in the three primary energy–producing pathways.

REFERENCES

1. Achten J, Gleeson M, Jeukendrup AE. Determination of the exercise intensity that elicits maximal fat oxidation. *Med Sci Sports Exerc.* 2002;34: 92–7.

2. Adams GR, Haddad F, Baldwin KM. Time course of changes in markers of myogenesis in overloaded rat skeletal muscles. *J Appl Physiol.* 1999;87:1705–12.

3. Adopo E, Peronnet F, Massicotte D, Brisson GR, Hillaire-Marcel C. Respective oxidation of exogenous glucose and fructose given in the same drink during exercise. *J Appl Physiol.* 1994;76: 1014–19.

4. Alberts DS, Martinez ME, Roe DJ. Lack of effect of a high-fiber cereal supplement on the recurrence of colorectal adenomas: Phoenix Colon Cancer Prevention Physician's Network. *N Engl J Med.* 2000;342:1156–62.

5. American College of Sports Medicine. *ACSM's Exercise Management for Persons with Chronic Diseases and Disabilities.* 3rd Ed. Champaign (IL): Human Kinetics; 2009.

6. American College of Sports Medicine. Physical activity and bone health. *Med Sci Sports Exerc.* 2004;36: 1985–96.

7. Barnard RJ, Roberts CK, Varon SM, Berger JJ. Diet-induced insulin resistance precedes other aspects of the metabolic syndrome. *J Appl Physiol.* 1998;84:1311–5.

8. Bergman BC, Wolfel EE, Butterfield GE, et al. Active muscle and whole body lactate kinetics after endurance training in men. *J Appl Physiol.* 1999;87:1684–96.

9. Birkeland KI, Hemmersbach P. The future of doping control in athletes. *Sports Med.* 1999;28:25–33.

10. Birkeland KI, Stray-Gundersen J, Hemmersbach P, Hallen J, Haug E, Bahr R. Effect of rhEPO administration on serum levels of sTfR and cycling performance. *Med Sci Sports Exerc.* 2000;32:1238–43.

11. Blair SN, Kampert JB, Kohl HW, et al. Influences of cardiorespiratory fitness and other precursors on cardiovascular disease and all-cause mortality in men and women. *J Am Med Assoc.* 1996;276: 205–10.

12. Bobbert MF, Ettema G, Huijing PA. The force-length relationship of a muscle-tendon complex: Experimental results and model calculations. *Eur J Appl Physiol.* 1990;61:323–9.

13. Brooks GA. Intra- and extra- cellular lactate shuttles. *Med Sci Sports Exerc.* 2000;32:790–9.

14. Brooks GA, Fahey TD, White TP, Baldwin KM. *Exercise Physiology: Human Bioenergetics and Its Applications.* Mountain View: Mayfield; 2000.

15. Buckely WE, Yesalis CE, Friedl KE, Anderson WA, Streit AL, Wright JE. Estimated prevalence of anabolic steroid use among male high school seniors. *JAMA.* 1988;260:3441–5.

16. Clarkson PM. Eccentric exercise and muscle damage. *Int J Sports Med.* 1997;18:S314–7.

17. Coggan AR, Coyle EF. Reversal of fatigue during prolonged exercise by carbohydrate infusion or ingestion. *J Appl Physiol.* 1987;63:2388–95.

18. Coggan AR, Coyle EF. Effect of carbohydrate feeding during high-intensity exercise. *J Appl Physiol.* 1988; 65:1703–9.

19. Coggan AR, Spina RJ, Kohrt WM, Bier DM, Holloszy JO. Plasma glucose kinetics in a well-trained cyclist fed glucose throughout exercise. *Int J Sport Nutr.* 1991; 1:279–88.

20. Cooper R, Cutler J, Desvigne-Nickens P, et al. Trends and disparities in coronary heart disease, stroke, and other cardiovascular diseases in the United States - Findings of the National Conference on Cardiovascular Disease Prevention. *Circulation.* 2000;102:3137–47.

21. Coyle EF, Hamilton MT, Gonzalez-Alonso J, Montain SJ, Ivy JL. Carbohydrate metabolism during intense exercise when hyperglycemic. *J Appl Physiol.* 1991;70:834–40.

22. Crist DM, Mackinnon LT, Thompson RF, Atterborn HA, Egan PA. Physical exercise increases natural cell-mediated tumor cytotoxicity in elderly women. *Gerontology.* 1989;35:66–71.

23. De Meersman RE. Respiratory sinus arrhythmia alteration following training in endurance athletes. *Eur J Appl Physiol.* 1992;64:434–6.

24. Dorn J, Vena J, Brasure J, Freudenheim J, Graham S. Lifetime physical activity and breast cancer risk in pre- and postmenopausal women. *Med Sci Sports Exerc.* 2003;35:278–85.

25. Duchman SM, Ryan AJ, Schedl HP, Summers RW, Bleiler TL, Gisolfi CV. Upper limit for intestinal absorption of a dilute glucose solution in men at rest. *Med Sci Sports Exerc.* 1997;29:482–8.

26. DuRant R. Use of multiple drugs among adolescents who use anabolic steroids. *N Engl J Med.* 1993; 328:922.

27. Evans SL, Davy KP, Stevenson ET, Seals DR. Physiological determinants of 10-km performance in highly trained female runners of different ages. *J Appl Physiol.* 1995;78:1931–41.

28. Evenson KR, Stevens J, Cai J, Thomas R, Thomas O. The effect of cardiorespiratory fitness and obesity on cancer mortality in women and men. *Med Sci Sports Exerc.* 2003;35:270–7.

29. Ferry A. Exercise and autoimmune diseases. In: Hoffman-Goetz L, editor. *Exercise and Immune Function.* Boca Raton (FL): CRC Press, Inc.; 1996. p. 163–78.

30. Ferster CB, Nurnberger JI, Levitt EB. The control of eating. *J Math.* 1962;1:87–109.

31. Fitts RH. Cellular mechanisms of muscular fatigue. *Physiol Rev.* 1994;74:49–94.

32. Fitzgerald L. Overtraining increases the susceptibility to infection. *Int J Sports Med.* 1991;12:S5–8.

33. French SA, Fulkerson JA, Story M. Increasing Weight-bearing physical activity and calcium intake for bone mass growth in children and adolescents: A review of intervention trials. *Prev Med.* 2000;31:722–31.

34. Fuchs CS, Giovannucci EL, Colditz GA. Dietary fiber and the risk of colorectal cancer and adenoma in women. *N Engl J Med.* 1999;340:169–76.

35. Georgopoulos D, Matamis D, Routsi C, et al. Recombinant human erythropoietin therapy in critically ill patients: A dose-response study. *Crit Care.* 2005; 9:R508–15.

36. Goldsmith RL, Bigger JT, Bloomfield DM, Steinman RC. Physical fitness as a determinant of vagal modulation. *Med Sci Sports Exerc.* 1997;29:812–7.

37. Goldsmith RL, Bigger JT, Steinman RC, Fleiss JL. Comparison of 24-hour parasympathetic activity in endurance-trained and untrained young men. *J Am Coll Cardiol.* 1992;20:552–8.

38. Green HJ. Muscle power: Fibre type recruitment, metabolism and fatigue. In: Jones NL, McCartney N, McComas AJ, editors. *Human Muscle Power.* Champaign (IL): Human Kinetics; 1986. p. 65–79.

39. Guyton AC, Hall JE. *Textbook of Medical Physiology.* Oxford (UK): Elsevier; 2006.

40. Hagberg JM, Moore GE, Ferrell RE. Specific genetic markers of endurance performance and VO_{2max}. *Exerc Sport Sci Rev.* 1991;29:15–9.

41. Hargreaves M. Metabolic responses to carbohydrate and lipid supplementation during exercise. In: Maughan RJ, Shirreffs SM, editors. *Biochemistry of Exercise IX.* Champaign (IL): Human Kinetics; 1996. p. 421–9.

42. Harrison BC, Robinson D, Davison BJ, Foley B, Seda E, Byrnes WC. Treatment of exercise-induced muscle injury via hyperbaric oxygen therapy. *Med Sci Sports Exerc.* 2001;33:35–42.

43. Haub MD, Potteiger JA, Jacobsen DJ, Nau KL, Magee LM, Comeau MJ. Glycogen replenishment and repeated short duration high intensity exercise: Effect of carbohydrate ingestion. *Int J Sport Nutr Exerc Metab.* 1998;9:406–15.

44. Heaney RP. The role of calcium in prevention and treatment of osteoporosis. *Physician Sports Med.* 1987; 15:83–8.

45. Heaney RP. Calcium, dairy products, and osteoporosis. *J Am Coll Nutr.* 2000;19:88S–99.

46. Heck H, Mader A, Hess G, Mucke S, Muller R, Hollman W. Justification of the 4-mmol/lactate threshold. *Int J Sports Med.* 1985;6:117–30.

47. Helmrich SP, Ragaland DR, Leung RW, Paffenbarger RS. Physical activity and reduced occurrence of non-insulin-dependent diabetes mellitus. *N Engl J Med.* 1991;225:147–52.

48. Hoffman-Goetz L. *Exercise and Immune Function.* Boca Raton (FL): CRC Press, Inc.; 1996.

49. Hoffman-Goetz L, Husted J. Exercise, immunity, and colon cancer. In: Hoffman-Goetz L, editor. *Exercise and Immune Function.* Boca Raton (FL): CRC Press, Inc.; 1996. p. 179–97.

50. Horowitz JF. Regulation of lipid mobilization and oxidation during exercise in obesity. *Exerc Sport Sci Rev.* 2001;29:42–6.

51. Hough DO, Dec KL. Exercise-induced asthma and anaphylaxis. *Sports Med.* 1994;18:162–72.

52. Joint National Committee on Prevention DEaToHBP. The seventh report of the Joint National Committee on Prevention, Detection, Evaluation, and Treatment of High Blood Pressure (JNC VII). *Hypertension.* 2003; 157:2413–46.

53. Kaaks R, Riboli E. Colorectal cancer and intake of dietary fibre: A summary of the epidemiological evidence. *Eur J Clin Nutr.* 1995;49:S10–7.

54. Kadi F, Eriksson A, Holmner S, Thornell LE. Effects of anabolic steroids on the muscle cells of strength-trained athletes. *Med Sci Sports Exerc*. 1999;31: 1528–34.

55. Kammerer RC. Drug testing and anabolic steroids. In: Yesalis CE, editor. *Anabolic Steroids in Sport and Exercise*. Champaign (IL): Human Kinetics; 2000. p. 283–308.

56. Kanis JA, Melton LJ III, Christiansen C, Johnston CC, Khaltaev N. The diagnosis of osteoporosis. *J Bone Miner Res*. 1994;9:1137–41.

57. Kelley G. Mechanical overload and skeletal muscle fiber hyperphasia: A meta-analysis. *J Appl Physiol*. 1996;81:1584–8.

58. Kelso TB, Hodgson DR, Visscher AR, Gollnick PD. Some properties of different skeletal muscle fiber types: Comparison of reference bases. *J Appl Physiol*. 1987;62:1436–41.

59. Kovan JR, Moeller JL. Respiratory system. In: McKeag DB, Moeller JL, editors. *ACSM's Primary Care Sports Medicine*. Philadelphia (PA): Lippincott, Williams & Wilkins; 2007. p. 165–71.

60. Krakoff LR. Diuretics for Hypertension. *Circulation*. 2005;112:e127–9.

61. Kuipers H, Keizer HA, Verstappen FTJ, Costill DL. Influence of a prostaglandin-inhibiting drug on muscle soreness after eccentric work. *Int J Sports Med*. 1985; 6:336–9.

62. Larsson L, Tesch PA. Motor unit fibre density in extremely hypertrophied skeletal muscles in man: Electrophysiological signs of muscle fibre hyperplasia. *Eur J Appl Physiol*. 1986;55:130–6.

63. Laskin JJ, Anderson M. Cerebral Palsy. In: *ACSM's Resources for Clinical Exercise Physiology*. 2002; p. 16–28.

64. Levine BD, Stray-Gundersen J. "Living high-training low": Effect of moderate-altitude acclimatization with low-altitude training on performance. *J Appl Physiol*. 1997;83:102–12.

65. Lipkin M, Reddy B, Newmark H, Lamprecht SA. Dietary factors in human colorectal cancer. *Annu Rev Nutr*. 1999;19:545–86.

66. MacDougall JD, Sale DG, Alway SE, Sutton JR. Muscle fiber number in biceps brachii of bodybuilders and control subjects. *J Appl Physiol*. 1984;57: 1399–403.

67. MacLennan R, Macrae F, Bain C. Randomized trial of intake of fat, fiber, and beta carotene to prevent colorectal adenomas: The Australian Polyp Prevention Project. *J Natl Cancer Inst*. 1995;87:1760–6.

68. Maddalozzo GF, Snow CM. High intensity resistance training: Effects on bone in older men and women. *Calcif Tissue Int*. 2000;66:399–404.

69. Mai V, Flood A, Peters U, Lacey N, Schairer C, Schatzkin A. Dietary fibre and risk of colorectal cancer in the Breast Cancer Detection Demonstration Project (BCDDP) follow-up cohort. *Int J Epidemiol*. 2003; 14:234–9.

70. Margolis S, Klag MJ. Hypertension. *Arch Intern Med*. 1995;155:4–44.

71. Mark AL, Correia M, Morgan DA, Shaffer RA, Haynes WG. Obesity induced hypertension: New concepts from the emerging biology of obesity. *Hypertension*. 1999;33:537–41.

72. Mazzeo RS. Exercise, immunity, and aging. In: Hoffman-Goetz L, editor. *Exercise and Immune Function*. Boca Raton (FL): CRC Press, Inc.; 1996. p. 199–241.

73. McConell GK, Fabris S, Proietto J, Hargreaves M. Effect of carbohydrate ingestion on glucose kinetics during exercise. *J Appl Physiol*. 1994;77:1537–41.

74. McCubbin JA, Shasby G. Effects of isokinetic exercise on adolescents with cerebral palsy. *Adapt Phys Activ Q*. 1985;2:56–64.

75. McCullough ML, Feskanich D, Rimm EB, et al. Adherence to the Dietary Guidelines for Americans and risk of major chronic disease in men. *Am J Clin Nutr*. 2000;72:1223–31.

76. McCullough ML, Feskanich D, Stampfer MJ, et al. Adherence to the Dietary Guidelines for Americans and risk of major chronic disease in women. *Am J Clin Nutr*. 2000;72:1214–22.

77. McCullough ML, Robertson AS, Chao A. A prospective study of whole grains, fruits, vegetables and colon cancer risk. *Cancer Causes Control*. 2003;14:959–70.

78. McKeown-Eyssen GE, Bright-See E, Bruce WR. A randomized trial of low fat high fibre diet in the recurrence of colorectal polyps: Toronto Polyp Prevention Group. *J Cancer Epidemiol*. 1994;47:525–36.

79. Mekjavic IB, Exner JA, Tesch PA, Eiken O. Hyperbaric oxygen therapy does not affect recovery from delayed onset muscle soreness. *Med Sci Sports Exerc*. 2000;32:558–63.

80. Minino AM, Heron MP, Murphy SL, Kochanek KD. Deaths: Final data for 2004. U.S. Department of Health and Human Services. 2007;55(19):1–120.

81. Muscolino JE. *Kinesiology: The Skeletal System and Muscle Function*. St. Louis (MO): Mosby Elsevier; 2006.

82. National Collegiate Athletic Association Research Staff. NCAA study of substance use habits of college student athletes. National Collegiate Athletic Association. 2001;1–48.

83. Nieman DC. Exercise, infection, and immunity. *Int J Sport Med*. 1994;15:S131–41.

84. Nieman DC, Johanssen LM, Lee JW. Infectious episodes in runners before and after a roadrace. *J Sports Med Phys Fitness*. 1996;29:289–96.

85. Nieman DC, Nehlsen-Cannarella SL, Markoff PA, et al. The effects of moderate exercise training on natural killer cells and acute upper respiratory tract infections. *Int J Sports Med*. 1990;11:467–73.

86. O'Connell DG, Barnhart R, Parks L. Muscular endurance and wheelchair propulsion in children with cerebral palsy or myelomeningocele. *Arch Phys Med Rehab*.1992;73:709–11.

87. Olney S, MacPhail H, Hedden D, Boyce W. Work and power in hemiplegic cerebral palsy gait. *Phys Ther*. 1990;70:431–8.

88. Park Y, Hunter DJ, Spiegelman D, et al. Dietary fiber intake and risk of colorectal cancer: A pooled analysis of prospective cohort studies. *JAMA*. 2005; 94:2849–57.

89. Pedersen BK, Nieman DC. Exercise immunology: Integration and regulation. *Immunol Today*. 1998;1–3.

90. Platz EA, Giovannucci E, Rimm EB. Dietary fiber and distal colorectal adenoma in men. *Cancer Epidemiol Biomarkers Prev*. 1997;6:661–70.

91. Potteiger JA. Aerobic endurance training. In: Baechle TR, Earle RW, editors. *Essentials of Strength Training and Conditioning.* Champaign (IL): Human Kinetics; 2000. p. 495–509.

92. Powers SK, Howley ET. *Exercise Physiology: Theory and Application to Fitness and Performance.* Dubuque: Brown & Benchmark; 2007.

93. Prentice WE. *Arnheim's Principles of Athletic Training: A Competency-based Approach.* New York (NY): McGraw-Hill Companies; 2006.

94. Richardson CR, Kriska AM, Lantz PM, Hayward RA. Physical activity and mortality across cardiovascular disease risk groups. *Med Sci Sports Exerc.* 2004; 36:1923–9.

95. Sanjoaquin MA, Appleby PN, Thorogood M, Mann JI, Key TJ. Nutrition, lifestyle and colorectal cancer incidence: A prospective investigation of 10998 vegetarians and non-vegetarians in the United Kingdom. *Br J Cancer.* 2004;90:118–21.

96. Schatzkin A, Lanza E, Corle D. Lack of effect of a low-fat, high-fiber diet on the recurrence of colorectal adenomas. *N Engl J Med.* 2000;342:1149–55.

97. Sesso HD, Paffenbarger RS, Ha T, Min Lee I. Physical activity and cardiovascular disease risk in middle-aged and older women. *Am J Epidemiol.* 1999;150:408–16.

98. Shephard RJ. *Physical Activity, Training and the Immune Response.* Carmel (IN): Cooper Publishing Group; 1997.

99. Sherwood L. *Fundamentals of Physiology: A Human Perspective.* Belmont (CA): Thompson Publishing; 2006.

100. Slattery ML, Schumacher MC, Smith KR, West DW, Abd-Elghany N. Physical activity, diet, and risk of colon cancer in Utah. *Am J Epidemiol.* 1988; 128:998–99

101. Staron RS, Malicky ES, Leonardi MJ, Falkel JE, Hagerman FC, Dudley GA. Muscle hypertrophy and fast fiber type conversions in heavy resistance-trained women. *Eur J Appl Physiol.* 1989;60:71–9.

102. Stepto NK, Martin DT, Fallon KE, Hawley JA. Metabolic demands of intense aerobic interval training in competitive cyclists. *Med Sci Sports Exerc.* 2001; 33:303–10.

103. Storms W. Exercise-induced asthma: Diagnosis and treatment for the recreational or elite athlete. *Med Sci Sports Exerc.* 1999;31:S33–8.

104. Terry P, Giovannucci E, Michels KB. Fruit, vegetables, dietary fiber, and risk of colorectal cancer. *J Natl Cancer Inst.* 2001;93:525–33.

105. Urhausen A, Coen B, Weiler B, Kindermann W. Individual anaerobic threshold and maximum lactate steady state. *Int J Sports Med.* 1993;14:134–9.

106. van Baak MA. Exercise training and substrate utilisation in obesity. *Int J Obes Relat Metab Disord.* 1999; 23(Suppl 3):S11–7.

107. Westerblad H, Allen DG, Lannergren J. Muscle fatigue: Lactic acid or inorganic phosphate the major cause? *News Physiol Sci.* 2002;17:17–21.

108. Windsor R, Dumitru D. Prevalence of anabolic steroid use by male and female athletes. *Med Sci Sports Exerc.* 1989;21:494.

109. Yesalis CE. *Anabolic Steroids in Sport and Exercise.* Champaign (IL): Human Kinetics; 2000.

110. Zimmet P, Boyko EJ, Collier GR, Courten M. Etiology of the metabolic syndrome: Potential role of insulin resistance, leptin resistance, and other players. *Ann N Y Acad Sci.* 25–44.

CHAPTER

Exercise Physiology

After completing this chapter you will be able to:

1. Define exercise physiology and provide examples of the relationship between exercise physiology and exercise science.

2. Identify the important historic events in the development of exercise physiology as a scientific discipline.

3. Discuss the differences between the acute and chronic responses to exercise.

4. Describe some of the important areas of study in the field of exercise physiology.

Exercise physiology is the study of the functional and physiologic responses and adaptations that occur during and following physical activity and exercise. Primarily concerned with the various systems of the body (see Chapter 2), exercise physiology is the study of how the systems individually and collectively respond to acute and chronic bouts of physical activity and exercise. The use of an integrated systems approach allows students to understand the role that physical activity and exercise play in improving health and reducing the risk of disease. Recently, a field of study called inactivity physiology has increased in popularity and is also often studied by exercise science professionals. Inactivity physiology is concerned with responses of the systems of the body to insufficient amounts, little, or no physical activity.

Exercise physiology is also used to enhance performance in sport and athletic competition by improving ways in which the systems of the body respond to training and competition. Athletes, coaches, and other exercise science professionals use the basic and advanced training principles of exercise physiology to enhance the function of the various systems of the body. The identification of those factors affecting performance and subsequent improvement as a response to training is the hallmark of using exercise physiology to improve performance. In some instances, exercise physiology is used synonymously with exercise science and many individuals often use the terms interchangeably. However as indicated in Chapter 1, exercise science is a broad term correctly used to describe the disciplines, subdisciplines, and areas of study that have movement as a central theme.

College and university academic programs are often structured to prepare students to function as exercise physiologists in clinical, fitness, sport, or research environments. Students who are trained to work in clinical environments, such as cardiovascular and pulmonary rehabilitation, will receive more educational training in the clinical aspects of exercise physiology (see Chapter 4). Training for a professional career in fitness and sport-oriented environments will include more experiences in understanding how untrained and trained persons will respond to the demands of regular exercise and training for athletic competition. Individuals preparing for a career in research will be exposed to more preparation in research design and methods, and data analysis procedures. This career track typically requires additional education in the form of a master's or doctoral degree and may involve working with whole animal and human models or with animal and human tissue samples. Regardless of the career track, preparation for a professional career in exercise physiology necessitates the study of the body's systems and how they respond to acute and chronic physical activities and exercises.

Exercise physiology Study of the functional responses and adaptations that occur during and following physical activity and exercise.

HISTORIC DEVELOPMENT OF EXERCISE PHYSIOLOGY

Although exercise physiology is relatively new as a defined body of knowledge, individuals have been interested in the physiologic responses to physical activity and exercise since the time of the early Greeks (17). The early historic events in medicine, physiology, exercise, and sport that have helped define exercise physiology have also influenced the development of other disciplines in exercise science as well. Many of those important historic events are described in Chapter 1, and the reader is directed to review that information for a broad overview. The material contained in this section should be considered a supplement to Chapter 1 and will contain only information specific to the recent historic development of exercise physiology.

Early Twentieth-Century Influences

One of the most significant events for the emergence of exercise physiology as a scientific discipline was the establishment in 1891 of the Department of Anatomy, Physiology, and Physical Training within the Lawrence Scientific School at Harvard University (97,98). Faculty and leaders in the department implemented a demanding 4-year science-based curriculum that included both theory and laboratory courses in exercise physiology (73,85,97,98). Expansion of this concept of coupling laboratory experiments with course content in exercise and physical training also occurred at Springfield College in Massachusetts and George Williams College in Chicago, Illinois (97). Despite the curricular offerings in exercise physiology at these universities, there was insufficient evidence that exercise physiology had established itself as an academic discipline until the opening of the Harvard Fatigue Laboratory in 1927 (Figure 3.1) (97).

The Harvard Fatigue Laboratory's primary purpose was to study the physiologic, psychological, and sociologic responses of industry workers to stressful stimuli (28,65). The founders of the laboratory included fatigue in the name because it was believed the term would help attract the interest and funding of business

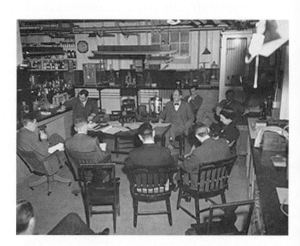

FIGURE 3.1 ▼ The Harvard Fatigue Laboratory (ca. 1946). (Photo from Baker Library Historical Collections, Harvard Business School.)

leaders and because the concept of fatigue could be understood by many individuals without being explained or defined (28). The Harvard Fatigue Laboratory attracted high quality scientists from around the world and produced scholars and professionals who would be instrumental in shaping exercise physiology as a scientific discipline. Paradoxically, the closure of the Harvard Fatigue Laboratory in 1947 was instrumental in facilitating the establishment of other exercise physiology laboratories across the United States. Many of the founders of these new laboratories were well-known individuals who had close connections to the Harvard Fatigue Laboratory and helped further expand the development of exercise physiology (24,98).

Late Twentieth-Century Influences

Beginning in the 1940s, there were a number of significant events that significantly shaped the discipline of exercise physiology. During this time period, several peer-reviewed journals published data from experiments involving the physiologic responses to exercise (98). By the late 1940s, a sufficient body of knowledge existed in exercise physiology to merit formal instructional course offerings by colleges and universities. The further development of exercise physiology occurred in response to a number of social, political, and professional factors. Poor performance by American school children on fitness tests and the competition between the United States and the Soviet Union to put a man in space and later land a man on the moon heightened the focus on fitness and performance of the American population. Other instrumental factors included the passage of funding for health-related research, facilities, and educational training programs by the National Institutes of Health; the interest of the American Physiological Society (APS) in exercise related research; the publication of the *Journal of Applied Physiology* by the APS; and the formation of the American College of Sports Medicine and its peer-reviewed journal *Medicine and Science in Sports and Exercise* (97). The interest in exercise and fitness of many of the early leaders of the ACSM resulted in an increased emphasis on the study of the physiologic responses to exercise (23,24).

Throughout the 1960s and 1970s, exercise physiology continued to expand and evolve. As interest in exercise physiology continued to grow, college curricula changed from traditional programs in physical education to more science-related courses and activities. Undergraduate students enrolled in courses in biochemistry and physiology, and participated in a variety of laboratory activities. This change better prepared students to enter professional careers that required a knowledge base in exercise physiology. Students now had an option to pursue a career in exercise physiology rather than be trained as physical education teachers (97). This trend continues today as many physical education programs require little formal course preparation in physiology and exercise physiology. Conversely, expanded curricula in exercise physiology include topics such as exercise testing and prescription, exercise management of chronic disease, advanced study in cellular functions and mechanisms, and genetics though requiring little or no coursework in teacher training.

Since the establishment of the ACSM, numerous organizations have emerged to provide support for other professionals with an interest in exercise physiology.

Table 3.1	Some Significant Historic Events in the Development of Exercise Physiology
YEAR	**EVENT**
1891	Establishment of the Department of Anatomy, Physiology, and Physical Training at Harvard University
1927	Opening of the Harvard Fatigue Laboratory at Harvard University
1948	Publication of the *Journal of Applied Physiology* by the American Physiological Society
1954	Formation of the American College of Sports Medicine
1969	Initial publication of *Medicine and Science in Sports and Exercise*
1978	Establishment of the NSCA
1985	Formation of the AACVPR
1997	Establishment of the American Society of Exercise Physiologists
2007	Acceptance of the ACSM into the Federation of American Societies for Experimental Biology

In 1997, the establishment of the American Society of Exercise Physiologists (ASEP) arose from the belief in the need for an organization to solely promote exercise physiology as a profession (see Chapter 11). Although ASEP remains the only organization with exercise physiology in its name, there are numerous other organizations such as the National Strength and Conditioning Association (NSCA) and the American Association of Cardiovascular and Pulmonary Rehabilitation (AACVPR) that have promoted the study and development of exercise physiology in health, physical activity, fitness, sport, and athletic performance. Table 3.1 identifies some of the important historic events in the development of exercise physiology.

Exercise physiology continues to expand as a discipline and organize as a profession. Students of undergraduate programs with an emphasis in exercise physiology coursework can enter professional careers as certified personal trainers, health fitness instructors, exercise specialists, and strength and conditioning coaches. These professions clearly indicate the role that practical applications of exercise physiology have to healthy and diseased populations. Students can further their educational training by enrolling in master's and doctoral degree programs to become college and university teachers and researchers in public and private settings. Students of exercise physiology are also very successful in entering into professional programs and schools of medicine, dentistry, chiropractic, physician assistant, and physical and occupational therapy. The role of exercise physiology will continue to be important in our society as we continue to identify how physical activity and exercise can improve health and reduce disease risk and as we continue to seek improvements in sport and athletic performance.

> ➤ *Thinking Critically*
>
> *In what ways has exercise physiology contributed to a broader understanding of the role physical activity and exercise play in the promotion of physical fitness and health, as well as the understanding of successful sport and athletic performance?*

THE BASIS OF STUDY IN EXERCISE PHYSIOLOGY

Two primary areas of study in exercise physiology are how the body responds to acute episodes of physical activity and exercise and how regular physical activity and exercise results in chronic adaptations of the various systems of the body. **Homeostasis** describes the condition of the systems of the body when the body is in a resting state. When the body is subjected to a stress, such as physical activity or exercise, the body's state of homeostasis is disrupted. When the body encounters work, physical activity or exercise, numerous changes occur that affect every system of the body. Understanding homeostasis is critical to understanding the acute responses and chronic adaptations to physical activity and exercise. When homeostasis is disrupted as a result of physical activity or exercise, the various systems of the body respond by either increasing or decreasing their level of activity. This coordinated response of the systems allows the body to meet the challenges of physical activity or exercise and works to return the body to homeostasis. Repeated challenges of appropriate intensity and duration to homeostasis result in chronic adaptations to the body.

Acute Responses to Physical Activity and Exercise

The **acute responses** of the systems of the body are those actions that occur in response to a single bout of physical activity or exercise. When an individual engages in physical activity or exercise, there are numerous challenges to homeostasis and almost every system of the body is involved to some degree. For example, during a brisk walk on a warm summer day, there are increases in the demand for energy production in the working muscle, a need for greater blood flow through the cardiovascular and pulmonary systems, and a rise in body temperature. In a healthy individual, the various systems of the body respond in a coordinated fashion to meet the demands of the body during exercise and return the body to homeostasis following the completion of exercise. In this example, there would be an increase in glucose and fatty acid uptake by working skeletal muscle, an increase in heart rate and stroke volume by the heart, and increase in the rate and depth of breathing by the lungs, and an increase in skin blood flow to assist with temperature regulation. Exercise science professionals must have a solid understanding of how the body systems respond to acute bouts of physical activity and exercise so that safe and effective physical activity and exercise programs can be prescribed for the individuals with which they are working. Table 3.2 illustrates how some of the major systems of the body respond to a single bout of exercise. Research and the study of the acute responses of the body during physical activity, exercise, sport, and athletic performance has allowed for a much greater understanding of how the systems of the body control the body's internal environment and response to increased challenges to homeostasis.

Homeostasis The maintenance of relatively stable internal physiologic conditions.

Acute responses Changes in the systems of the body that occur in response to a single bout of physical activity or exercise.

Table 3.2	Acute Responses of the Body to a Single Bout of Exercise
BODY SYSTEM	**ACUTE RESPONSES**
Cardiovascular system	Increases in heart rate, stoke volume, cardiac output, blood pressure, and a redirection of blood flow to the working tissues of the body
Pulmonary system	Increases in air movement into and out of the lungs and increased blood flow through the lungs
Muscular system	Increases in force production, utilization and production of energy, and heat production
Endocrine system	Increases in the release of epinephrine and norepinephrine

Table 3.3	Examples of Research in the Acute Responses of Some Body Systems to Exercise
BODY SYSTEM	**ACUTE RESPONSE**
Cardiovascular system	What factors regulate the local control of blood flow to working muscle?
Pulmonary system	Does pulmonary ventilation limit maximal effort exercise?
Muscular system	What factors contribute to a loss of force production in skeletal muscle during exercise?
Endocrine system	How do different levels of carbohydrate, fat, and protein intake affect the release of the hormones insulin and glucagon?

Table 3.3 provides examples of areas of research in how the different systems of the body respond in an acute manner to physical activity or exercise.

Chronic Adaptations to Physical Activity and Exercise

The term **chronic adaptations** to physical activity and exercise refers to the adaptations that occur in the systems of the body with repeated regular physical activity and exercise. If the physical activity or exercise is performed on a regular basis and is of sufficient intensity, duration, and frequency there will be positive adaptations of the systems of the body. These adaptations, often called training responses, occur with the primary purpose of improving the body's response to the challenges imposed by the physical activity or exercise. Table 3.4 provides

Chronic adaptations Changes in the systems of the body that occur in response to repeated regular physical activity and exercise.

Table 3.4	Chronic Adaptations of Some Body Systems to Physical Activity and Exercise	
BODY SYSTEM	**CHRONIC ADAPTATIONS**	
Cardiovascular system	Increases in stoke volume and cardiac output and decreases in heart rate at the same absolute workload	
Pulmonary system	Improved air movement into and out of the lungs and increased blood flow through the lungs at the same absolute workload	
Muscular system	Increased energy production from fat and decreased lactic acid formation at the same absolute workload	
Endocrine system	Decreased release of epinephrine and norepinephrine at the same absolute workload	

Table 3.5	Examples of Research in the Study of Chronic Adaptations to Some Body Systems in Response to Regular Physical Activity and Exercise	
BODY SYSTEM	**CHRONIC ADAPTATIONS**	
Cardiovascular system	What factors influence the reduction in blood pressure in hypertensive individuals following exercise training?	
Pulmonary system	How does exercise training improve blood flow through the entire lung?	
Muscular system	How does regular exercise influence the uptake of glucose by skeletal muscle in persons with diabetes?	
Endocrine system	What hormones cause the shift in energy metabolism following training in athletes?	

some examples of the responses of the systems of the body to chronic physical activity and exercise.

In general, the chronic adaptations to exercise improve various functions of the body while at rest and during submaximal and maximal exercise. For example, if an individual participates in a regular walking program for exercise there will be adaptations to the systems of the body that result from the chronic exercise. For a given level of exercise intensity, regular walking would result in the greater use of fat as an energy source, a lower heart rate and higher stroke volume, better exchange of oxygen and carbon dioxide in the lungs, and an improved regulation of body temperature. It is important to note that as with the acute responses to exercise, the chronic adaptations are highly variable and strongly influenced by the type of physical activity and exercise performed. Table 3.5 provides some examples of areas of study in the chronic adaptations of the different systems of the body as they respond to regular physical activity and exercise. Exercise physiology is grounded in the study and understanding

> **Thinking Critically**
> *Why do athletes and coaches need to be knowledgeable about the acute responses and chronic adaptations to endurance exercise and resistance exercise training?*

of the acute responses and chronic adaptations to physical activity and exercise. Much of the knowledge base in the study of exercise physiology and exercise science in general is the result of research and observation into the acute responses and chronic adaptations of the systems of the body to physical activity and exercise.

AREAS OF STUDY IN EXERCISE PHYSIOLOGY

Working as an exercise specialist, personal trainer, strength and conditioning coach, or a clinical exercise physiologist in an allied health profession requires individuals to draw upon their educational background and experiences to perform their job to the best level possible. Exercise physiology contributes to a complete understanding of health, physical activity, exercise, sport, and athletic performance through a wide variety of areas too numerous to cover them all adequately in an introductory exercise science textbook. The areas discussed in the following sections are some of the primary interest areas in exercise physiology. The areas selected are by no means meant to infer an inclusive list or indicate greater importance than a topic area not covered but are meant to provide a sampling of areas in which the knowledge of exercise physiology is generated and used. It is hoped that as you read through these sections, you will gain a better understanding of how the various systems interact to control the body functions and how various aspects of physical activity and exercise influence these responses.

Factors Controlling Substrate Metabolism

Exercise scientists and other allied health professionals have long been interested in the different factors that control energy production in the body during exercise. The energy sources, often called **substrates**, used by the body are carbohydrates, fats, and proteins. Understanding how the body tissues use these macronutrients to provide energy is critical to providing advice on how to enhance physical activity and exercise and for providing recommendations to improve sport and athletic performance. At rest and in a **postabsorptive state**, the tissues of the body rely on fat and carbohydrate as the primary sources of energy, with little energy provided from protein (54). However, the percentage of energy supplied to the body from carbohydrates, fats, and protein can be influenced by numerous factors. For example, eating meals of different macronutrient content can alter the energy sources utilized during rest and exercise. Meals high in carbohydrate content can increase glucose and glycogen utilization and enhance exercise performance whereas meals low in carbohydrate content can decrease carbohydrate utilization and often adversely affect exercise

---

Substrates A source of energy for the cells of the body.

Postabsorptive state The condition following the complete absorption of a meal.

Crossover point The point where the body receives more of its energy from carbohydrate rather than fat.

performance (34,94). Food restriction, either through dieting or starvation or prolonged exercise can alter substrate utilization by promoting a greater contribution of energy supplied from protein (94,99).

The intensity and duration of physical activity and exercise are two primary factors affecting substrate utilization. During low-intensity physical activity and exercise, fat is the primary substrate for energy production. As physical activity or exercise intensity increases, there is a greater reliance on carbohydrate as an energy source. When exercise intensity reaches close to 100% of maximal oxygen consumption (VO_{2max}), almost 100% of the energy is provided by the metabolism of carbohydrates (20,52). There is an exercise intensity that results in a point being reached when there is a shift from fat to carbohydrate as the predominant energy substrate. This point has been labeled the **crossover point** (20). During exercise, there are several factors that cause the shift in substrate utilization to occur. As exercise intensity increases, more fast glycolytic fibers are recruited to power muscular contraction and these fibers rely predominately on carbohydrate as the energy substrate (52). The second factor directly affecting the shift in substrate utilization is an increase in the concentration of the hormone epinephrine. As the exercise intensity increases, the sympathetic nervous system and the adrenal medulla increase the release of epinephrine into the circulation. Epinephrine increases carbohydrate metabolism by increasing muscle glycogen breakdown and inhibiting the release of fat from adipose tissue (52). Improvements in cardiorespiratory fitness as a result of increased levels of regular physical activity or exercise result in a shift in substrate utilization so that greater fat utilization occurs at higher exercise intensities. This results in less carbohydrate and more fat being used during physical activity or exercise (19). Figure 3.2 provides an illustration of the role of exercise intensity on substrate utilization and the crossover point.

During long-duration physical activity or exercise, there is a gradual increase in the utilization of fat as an energy substrate. This results in a decrease in the use of carbohydrates as a fuel source (53). There are several factors that cause the shift in fuel utilization during prolonged exercise to occur. The use of fat as an energy source in skeletal muscle depends in part on the mobilization of fat from adipose tissue and delivery of fat by the circulatory system to working skeletal muscle (19).

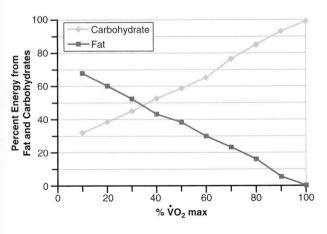

FIGURE 3.2 ▼ Effect of exercise intensity on substrate utilization and the crossover point (Source: Powers SK, Howley ET. *Exercise Physiology: Theory and Application to Fitness and Performance.* Dubuque: Brown & Benchmark; 2007, p. 56, Chapter 4, Figure 4.11.)

Table 3.6	Some Factors Affecting Fuel Utilization During Exercise
FACTOR	**GENERAL RESPONSE**
Increased exercise intensity	Increased use of carbohydrate
Increased exercise duration	Increased use of fat
Epinephrine and norepinephrine	Increased use of carbohydrate
Glucagon	Increased use of fat
Lactic acid	Decreased use of fat

The mobilization of fat from adipose is controlled by enzymes called lipases. The activity level of these enzymes is influenced by the hormones epinephrine, norepinephrine, and glucagon. During long-duration exercise, the concentration of these hormones in the blood increases resulting in an increase in fatty acid release into the circulation. The delivery of the fats to the working tissues occurs as a result of increased blood flow to the muscles that are active during physical activity and exercise (52,53). Fat mobilization can be inhibited by high blood levels of lactic acid and the hormone insulin. If during long-duration exercise there is an increase in the exercise intensity so that blood lactic acid levels increase, this could result in a decrease in fat mobilization and utilization as a fuel substrate (19). Insulin also inhibits fat mobilization, but generally during long-duration exercise there is a decline in blood insulin levels (19). Table 3.6 identifies some of the prominent factors affecting fuel utilization during exercise.

Implications for Physical Activity and Exercise

The control of factors affecting substrate metabolism has implications for exercise science professionals designing physical activity and exercise programs. For example, if the intention is to decrease body weight and body fat then physical activity and exercise that promotes the use of fat as the substrate should be emphasized. It is often recommended that exercise intensity be kept low to promote the use of fat as a fuel substrate because there is a greater percentage of fat utilized at low intensities. However, this recommendation does not take into account the total amount of energy expended during the exercise session. At higher exercise intensities, more total fat could be used as a fuel source even though the percentage of fat being utilized may be less than that which occurs at a lower intensity of exercise (89). Another consideration is whether the consumption of a pre-exercise meal or beverage high in carbohydrate is necessary. If a meal or glucose beverage is consumed too close to the start of exercise, there will likely be an increase in the insulin concentration in the blood, which will decrease the mobilization of fat and result in a reduction in the use of fat as a fuel substrate (57).

Hypoglycemic A condition of abnormally low blood glucose levels.

Implications for Sport and Athletic Performance

Athletes who participate in sports or athletic competitions that are of prolonged duration (e.g., triathlons, long-distance running and cycling) must be careful about maintaining blood glucose and muscle glycogen concentrations during exercise. During long-duration exercise performed at moderate to high intensity, there is a significant reliance on muscle glycogen as the carbohydrate energy source. During prolonged exercise that lasts 3 to 4 hours or longer, both blood glucose and muscle glycogen contribute to energy production in an equal percentage. As muscle glycogen concentration decreases, the use of blood glucose increases so that when an athlete is nearing a level of muscle glycogen depletion blood glucose may be the predominate source of carbohydrate as a fuel (31).

If blood glucose concentration is not maintained during long-duration exercise, the athlete could become **hypoglycemic** which may lead to fatigue, a decrease in performance, and possible serious medical conditions. Consequently, it is important to maintain blood glucose concentrations during exercise (89). The timing and type of carbohydrate consumption are two factors that are critical for helping to maintain blood glucose concentrations during long-duration exercise. It is suggested that a carbohydrate feeding of between 1 and 5 g of carbohydrate per kilogram body mass should occur between 1 and 4 hours prior to the start of exercise (94). Although this procedure results in an increased use of carbohydrate as a substrate early in the exercise bout, the additional carbohydrate consumed will help maintain blood glucose for a longer period of time during exercise (94). Carbohydrate should also be consumed during exercise (Figure 3.3)

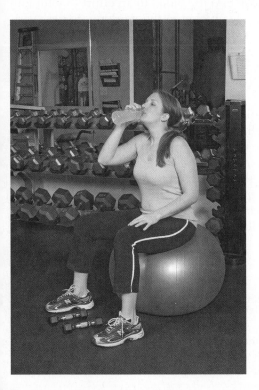

FIGURE 3.3 ▼ Carbohydrate consumption during exercise. (From *ACSM's Resource for the Personal Trainer*, 3rd ed. Baltimore (MD): Lippincott Williams & Wilkins; 2010.)

> ➤ *Thinking Critically*
> *Why would consumption of carbohydrate prior to and during exercise have different effects on an individual exercising to improve health versus an individual competing in a prolonged athletic competition?*

and this procedure has been shown to delay the onset of fatigue and improve long-duration exercise performance (108). The best type of carbohydrate to consume during exercise is glucose, sucrose, or **glucose polymer solutions** at a concentration of approximately 6% to 8% (94). Exercise scientist professionals continue to examine ways to improve athletic performance and decrease the potential for the adverse effects of muscle glycogen depletion and hypoglycemia through the ingestion of glucose and glucose polymer beverages, and energy bars prior to and during exercise.

Muscle Control of Glucose Uptake

The control of blood glucose uptake by tissues of the body at rest and during physical activity and exercise has important implications for overall health and athletic performance, and is of considerable interest to exercise science professionals. The body closely regulates energy utilization so that as skeletal muscle uses energy during physical activity or exercise there is an increase in energy production by the tissues. As the need for energy increases, there are a variety of changes that occur in the body. For example, the use of carbohydrates as an energy source in muscle results in the breakdown and utilization of muscle glycogen and an increase in the uptake of glucose from the blood into the individual muscle cells. There is also an increase in liver glycogen breakdown into glucose with the subsequent release of the glucose into the blood in an effort to maintain blood glucose concentration and to provide glucose to the working tissues. Various hormones, including epinephrine, norepinephrine, and glucagon, stimulate the breakdown (19).

The movement of glucose from the blood into the cell depends on the interaction of the hormone insulin and a glucose transport protein. Insulin is released from the pancreas to help control blood glucose levels in the body and help glucose enter into the cells of the body. Glucose enters the cells by interacting with a glucose transport protein on the cell membrane. There are several glucose transport proteins, but the one specific to skeletal muscle is called the **glucose transport protein 4** or Glut 4. When a muscle cell needs glucose, it increases the number of the Glut 4 proteins in the cell membrane (32). Several factors stimulate an increase in Glut 4 proteins including insulin, increased blood flow to skeletal muscle, increased glucose concentration, and muscle contractions (92). Figure 3.4 illustrates the process by which insulin facilitates the Glut 4 transport protein to take glucose into the cell.

Glucose polymer solution A beverage that contains multiple glucose molecules linked together in solution.

Glucose transport protein 4 A type of protein molecule that works with insulin to facilitate glucose uptake by skeletal muscle fibers.

Basal

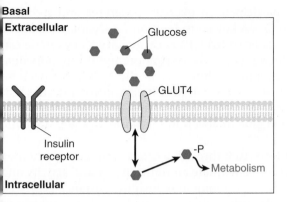

Insulin

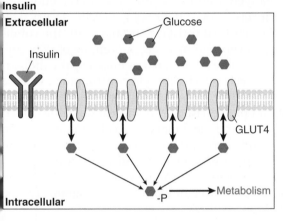

FIGURE 3.4 ▼ Insulin and Glut 4 facilitate glucose uptake by cells of the body.

Once glucose enters a muscle fiber, it can be stored as muscle glycogen or immediately used to produce energy. The stored muscle glycogen can be broken down for energy by chemical compounds, called enzymes, in the muscle fiber. The muscle glycogen and blood glucose are metabolized through a series of chemical reactions and provide energy to support the functions of the contracting muscle fibers. As mentioned previously, the exercise intensity is one of the strongest factors influencing the use of carbohydrate as a fuel source. As exercise intensity increases, the reliance on carbohydrates as an energy source increases (Figure 3.1).

Implications for Physical Activity and Exercise

The role of physical activity and exercise in regulating glucose metabolism is of importance in promoting health and wellness. Diabetes mellitus is a disease condition whereby insufficient insulin is produced by the pancreas (type 1) or the insulin does not promote the uptake of glucose by the cell (type 2). At one time, it was believed that individuals with type 1 diabetes mellitus should not participate in physical activity, exercise, sport, or athletic competition because these individuals have difficulty controlling their blood glucose concentration. However, with a better understanding of the role of glucose transport proteins in controlling blood glucose, individuals with type 1 diabetes who are otherwise healthy are now encouraged to participate in exercise programs and sports to improve their health and wellness (7). A key consideration for the type 1 diabetic is whether the individual is in metabolic control. Physical activity and exercise can have a dramatic impact on the blood glucose concentration and if the individual is not careful about regulating diet and the intensity of the activity or exercise then hypoglycemia and **insulin shock** can occur. Metabolic control indicates that the individual is on a regular schedule of diet, insulin, and physical activity that allows for the maintenance of blood glucose levels in the normal range with little fluctuation (70,91).

Type 2 diabetes mellitus manifests itself through a series of processes whereby the body becomes resistant to insulin. Inadequate amounts of physical activity and poor nutritional habits can lead to the development of insulin resistance (12,101). This condition is characterized by relatively well-maintained insulin secretion and normal to elevated plasma insulin levels. Type 2 diabetes generally occurs later in life and there are usually several other health risks associated with the condition including hypertension, high blood cholesterol levels, abdominal obesity, and physical inactivity (6). Physical activity and exercise are beneficial to the individual with type 2 diabetes as increased levels of activity help control blood glucose concentration and also have a positive effect on the associated health risks (6). The combination of a regular program of exercise and modification to the nutritional intake may allow the individual with type 2 diabetes to eliminate the need for **exogenous insulin** or the oral medications used to stimulate insulin secretion by the pancreas (6). Exercise science professionals involved in the prescription of physical activity and exercise must be aware of the process by which glucose is taken up and used for energy so that effective individualized programs can be developed for healthy and diseased individuals.

Implications for Sport and Athletic Performance

Success in certain types of sport and athletic performance is dependent on the ability of the body and muscle fibers to produce energy very quickly. Those athletic events that are characterized by short duration and high-intensity periods of activity (e.g., sprinting, football, volleyball) depend heavily on the ability to rapidly use carbohydrates (primarily muscle glycogen) as an energy source. Exercise scientists, strength and conditioning coaches, sports coaches, and athletes have long been interested in improving energy production from carbohydrates and delaying the onset of fatigue that occurs from a buildup of lactic acid in the muscle: a by-product of carbohydrate metabolism.

The formation of lactic acid in skeletal muscle is a complex process. During rest and low-intensity exercise, most of the energy is produced by using oxygen in the **aerobic metabolism** of carbohydrates and fats. Although there is a small amount of lactic acid being produced in the muscle, it is quickly cleared by a number of processes in the body. As the exercise intensity increases, there is an increase in the production of lactic acid and at the same time an increase in the removal of lactic acid from the tissues. There is, however, an exercise intensity whereby lactic acid accumulates in the muscle and blood. As lactic acid (or more accurately the negatively charged lactate ion and its associated positively charged hydrogen ion) increases in concentration, it contributes to fatigue in the contracting muscle.

The fatigue in the muscle is likely caused by the increased acidity that affects various enzymes involved in energy production or interferes with the muscle's contractile process (103).

The development of various training programs designed to increase energy production from aerobic sources and decrease the fatiguing effects of lactic acid has long been a goal of coaches and athletes. In aerobic endurance events, the successful competitor among athletes with similar VO_{2max} values is usually the person who can maintain aerobic energy production at the highest percentage of his or her VO_{2max}, without accumulating large amounts of lactic acid in the muscle and blood (74). Although many terms are used to describe this phenomenon, the lactate threshold is the one most commonly seen in the literature. The lactate threshold is that exercise intensity at which a specific blood lactate concentration is observed or where blood lactate concentration begins to increase above resting levels (102). Research has shown that an athlete's lactate threshold appears to be a strong predictor of aerobic endurance performance (35,36). The maximal lactate steady state is another term that also appears in the aerobic training literature. The maximal lactate steady state is the exercise intensity where maximal lactate production equals maximal lactate clearance within the body (13). Many experts consider the maximal lactate steady state exercise intensity to be a better indicator of aerobic endurance performance than either maximal oxygen consumption or the lactate threshold (13,48). What is clear from this information is that aerobic endurance athletes must improve their ability to decrease the production of lactic acid and increase the removal of lactic acid from the muscle and blood. This requires the athlete to train at elevated levels of blood and muscle lactate to maximize training-induced improvements that decrease lactic acid production and increase lactic acid clearance by the body (87). The development of and use of nutritional ergogenic aids, such as sodium bicarbonate and sodium citrate, to help minimize the effects of lactic acid buildup during high-intensity exercise is also of interest to exercise science professionals. Both sodium bicarbonate and sodium citrate help maintain the normal pH levels of the body as lactic acid concentrations increase (88).

Skeletal Muscle Physiology

Skeletal muscle has a number of important functions in the human body (see Chapter 2). As a result, exercise scientists have been studying skeletal muscle to gain a better understanding of how muscle performs various functions during exercise and sport performance. Skeletal muscle fibers develop from **embryonic myotubes** into mature muscle fibers and this development is influenced by various growth-promoting factors (55). As the fibers develop, various regulatory

---

Insulin shock Acute hypoglycemia usually resulting from an excessive insulin and characterized by sweating, trembling, dizziness, and, if left untreated, convulsions and coma.

Exogenous insulin Insulin administered from outside the body.

Aerobic metabolism The production of energy through the use of oxygen in the cell.

Embryonic myotubes Immature structures that can potentially convert into muscle fibers.

and contractile proteins are arranged in a systematic pattern that allows the fiber to generate force upon stimulation from a motor neuron (55). Skeletal muscle fibers are a **heterogeneous group** of fibers with distinct contractile and metabolic characteristics (69) (see Chapter 2, Table 2.3). Each of these fiber types has characteristics that allow them to perform distinct functions and respond in different ways during muscle contraction. Skeletal muscle fibers are unique to individuals and specific muscle groups. Generally, muscle fiber types cannot be changed unless there is a dramatic change in the physical activity or exercise habits of an individual. In this instance, the muscle fiber types will take on characteristics that help the muscle meet the requirements of the physical activity or exercise.

Implications for Physical Activity and Exercise

Skeletal muscle plays an important role in promoting health and wellness for a wide age range of individuals. Exercise science professionals have long been interested in identifying the most appropriate resistance exercise program to enhance muscular strength development and improve muscular fitness, balance, coordination, and other measures of motor performance (95). Through years of research, much has been learned about the various components needed for a successful resistance exercise program. Some of the characteristics affecting strength development are shown in Figure 3.5. Resistance exercise training causes muscle fiber hypertrophy (40,80) as a result of increased protein synthesis (86). Increases in muscular strength (90) and muscular power (104) are observed following participation in resistance training programs. The importance of muscular strength

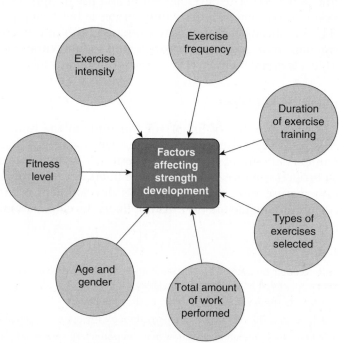

FIGURE 3.5 ▼ Factors affecting strength development (95).

in older adults is critical for maintaining normal functional ability and often independence (60). As long as certain training principles are met, older adults can increase muscular size and strength following resistance exercise training (21,43). Although much is known about how individuals respond to resistance exercise programs, there are still many unanswered questions in the areas of gender differences in response to training, the appropriate volume of training to reduce the risk of lifestyle-related diseases, and the role of resistance exercise in treating individuals with disease conditions.

Implications for Sport and Athletic Performance

The muscle fiber type is an important consideration for athletes in specific sports because of the unique functional and metabolic characteristics of the fibers. The use of the **muscle biopsy** (in combination with the **skinned fiber technique**) has allowed exercise scientists to identify differences in fiber types between individuals. In sedentary men and women, between 45% to 55% of the total percentage of fibers are slow twitch fibers (41). Specific distribution patterns of fiber types are evident among highly successful athletes (33,96). Slow twitch muscle fibers predominate in the active muscle of successful aerobic endurance-trained athletes, whereas fast twitch muscle fibers predominate in the active muscle of successful sprint- and resistance-trained athletes (33,96). Of particulate interest to exercise science professionals, coaches, and athletes is whether muscle fiber types can be altered with training. It would appear that an appropriate duration, frequency, and intensity of training can alter the characteristics of the fiber types in the muscles that are being trained. In general, low-intensity endurance training results in fast twitch fibers altering their functional and metabolic characteristics to become more like slow twitch fibers. Conversely, high-intensity sprint training and resistance exercise training causes the functional and metabolic characteristics of slow twitch fibers to become more like fast twitch fibers. Training may or may not convert fibers from one type to another, but training does alter the characteristics of the fibers to support the type of training performed (72).

Bone Metabolism

The skeletal system is a very important and dynamic system of the body. Though most individuals have good bone health, there are several individuals in both the general population and the athletic population that are at increased risk for poor bone health (71). As a result, exercise science professionals have been interested in how physical activity and exercise influence bone metabolism. Osteoporosis is

---

Heterogeneous group A collection composed of parts having dissimilar characteristics or properties.

Muscle biopsy A needle technique used to collect tissue samples from a muscle.

Skinned fiber technique A laboratory technique that allows for easy control of the external environment of a muscle fiber.

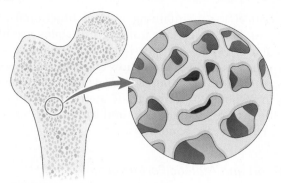

A Normal bone

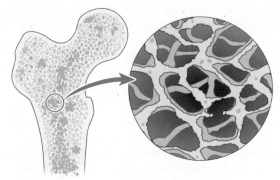

B Osteoporosis

FIGURE 3.6 ▼ Normal bone and osteoporotic bone.

a disease condition characterized by low bone mineral density. Figure 3.6 provides radiographs of normal bone and osteoporotic bone.

Older adults, especially females are at an increased risk for developing osteoporosis (71). Female athletes participating in high-volume training are also at increased risk of developing low bone mineral density and possibly osteoporosis (71,84). Of concern to those individuals with low bone mineral density and osteoporosis is the increased risk of bone fracture that is associated with repeated force or trauma (71). There are two generally accepted strategies for making the skeleton more resistant to fracture: (a) maximizing the amount of bone mineral density in the first three decades of life and (b) minimizing the decline in bone mineral density after the age of 40 years (71). The efforts of various exercise science professionals is very important for helping individuals develop physical activity and exercise programs, as well as good nutritional habits that will improve bone health.

Implications for Physical Activity and Exercise

Exercise science and allied health professionals have expanded considerably the information about the role of physical activity in maintaining good bone health. Mechanical loading is the application of force to the tissues of the body and is an important consideration in bone health. Mechanical loading forces that are unique, variable, and dynamic in nature result in changes to the skeletal system that increase bone mineral density (22,71). It is clear that the intensity, duration, and frequency of the mechanical loading is important for maximizing bone formation, but further research is needed to determine if a specific threshold exists (71). Other factors that appear to play an important role in the development of poor bone health are calcium insufficiency (75) and estrogen deficiency (110). Maximizing bone mass in children, adolescents, and young adults is critical as peak bone mass is thought to be attained by the end of the third decade of life (71). Though the optimal type, frequency, intensity, and duration have yet to be conclusively determined, it is clear that both physical activity and exercise are critical for maximizing bone mineral density (71).

Starting at the age of about 40 years, bone mass decreases by about 0.5% or more per year, regardless of gender or ethnicity. The rate of loss varies by skeletal region and is potentially influenced by genetics, nutrition, hormonal status, and regular physical activity (71). It would appear that certain types of physical activity and exercise are more beneficial for preserving bone mass. Activities with higher intensity mechanical loading forces, such as brisk walking, stair climbing, and jogging, seem to provide a better response of the skeletal system for increasing bone mass (30,37,71). Regular physical activity may also reduce fracture risk by either increasing the bone mineral content, decreasing the bone mineral loss, or increasing muscular strength and balance and consequently reducing the risk of falling (5,71).

Implications for Sport and Athletic Performance

Female athletes displaying certain characteristics and participating in particular sports are at an increased risk for developing osteoporosis (84). Young female athletes who exhibit disordered eating, **amenorrhea**, and bone mineral loss are characterized as having the female athlete triad (84). Disordered eating is characterized by a wide range of harmful and often ineffective eating behaviors used in attempts to achieve weight loss or a lean appearance. Short- and long-term morbidity, decreased performance, amenorrhea, and even mortality are outcomes of disordered eating (58,62,84). Amenorrhea is the absence of a regular menstrual cycle and can be classified as primary or secondary. **Hypothalamic amenorrhea** results in decreased ovarian hormone production and **hypoestrogenimia** similar to menopause. This condition is associated with both exercise and the eating disorder known as anorexia nervosa. Both hypothalamic amenorrhea and menopause are associated with decreased bone mineral density (25,84). The combination of disordered eating, amenorrhea, and osteoporosis form the foundation of the female athlete triad as depicted in Figure 3.7.

Adolescents and young women who participate in sports or athletic competitions in which low body weight is emphasized for enhanced performance or appearance are at a high risk for developing the female athlete triad. If a female develops the triad, the combination of poor eating habits resulting in inadequate calcium

Amenorrhea Abnormal Suppression or absence of menstruation.
Hypothalamic amenorrhea Condition in which there is an absence of a normal menstrual cycle that is caused by a disorder of the hypothalamus.
Hypoestrogenimia Low levels of the female hormone estrogen.

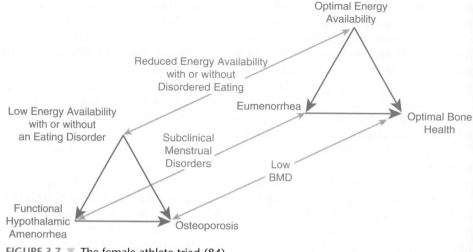

FIGURE 3.7 ▼ The female athlete triad (84).

intake and low estrogen levels from amenorrhea can result in a significant loss of bone mineral content (84,89). Exercise science and allied healthcare professionals continue to work to establish better prevention, detection, and treatment programs for girls and women who display characteristics of the female athlete triad.

Energy Balance and Weight Control

Body weight is of critical importance for promoting overall good health and optimizing performance in certain sports and athletic competitions. Although many individuals are able to regulate and control their body weight with relative ease, there are countless others who struggle with trying to prevent excess weight gain, achieve significant weight loss, or in some instances achieve weight gain. Body weight control can be best described using the energy balance equation. This equation describes the changes that occur to body weight when there are alterations to energy intake and energy expenditure.

FACTOR		FACTOR	OUTCOME
Energy intake	=	Energy expenditure	Stable body weight
Energy intake	>	Energy expenditure	Increase in body weight
Energy intake	<	Energy expenditure	Decrease in body weight

Upon initial observation of the energy balance equation, it would appear that understanding and achieving a desired body weight is a fairly simple process. However, there are numerous genetic, environmental, physiologic, and behavioral factors that could potentially influence energy intake or energy expenditure causing the equation to become unbalanced and lead to weight gain or weight loss. Factors affecting energy intake and energy expenditure of individuals are shown in Figure 3.8 (54).

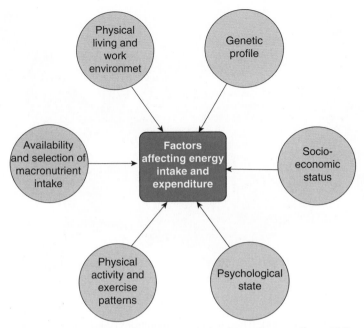

FIGURE 3.8 ▼ Factors affecting energy intake and expenditure (54).

It is likely that a number of these factors are interrelated and contribute to weight gain or weight loss in individuals. Exercise science professionals work in conjunction with other allied health professionals to identify the factors promoting weight gain and the most successful methods for losing weight and maintaining a healthy body weight.

Implications for Physical Activity and Exercise

Understanding energy balance and weight control is critical for promoting good health and fitness. The United States and many other countries have seen a rapid and large increase in the number of overweight and obese individuals over the last several decades so that more individuals are overweight or obese than ever before (46,47). Figure 1.3 shows the change in the percentage of overweight and obese individuals in the United States during the last 30 years. A multitude of environmental and individual factors have been suggested as contributing to this rapid weight gain (63). Furthermore, there is likely to be no one-intervention strategy or treatment program that will assist individuals with weight loss and the prevention of weight gain.

Research has shown us that obesity is associated with an increased risk and prevalence of chronic diseases and health conditions such as cancer (49,50), heart disease (68), **hyperinsulinemia** (56,79), **hyperlipidemia** (11), and

Hyperinsulinemia The presence of excess insulin in the blood.
Hyperlipidemia The presence of excess fat or lipids in the blood.

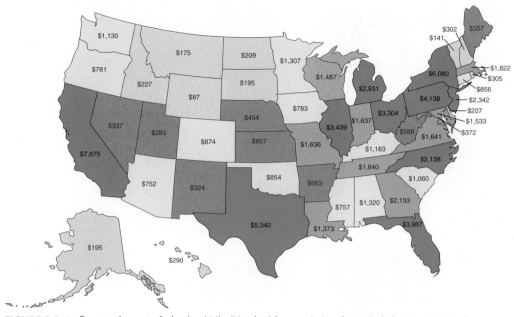

FIGURE 3.9 ▼ Economic cost of obesity (44). (Used with permission from Finkelstein EA, Fiebelkorn IC, Wang G. State-level estimates of annual medical expenditures attributable to obesity. *Obes Res.* 2004;12:18–24.)

hypertension (45). Obesity also decreases the quality of life (42) and has a significant economic cost to our healthcare system (3). Figure 3.9 illustrates the state-level estimates of adult obesity–attributable medical expenditures (44). Major health initiatives are designed to reduce the number of overweight and obese individuals in the United States (100) and other countries (107). Achieving the target goals can only be accomplished by identifying those interventions most appropriate for promoting weight loss and the prevention of weight gain (67).

There are several factors to be considered when examining the relationship of obesity to health and fitness. Body mass index (BMI) is a measure of body fat based on the individual's height and weight (BMI = body weight/height^2). The level of BMI at which there is an increased risk of morbidity and mortality is not clearly defined (67). It has been recommended by the National Institutes of Health that weigh loss is indicated in adults with a BMI ≥ 25 kg·m^{-2} (83). The pattern of body fat distribution in overweight and obese individuals may also contribute to an increased health risk. Specifically, an increased level of intra-abdominal fat is positively associated with hyperinsulinemia, **hypercholesterolemia**, and hypertension (38,39). Weight loss in overweight and obese individuals does not have to be large to positively affect health. A 5% to 10% reduction of body weight can significantly improve health by decreasing blood lipids, blood pressure, and factors related to the onset of type 2 diabetes (51,67,105), however, long-term health benefits may be maximized with sustained weight loss of greater than or equal to 10% of initial body weight (67).

Hypercholesterolemia The presence of excess cholesterol in the blood.

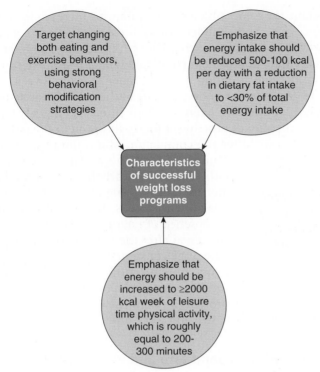

FIGURE 3.10 ▼ Characteristics of successful weight loss programs (67).

Weight loss intervention programs incorporate various strategies to promote safe and effective loss of body weight. Although it remains unclear what the best short- and long-term programs for weight loss might be for individuals of various ethnic backgrounds, gender, and different levels of body weight and body fat, several characteristics of successful weight loss programs have been identified (67). These characteristics are provided in Figure 3.10.

Implications for Sport and Athletic Performance

The maintenance of energy balance and regulation of body weight for various groups of athletes is critical for ensuring success in competition. Of particular importance is the maintenance and/or increase of lean body mass in both endurance- and resistance-trained athletes. The maintenance of lean body mass is strongly influenced by the energy expenditure during training and the energy intake in the form of macronutrient consumption (54,78). It is clear that both endurance- and resistance-trained athletes have greater dietary protein needs than the current dietary reference intake (DRI) for persons over 18 years of age. The DRI for protein is currently set at 0.8 g protein per kilogram body weight per day (54). However, the recommended requirements for dietary protein intake are higher in active individuals (78). It is recommended that endurance athletes should consume between 1.2 and 1.4 g of protein per kilogram body weight per day and resistance-trained athletes should consume between 1.4 and 1.7 g of protein per kilogram body mass per day (76,77).

It is important for some athletes to maintain or increase lean body mass for either appearance (e.g., body builders) or for force production (e.g., weight lifting, sprinting, American football). To increase lean muscle mass, an appropriate intake of dietary carbohydrate and protein combined with a resistance training program is essential. Considerable attention has been made by exercise science professionals in an effort to gain a better understanding of the role of muscle protein metabolism after resistance-training exercise. High intensity, high-volume resistance exercise increases the rate of protein synthesis and protein breakdown in skeletal muscle for several hours after the completion of a training session (86,106). To minimize protein loss and increase protein synthesis, both protein and carbohydrate should be consumed after training. During this period, the rate of protein breakdown exceeds the rate of protein synthesis in the absence of energy intake (18,86). When food is consumed after the completion of a training session, the energy consumed helps create an **anabolic** environment in the muscle that favors protein synthesis (82). The enhanced protein synthesis promotes the repair of tissues damaged during exercise and helps facilitate the development of new proteins in the muscle (106). These two factors usually lead to increases in muscle size and force production.

> ➤ *Thinking Critically*
> *What information might be valuable to know when prescribing an exercise training program for an individual trying to lose weight or gain weight?*

Assessment of Energy Expenditure and Physical Activity

An accurate assessment of energy expenditure during physical activity and exercise is important for promoting health and understanding factors that influence athlete performance. Exercise science professionals working with other highly skilled professionals from chemistry, engineering, and computer technology have developed a number of accurate and reliable assessment tools for determining energy expenditure under a variety of conditions. The assessment methods of energy expenditure and physical activity include those which are very invasive (e.g., muscle biopsy) and complex (e.g., doubly labeled water) to those less-invasive (e.g., heart rate telemetry) and simple (e.g., pedometers). Figure 3.11 shows the invasive muscle biopsy procedure used to determine concentrations

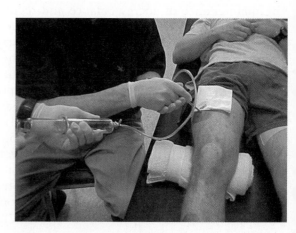

FIGURE 3.11 ▼ Muscle biopsy of the vastus lateralis.

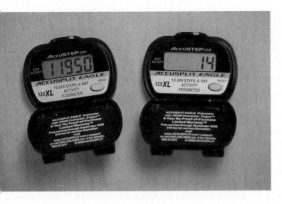

FIGURE 3.12 ▼ Commonly used pedometers for the assessment of physical activity levels.

of intramuscular metabolites, whereas Figure 3.12 shows pedometers that can be worn on clothing for the assessment of physical activity.

In some instances, the assessment of energy expenditure can be used to answer basic research questions such as how metabolic pathways are controlled in skeletal muscle. The assessment of energy expenditure also has many practical applications. For example, knowing the amount of energy expended during a particular activity can be useful for an exercise science professional developing an exercise program to promote weight loss or identifying the fitness requirement for a particular job skill.

Most assessments of energy expenditure are considered indirect. Though it is possible to directly measure energy expenditure, the process is difficult and expensive. Indirect assessments of energy expenditure generally involve a measure of some physiologic variable and then a determination of energy expenditure is derived from a mathematical prediction equation. For example, the assessment of energy expenditure by respiratory gas analysis involves the use of technical equipment for the measurement of pulmonary ventilation (i.e., air flow into and out of the lungs), and the concentration of oxygen and carbon dioxide in the expired air. In this type of assessment, energy expenditure is most accurately measured if the total oxidation of carbohydrates, fats, and protein is determined. Other assessment methods of energy expenditure that require the measurement of a physiologic variable include the doubly labeled water method, which requires collection of urine or saliva and the heart rate–monitoring method that requires an accurate and continuous measurement of heart rate. These assessment methods are accurate but labor intensive and often costly (81).

The assessment of physical activity in large groups of individuals is generally accomplished through the use of physical activity questionnaires, pedometers, and accelerometers. Each of these methods of assessment has been validated for accuracy, usually against a method that requires the measurement of a physiologic variable (e.g., respiratory gas exchange or doubly labeled water). The assessment of physical activity using a questionnaire requires an individual to accurately recall or record the activities of the day or week. The use of pedometers and accelerometers are less reliant on individual compliance and are being used more

Anabolic The process where larger molecules or compounds are built from smaller molecules or compounds.

Table 3.7	Some Examples of Energy and Physical Activity Assessment Methods
ASSESSMENT METHOD	**GENERAL COMMENTS**
Muscle biopsy	Very invasive, limited to small numbers of subjects
Doubly labeled water	Very expensive, limited to small numbers of subjects, requires frequent visits to a laboratory
Respiratory gas exchange	Expensive, limited primarily to a laboratory environment, although portable units are becoming more common
Physical activity questionnaires	Inexpensive, can be used for large numbers of individuals
Pedometers and accelerometers	Inexpensive, allows for free movement of the individual

commonly to assess levels of physical activity and energy expenditure (4,59,81). Table 3.7 provides a summary of energy assessment methods. A more complete description of these assessment methods can be found in Chapter 10.

Implications for Physical Activity and Exercise

The use of the various methods to assess energy expenditure and physical activity has allowed for the development of a compendium of physical activities that provides an estimate of energy expenditure during the performance of different activities (2). This compendium can be very useful for exercise science professionals when developing exercise prescriptions for promoting health and fitness. The ACSM Position Stand titled "Appropriate physical activity intervention strategies for weight loss and prevention of weight regain for adults" recommends that long-term weight loss is best accomplished if individuals perform 200 to 300 minutes of moderate intensity physical activity per week (67). For exercise science professionals developing an exercise program for a client to meet this goal it is beneficial to have a reference of physical activity energy expenditure to which they can go. Furthermore, individuals who are involved in weight loss programs may experience more success if they have an understanding of how much energy is expended in different activities. Additionally, the accurate assessment of energy expenditure and physical activity can be beneficial to exercise science professionals and researchers testing the effectiveness and **efficacy** of weight loss programs.

Implications for Sport and Athletic Performance

The assessment of energy expenditure can also be useful for enhancing performance in certain sports and athletic competitions. The determination of which energy system predominates in the supply of energy to contracting muscles is

Efficacy The power or capacity to produce a desired effect.

important for understanding basic research questions involving the control of energy pathways and also for developing effective training programs. For example, the development of the muscle biopsy procedure has allowed for the accurate determination of how energy exchange occurs in skeletal muscle (14). Many exercise scientists have used muscle biopsies to study changes in muscle substrates, enzyme activities, and metabolite levels prior to, during, and following exercise. The use of the muscle biopsy procedure has facilitated a greater understanding of the enhancement of exercise performance following the use of supplemental nutritional aids (61). The classic muscle glycogen studies (1,14–16) would not have provided as much insight into the mechanisms by which altering dietary intake of carbohydrate (66) improves endurance performance without the measurement of intramuscular glycogen levels. The muscle biopsy procedure is often combined with other assessment techniques, such as blood collection and respiratory gas analysis, to help exercise science professionals gain a better understanding of energy metabolism during exercise training and competition.

Environmental Exercise

Individuals often perform physical activity and exercise in a variety of environmental conditions. Ensuring safety during exercise and optimizing athletic performance in challenging environmental conditions have been at the forefront of study in exercise physiology for many years. For example, the 1968 Olympic Games held in Mexico City brought attention to the influence of altitude on athletic performance when several records were set in the short-duration athletic events and performance in the longer distance athletic events was adversely affected. Since that time, exercise science professionals have been interested in factors affecting short- and long-duration exercise performance at altitude. Performing physical activity and exercise in hot and cold environmental temperature conditions impacts individuals in many ways and though we have considerable knowledge about the impact of these conditions on human responses, many individuals still suffer injuries during exercise in these environmental conditions.

Implications for Physical Activity and Exercise

Our body's core temperature (~37°C) is closely regulated within a few degrees of values that can lead to severe injury and death from being too hot or too cold. Heat-related health problems experienced by individuals include heat syncope, heat cramps, heat exhaustion, and heat stroke (8). Figure 3.13 shows the factors that affect an individual's response to exercise in the heat (8). When an individual performs physical activity or exercise in hot and/or humid conditions, there is an increased activity in the systems of the body that control temperature regulation. The main response is the cardiovascular system's increase in blood flow to the skin, which results in an increase in sweating. If fluids are not replaced, the increased sweat loss can lead to dehydration. When an individual becomes dehydrated, there is a reduction in physical work capacity and exercise performance, a faster time to physical exhaustion, and an increase in heat storage in the body (8,9,29), the latter of which increases the risk for heat-related health problems. Individuals who are physically unfit or who do not follow the guidelines for fluid

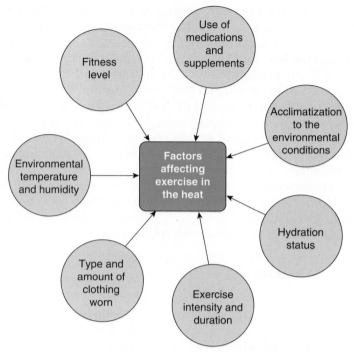

FIGURE 3.13 ▼ The factors that affect an individual's response to exercise in the heat (8)

replacement are at an increase risk of developing heat-related problems during physical activity or exercise in hot and/or humid conditions. Guidelines for athlete safety and the reduction of heat-related illness have been developed by a number of professional organizations including the ACSM (8,10,93) and the National Athletic Trainers Association (26) and are shown in Table 3.8. These guidelines and additional information can be found at the Web sites of the ACSM (www.acsm.org) and the National Athletic Trainers Association (www.nata.org).

Implications for Sport and Athletic Performance

Maintaining appropriate hydration status is critical for reducing the risk of heat-related injury and optimizing athletic performance (93). Factors such as environmental conditions, gender, age, and diet affect sweat and electrolyte losses during exercise, and therefore individual fluid replacement patterns should be developed. Athletes, coaches, and exercise science professionals should ensure that fluid replacement practice include prehydration to begin physical activity euhydrated; consuming fluids during exercise to prevent excessive dehydration; and replacing fluids and electrolytes after the completion of exercise. It is very important to match fluid and electrolyte intake with water loss to prevent dehydration. Conversely, overdrinking can lead to symptomatic exercise–associated **hyponatremia,** a condition that can lead to severe medical complications (93).

Table 3.8	Guidelines for Participant Safety and Reduction of Heat-related Illness (8,26)
Avoid the scheduling of athletic events and practices in extremely hot weather as much as possible	
Make sure athletes are gradually acclimatized to hot and humid environmental conditions	
Monitor athletes for signs and symptoms of heat strain	
Monitor athletes for adequate fluid replacement during and after training and competition	

Physical Activity and Exercise in Cold Environmental Conditions

Physical activity and exercise in cold environmental conditions can lead to decreases in performance and an increased risk of **hypothermia** (27). There are several factors that interact during physical activity and exercise in the cold that could potentially increase the physiologic strain and injury risk beyond that associated with similar levels of activity conducted under more temperate conditions (Figure 3.14) (27).

Heat is lost from the body through four processes: **conduction**, **convection**, **radiation**, and **evaporation** (89). The two most critical environmental factors interacting with the environmental temperature to promote heat loss in cold conditions are wind and water. The wind chill index indicates how fast heat would be lost at different wind speeds and temperatures (89). Water has a thermal conductivity that is about 25 times greater than air at the same temperature (64), so more heat is lost from the body through water than air. There are several measures that can be taken to minimize the effects of cold environmental conditions on physical activity and exercise performance and reduce the risk of cold injury. The physiologic responses to acclimatization to cold weather are very modest and depend on the severity of the exposures to the cold (27,109). To best prevent hypothermia, it is important to assess the level of cold by monitoring the environmental temperature, wind, and solar impact, as well as the rain immersion depth and altitude if applicable (27). The risk of performing physical activity or exercise in the cold is then assessed by analyzing what is to be performed and the clothing available to wear. It is also important to identify those individuals such as children and the aged who are at higher risk of hypothermia. The physical activity and exercise intensity and duration, experience, physical condition, general health, and nutritional status of the individual should also be considered to determine if an elevated risk of cold injury exists (27). Appropriate risk management can help

Hyponatremia An abnormally low concentration of sodium in the blood.
Hypothermia Abnormally low body temperature.
Conduction The process of heat loss through direct transfer to a cooler object.
Convection The process of heat loss to the air surrounding the body.
Radiation The process of heat loss through the air to solid cooler objects.
Evaporation The process of heat loss through sweat evaporating from the skin surface.

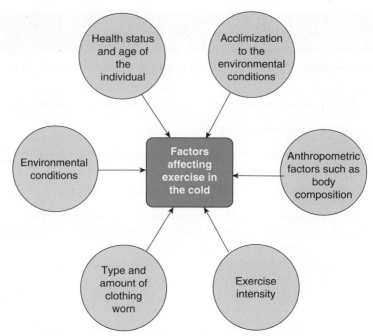

FIGURE 3.14 ▼ Factors affecting exercise in the cold (27).

prevent cold injuries such as frostbite and hypothermia from occurring during physical activity and exercise in the cold (27). Exercise science professionals work to ensure that physical activity, exercise, sports, and athletic competitions can be performed safely in cold environmental conditions.

OTHER AREAS OF STUDY

The discipline of exercise physiology encompasses several areas of study not mentioned in this chapter. For example, strength and conditional professionals are interested in the various responses of the body to different training and conditioning methods, such as periodization, high-intensity training, plyometrics, and concurrent strength and endurance training. Exercise science professionals are also interested in the hormonal regulation of metabolism, the measurement of work, power, and exercise efficiency, and the role of the cardiovascular and respiratory systems in promoting improvements in fitness. Exercise specialists and personal trainers work to develop exercise prescriptions for health and fitness in healthy and diseased individuals as well as special populations such as children, females, the aged, and the disabled. Exercise science professionals are interested in how genetic mechanisms control responses to exercise as well as regulate both aerobic capacity and physical activity levels. The interaction of nutrition and body composition on health and performance has also been studied extensively by exercise science professionals but there is still much to be learned in these areas.

> ### ➤ *Thinking Critically*
> *How might coursework in exercise science prepare an individual for a career as an exercise physiologist, exercise specialist, or strength and conditioning coach?*

I N T E R V I E W

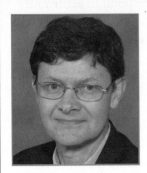

L. Bruce Gladden, PhD, FACSM, Professor of Exercise
Physiology in the Department of Kinesiology at Auburn University

Brief Introduction

I attended the University of Tennessee, Knoxville as an undergraduate, receiving a BS degree in zoology with a minor in chemistry. At the end of my undergraduate career, I planned to attend graduate school in physiology at another university. However, I participated in a research project in Dr Hugh Welch's Exercise Physiology Laboratory during the summer after graduation. After a few twists and turns, I entered the PhD program with Dr Welch as my supervisor.

➤ Why did you choose to become involved in your work as an exercise physiologist?

I became very excited about exercise physiology when I took my first class in exercise physiology during the last term of my senior year as an undergraduate.

➤ Which individuals or experiences were most influential in your career development?

My first exercise physiology class really got me excited. It was taught by Dr Hugh Welch, who ultimately became my advisor in graduate school. After completing my PhD work, I was a postdoctoral fellow for two years in Dr Wendell Stainsby's lab at the University of Florida. Hugh Welch taught me to calibrate, calibrate, calibrate! His emphasis was on being certain that your data were valid, accurate, and precise. Wendell Stainsby taught me the muscle preparation that I have used so much in my research career and emphasized that physiology is fun! Wendell's enthusiasm for research was contagious.

➤ What are your top two or three professional accomplishments?

In general, I am proud of my small contribution to the area of lactate metabolism. Specifically, my lab used an isolated muscle preparation in situ to demonstrate that skeletal muscle not only produces and releases lactate, but it also takes up and consumes lactate on a net basis. Contracting skeletal muscles avidly consume lactate when they are in a metabolic steady state. I suppose as a result of my work in the area, I was asked to write a chapter on lactate metabolism for the *American Physiological Society's Handbook of Physiology* (Section 12, Exercise). That was a great thrill for me. As a result of that chapter, and the support of Dr George Brooks, I was subsequently asked to write a topical review on lactate metabolism for the *Journal of Physiology*. That topical review has been among the top ten electronically accessed articles online for the *Journal of Physiology* for every month except one since it was first published in June of 2004.

➤ What advice would you have for a student exploring a career in exercise science?

My advice to undergraduate students who are interested in exercise science (specifically, exercise physiology) is to remember the "physiology" part of the subject area. Exercise physiologists are physiologists who specialize in the study of exercise. Accordingly, successful students will acquire a strong foundation in the basic sciences (particularly biology and chemistry). I have always wished that I had taken even more of those basic science courses during my undergraduate career.

SUMMARY

- Exercise physiology is the study of how the systems of the body respond to acute and chronic physical activity and exercise.
- Physical activity and exercise can elicit both subtle and profound challenges to the body's systems.
- Whether responding to an acute challenge or chronic exposure, the systems of the body respond in an attempt to return the body to homeostasis and ready the body for the next challenge.
- Exercise physiology uses a variety of approaches to answer questions and provide recommendations for improving health through physical activity and exercise.
- Areas of study in exercise physiology provide safe and effective training methods to enhance performance in sport and athletic competition.

FOR REVIEW

1. How was the Harvard Fatigue Laboratory important in the development of exercise physiology as a scientific discipline?

2. During the beginning of exercise, what are some of the acute responses of the cardiovascular, pulmonary, muscular, and endocrine systems of the body?

3. How does a regular exercise program result in chronic adaptations to the cardiovascular, pulmonary, muscular, and endocrine systems of the body?

4. What are some factors that control energy utilization during exercise?

5. Why should athletes participating in long-duration exercise be concerned about ingesting carbohydrates prior to and during exercise?

6. How do insulin and the Glut 4 transport proteins work to increase glucose uptake by the muscle cells?

7. What is the primary factor affecting glucose uptake in an individual with Type 2 diabetes?

8. What benefits does an older adult obtain from participation in a resistance training program?

9. What are the significant health implications of the female athlete triad?

10. List some of those diseases that have an increased risk of occurrence in an obese individual.

11. What are the recommendations for protein intake for an endurance athlete and a strength athlete?

(Continued)

12. What are the most commonly used ways to assess physical activity in large populations?

13. List five factors that affect an individual's response to exercise in the heat.

14. Explain why the wind chill index is an important factor in the regulation of body temperature in a cold environment.

REFERENCES

1. Ahlborg B, Bergstrom J, Ekelund LG, Hultman E. Muscle glycogen and muscle electrolytes during prolonged physical exercise. *Acta Physiol Scand.* 1967;70:129–42.
2. Ainsworth BE, Haskell WL, Whitt MC, et al. Compendium of physical activities: An update of activity codes and MET intensities. *Med Sci Sports Exerc.* 2000;32:S498–516.
3. Allison DB, Zannolli R, Venkat Narayan KM. The direct health care costs of obesity in the United States. *Am J Public Health.* 1999;89:1194–9.
4. Allor KM, Pivarnik JM. Stability and convergent validity of three physical activity assessments. *Med Sci Sports Exerc.* 2001;33:671–6.
5. American College of Sports Medicine. Osteoporosis and exercise. *Med Sci Sports Exerc.* 1995;27:i–vii.
6. American College of Sports Medicine. Exercise and type 2 diabetes. *Med Sci Sports Exerc.* 2000; 32(7): 1345–60.
7. American Diabetes Association and American College of Sports Medicine. Diabetes mellitus and exercise. *Med Sci Sports Exerc.* 2000;29:i–vi.
8. Armstrong LE, Casa DJ, Millard-Stafford ML, et al. Exertional heat illness during training and competition. *Med Sci Sports Exerc.* 2007;39:556–72.
9. Armstrong LE, Costill DL, Fink WJ. Influence of diuretic-induced dehydration on competitive running performance. *Med Sci Sports Exerc.* 1985;17:456–61.
10. Armstrong LE, Epstein Y, Greenleaf JE, et al. Heat and cold illness during distance running. *Med Sci Sports Exerc.* 1996;28:i–x.
11. Ashley FW, Kannel WB. Relation of weight change to changes in atherogenic traits: The Framingham Study. *J Chronic Dis.* 1974;27:103–14.
12. Barnard RJ, Roberts CK, Varon SM, Berger JJ. Diet-induced insulin resistance precedes other aspects of the metabolic syndrome. *J Appl Physiol.* 1998;84:1311–5.
13. Beneke R. Anaerobic threshold, individual anaerobic threshold, and maximal lactate steady state in rowing. *Med Sci Sports Exerc.* 1995;27:863–7.
14. Bergstrom J. Muscle electrolytes in man. Determination by neutron activation analysis on needle biopsy specimens. A study on normal subjects, kidney patients and patients with chronic diarrhoea. *Scand J Clin Lab Investig.* 1962;14:1–110.
15. Bergstrom J, Hermansen L, Hultman E, Saltin B. Diet, muscle glycogen and physical performance. *Acta Physiol Scand.* 1967;71:140–50.
16. Bergstrom J, Hultman E. Muscle glycogen synthesis after exercise: An enhancing factor localized to the muscle cells in man. *Nature.* 1966;210:309–11.
17. Berryman JW. Ancient and early influences. In: Tipton CM, editor. *Exercise Physiology: People and Ideas.* New York (NY): Oxford University Press; 2003. p. 1–38.
18. Biolo G, Maggi SP, Williams BD, Tipton KD, Wolfe RR. Increased rates of muscle protein turnover and amino acid transport after resistance exercise in humans. *Am J Physiol.* 1995;268:E514–20.
19. Brooks GA, Fahey TD, White TP, Baldwin KM. *Exercise Physiology: Human Bioenergetics and Its Applications.* Mountain View (CA): Mayfield; 2000.
20. Brooks GA, Mercier J. Balance of carbohydrate and lipid utilization during exercise: The "crossover" concept. *J Appl Physiol.* 1994;76:2253–61.
21. Brown AB, McCartney N, Sale DG. Positive adaptations to weight-lifting training in the elderly. *J Appl Physiol.* 1990;69:1725–33.
22. Burr DB, Robling AG, Turner CH. Effects of biomechanical stress on bones in animals. *Bone.* 2002;30:781–6.
23. Buskirk ER. From Harvard to Minnesota: Keys to our history. In: Holloszy JO, editor. *Exercise and Sport Sciences Reviews.* Baltimore (MD): Williams & Wilkins; 1992. p. 1–26.
24. Buskirk ER, Tipton CM. Exercise Physiology. In: Massengale JD, Swanson RA, editors. *The History of Exercise and Sport Science.* Champaign (IL): Human Kinetics; 2003. p. 367–438.
25. Cann CE, Martin MC, Genant HK, Jaffe RB. Decreased spinal mineral content in amenorrheic women. *JAMA.* 1984;251:626–9.
26. Casa DJ, Armstrong LE, Hillman S. National Athletic Trainer's Association position statement: Fluid replacement for athletes. *J Athl Train.* 2007; 35:212.
27. Castellani JW, Young AJ, Ducharme MB, et al. Prevention of cold injuries during exercise. *Med Sci Sports Exerc.* 2006;38:2012–29.

28. Chapman CB. The long reach of Harvard's Fatigue Laboratory, 1926–1947. *Perspect Biol Med.* 1990;34:17–33.

29. Cheuvront SN, Carter RC, Sawka MN. Fluid balance and endurance exercise performance. *Curr Sports Med Rep.* 2003;2:202–8.

30. Chow R, Harrison JE, Notarius C. Effect of two randomized exercise programmes on bone mass of healthy post-menopausal women. *Br Med J.* 1987;295:1441–4.

31. Coggan AR, Coyle EF. Carbohydrate ingestion during prolonged exercise: Effects on metabolism and performance. In: Holloszy JO, editor. *Exercise and Sport Sciences Reviews.* Philadelphia (PA): Williams & Wilkins; 1991. p. 1–40.

32. Cortright RN, Dohm GL. Mechanisms by which insulin and muscle contraction stimulate glucose transport. *Can J Appl Physiol.* 1997;22:519–30.

33. Costill DL, Fink WJ, Pollock ML. Muscle fiber composition and enzyme activities of elite distance runners. *Med Sci Sports.* 1976;8:96–102.

34. Coyle EF. Substrate utilization during exercise in active people. *Am J Clin Nutr.* 1995;61:968S–79S.

35. Coyle EF, Coggan AR, Hopper MK, Walters TJ. Determinants of endurance in well-trained cyclists. *J Appl Physiol.* 1988;64:2622–30.

36. Coyle EF, Feltner ME, Kautz SA, et al. Physiological and biomechanical factors associated with endurance cycling performance. *Med Sci Sports Exerc.* 1991;23: 93–107.

37. Dalsky GP, Stocke KS, Ehsani AA, Slatopolsky E, Lee WC, Birge SJ. Weight-bearing exercise training and lumbar BMC in postmenopausal women. *Ann Intern Med.* 1988;108:824–8.

38. Després JP, Couillard C, Gagnon J, et al. Race, visceral adipose tissue, plasma lipids, and lipoprotein lipase activity in men and women: The health, risk factors, exercise training, and genetics (HERITAGE) family study. *Arterioscler Thromb Vasc Biol.* 2000;20:1932–8.

39. Després JP, Moorjani S, Lupien PJ, Tremblay A, Nadeau A, Bouchard C. Regional distribution of body fat, plasma lipoproteins, and cardiovascular disease. *Arteriosclerosis.* 1990;10:497–511.

40. Dietz WH. Does energy expenditure affect changes in body fat in children. *Am J Clin Nutr.* 1998;67:190–1.

41. Edstrom L, Ekblom B. Differences in sizes of red and white muscle fibers in vastus lateralis of musculus quadriceps of normal individuals and athletes: Relation to physical performance. *Scand J Clin Lab Investig.* 1972;30:175.

42. Engel TJ, Crosby RD, Kolotkin RL, et al. Impact of weight loss and regain on quality of life: Mirror image or differential effect? *Obes Res.* 2003;11:1207–13.

43. Fiatarone MA, Marks EC, Ryan ND, Meredith CN, Lipsitz LA, Evans WJ. High-intensity strength training in nonagenarians. *JAMA.* 1990;263:3029–34.

44. Finkelstein EA, Fiebelkorn IC, Wang G. State-level estimates of annual medical expenditures attributable to obesity. *Obes Res.* 2004;12:18–24.

45. Flegal KM, Carroll MD, Kuczmarski RJ, Johnson CL. Overweight and obesity in the United States: Prevalence and trends, 1960–1994. *Int J Obes.* 1998;22:39–47.

46. Flegal KM, Carroll MD, Ogden CL, Johnson CL. Prevalence and trends in obesity among US adults, 1999–2000. *JAMA.* 2003;288:1723–7.

47. Flegal KM, Graubard BI, Williamson DF, Gail MH. Excess deaths associated with underweight, overweight, and obesity. *JAMA.* 2005;293:1861–7.

48. Foxdal P, Sjodin B, Sjodin A, Ostman B. The validity and accuracy of blood lactate measurements for the prediction of maximal endurance capacity. *Int J Sports Med.* 1994;15:89–95.

49. Garfinkel L. Overweight and mortality. *Cancer.* 1986;58:1826–9.

50. Giovannucci E, Ascherio A, Rimm EB, Colditz GA, Stampfer MJ, Willett WC. Physical activity, obesity, and risk for colon cancer and adenoma in men. *Ann Intern Med.* 1995;122:327–34.

51. Goldstein DJ. Beneficial health effects of modest weight loss. *Int J Obes.* 1992;16:397–415.

52. Gollnick PD. Metabolism of substrates: Energy substrate metabolism during exercise and as modified by training. *Fed Proc.* 1983;44:353–7.

53. Gollnick PD, Saltin B. Fuel for muscular exercise: Role of fat. In: Horton ES, Terjung RL, editors. *Exercise, Nutrition and Energy Metabolism.* New York (NY): MacMillan; 1988. p. 72–88.

54. Gropper SS, Smith JL, Groff JL. *Advanced Nutrition and Human Metabolism.* Belmont (CA): Wadsworth; 2004.

55. Guyton AC, Hall JE. *Textbook of Medical Physiology.* Oxford (UK): Elsevier; 2006.

56. Haffner SM, Mitchell BD, Hazuda HP, Stern MP. Greater influence of central distribution of adipose tissue on incidence of non-insulin-dependent diabetes in women than men. *Am J Clin Nutr.* 1991;53:1312–7.

57. Hargreaves M. Metabolic responses to carbohydrate and lipid supplementation during exercise. In: Maughan RJ, Shirreffs SM, editors. *Biochemistry of Exercise IX.* Champaign (IL): Human Kinetics; 1996. p. 421–9.

58. Harris RT. Bulimarexia. *Ann Intern Med.* 1983;99: 800–7.

59. Haskell WL. Assessment of physical activity. *Med Sci Sports Exerc.* 1993;25:60–70.

60. Haskell WL, Phillips WT. Exercise training, fitness, health, and longevity. In: Lamb DL, Gisolfi CV, editors. *Perspectives in Exercise Science and Sports Medicine: Exercise in Older Adults.* Carmel (IN): Cooper Publishing Group; 1995. p. 11–52.

61. Haub MD, Potteiger JA, Jacobsen DJ, Nau KL, Magee LM, Comeau MJ. Glycogen replenishment and repeated short duration high intensity exercise: Effect of carbohydrate ingestion. *Int J Sport Nutr Exerc Metab.* 1998;9:406–15.

62. Herzog DB, Copeland PM. Eating disorders. *N Engl J Med.* 1985;313:295–303.

63. Hill JO. Genetic and environmental contributions to obesity. *Am J Clin Nutr.* 1998;68:991–2.

64. Horvath SM. Exercise in a cold environment. In: Miller DI, editor. *Exercise and Sport Sciences Review.* Salt Lake City: Franklin Institute; 1981. p. 221–63.

65. Horvath SM, Horvath EC. *The Harvard Fatigue Laboratory: Its History and Contributions.* Englewood Cliffs (NJ): Prentice-Hall; 1973.

66. Ivy JL, Katz A, Cutler CL, Sherman WM, Coyle EF. Muscle glycogen synthesis after exercise: Effect of time of carbohydrate ingestion. *J Appl Physiol.* 1988;64:1480–5.

67. Jakicic JM, Clark KL, Coleman E, et al. Appropriate intervention strategies for weight loss and prevention of weight regain for adults. *Med Sci Sports Exerc.* 2001;33:2145–56.

68. Katzmarzyk PT, Gagnon J, Leon AS, et al. Fitness, fatness, and estimated coronary heart disease risk: The HERITAGE family study. *Med Sci Sports Exerc.* 2001;33:585–90.

69. Kelso TB, Hodgson DR, Visscher AR, Gollnick PD. Some properties of different skeletal muscle fiber types: comparison of reference bases. *J Appl Physiol.* 1987;62:1436–41.

70. Kemmer FW, Berger M. Exercise and diabetes mellitus: Physical activity as a part of daily life and its role in the treatment of diabetic patient. *Int J Sport Med.* 1983;4:77–88.

71. Kohrt WM, Bloomfield SA, Little KD, Nelson ME, Yingling VR, American College of Sports Medicine. Physical activity and bone health. *Med Sci Sports Exerc.* 2004;36:1985–96.

72. Kraemer WJ, Patton JF, Gordon SE, Harman EA, Deschenes MR, Reynolds K, Newton RU. Compatibility of high-intensity strength and endurance training on hormonal and skeletal muscle adaptations. *J Appl Physiol.* 1995;78:976–89.

73. Kroll WP. *Graduate Study and Research in Physical Education.* Champaign (IL): Human Kinetics; 1982.

74. Lamb DR. Basic principles for improving sport performance. *Sports Sci Exch.* 1995;8:1–5.

75. Lanyon LE, Rubin CT, Baust G. Modulation of bone loss during calcium insufficiency by controlled dynamic loading. *Calcif Tissue Int.* 1986;38:209–16.

76. Lemon PWR. Do athletes need more dietary protein and amino acids? *Int J Sport Nutr.* 1995;5:S39–61.

77. Lemon PWR. Effects of exercise on dietary protein requirements. *Int J Sport Nutr.* 1998;8:426–47.

78. Lemon PWR. Beyond the zone: protein needs of active individuals. *J Am Coll Nutr.* 2000;19: 513S–21S.

79. Lew EA, Garfinkel L. Variations in mortality by weight among 750,000 men and women. *J Clin Epidemiol.* 1979;32:563–76.

80. McCall GE, Byrnes WC, Dickinson A, Pattany PM, Fleck SJ. Muscle fiber hypertrophy, hyperplasia, and capillary density in college men after resistance training. *J Appl Physiol.* 1996;81:2004–12.

81. Melby CL, Ho RC, Hill JO. Assessment of human energy expenditure. In: Bouchard C, editor. *Physical Activity and Obesity.* Champaign (IL): Human Kinetics; 2000. p. 103–31.

82. Miller SL, Tipton KD, Chinkes DL, Wolf SE, Wolfe RR. Independent and combined effects of amino acids and glucose after resistance exercise. *Med Sci Sports Exerc.* 2003;35:449–55.

83. National Institutes of Health and National Heart, Lung and Blood Institute. Clinical guidelines on the identification, evaluation, and treatment of overweight and obesity: The evidence report. Washington (DC): US Government Press; 1998.

84. Nattiv A, Loucks AB, Manore MM, Sanborn CF, Sundgot-Borgen J, Warren MP. The female athlete triad. *Med Sci Sports Exerc.* 2007;29:i–x.

85. Park RJ. The rise and demise of Harvard's B.S. program in anatomy, physiology, and physical training: A case of conflicts of interest and scare resources. *Res Q Exerc Sport.* 1992;63:246–60.

86. Phillips SM, Tipton KD, Aarsland A, Wolf SE, Wolfe RR. Mixed muscle protein synthesis and breakdown after resistance exercise in humans. *Am J Physiol.* 1997;273:E99–107.

87. Potteiger JA. Aerobic endurance training. In: Baechle TR, Earle RW, editors. *Essentials of Strength Training and Conditioning.* Champaign (IL): Human Kinetics; 2000. p. 495–509.

88. Potteiger JA, Webster MJ, Nickel GL, Haub MD, Palmer RJ. The effects of buffer ingestion on metabolic factors related to distance running performance. *Eur J Appl Physiol.* 1996;72:365–71.

89. Powers SK, Howley ET. *Exercise Physiology: Theory and Application to Fitness and Performance.* Dubuque (IA): Brown & Benchmark; 2007.

90. Rhea MR, Alvar BA, Burkett LN, Ball SD. A meta-analysis to determine the dose response for strength development. *Med Sci Sports Exerc.* 2003;35:456–65.

91. Richter ER, Galbo H. Diabetes, insulin, and exercise. *Sports Med.* 1986;3:275–88.

92. Rose AJ, Richter EA. Skeletal muscle glucose uptake during exercise: How is it regulated? *Physiology.* 2005;20:260–70.

93. Sawka MN, Burke LM, Eichner ER, et al. Exercise and fluid replacement. *Med Sci Sports Exerc.* 2007;39:377–90.

94. Sherman WM. Carbohydrate feedings before and after exercise. In: Lamb DL, Williams MR, editors. *Perspectives in Exercise Science and Sports Medicine.* New York (NY): McGraw-Hill Companies; 1991.

95. Starkey DB, Pollock ML, Ishida Y, et al. Effect of resistance training volume on strength and muscle thickness. *Med Sci Sports Exerc.* 1996;28:1311–20.

96. Tesch PA, Karlsson J. Muscle fiber types and size in trained and untrained muscles of elite athletes. *J Appl Physiol.* 1985;59:1716–20.

97. Tipton CM. Exercise physiology, part II: A contemporary historical perspective. In: Massengale JD, Swanson RA, editors. *The History of Exercise and Sport Science.* Champaign (IL): Human Kinetics; 1997. p. 396–438.

98. Tipton CM. Contemporary Exercise physiology: Fifty years after the closure of the Harvard Fatigue Laboratory. In: Holloszy JO, editor. *Exercise and Sport Science Reviews.* Baltimore (MD): Williams & Wilkins; 1998. p. 315–39.

99. Tipton KD, Wolfe RR. Exercise-induced changes in protein metabolism. *Acta Physiol Scand.* 1998;162:377–87.

100. U.S. Department of Health and Human Services, Centers for Disease Control and Prevention and National Center for Chronic Disease Prevention and Health Promotion. Physical activity and health: A report of the Surgeon General; 1999. Atlanta, GA.

101. van Baak MA, Borghouts LB. Relationships with physical activity. *Nutr Rev.* 2000;58:S16–8.

102. Wells CL, Pate RR. Training for performance of prolonged exercise. In: Lamb DL, Murray R, editors. *Perspectives in Exercise Science and Sports Medicine.* Indianapolis: Benchmark Press, Inc.; 1995. p. 357–88.

103. Westerblad H, Allen DG, Lannergren J. Muscle fatigue: Lactic acid or inorganic phosphate the major cause? *News Physiol Sci.* 2002;17:17–21.

104. Wilson GJ, Newton RU, Murphy AJ, Humphries BJ. The optimal training load for the development of dynamic athletic performance. *Med Sci Sports Exerc.* 1993;25:1279–86.

105. Wing RR. Physical activity in the treatment of the adulthood overweight and obesity: Current evidence and research issues. *Med Sci Sports Exerc.* 1999;31:S547–52.

106. Wolfe RR. Protein supplements and exercise. *Am J Clin Nutr.* 2000;72:551S–7S.

107. World Health Organization. *Globalization and Health: Proceedings of a Conference at the Nuffield Trust,* 2005 May 19–20: London. 2006;14:4–13.

108. Wright DA, Sherman WM, Dernbach AR. Carbohydrate feedings before, during or in combination improve cycling endurance performance. *J Appl Physiol.* 1991;71:1082–8.

109. Young AJ. Homeostatic responses to prolonged cold exposure: Human cold acclimatization. In: Fregly MJ, Blatteis CM, editors. *Handbook of Physiology: Environmental Physiology.* Bethesda (MD): American Physiological Society; 1996. p. 419–38.

110. Zaman G, Cheng MZ, Jessop HL, White R, Lanyon LE. Mechanical strain activates estrogen response elements in bone cells. *Bone.* 2000;27:233–9.

Clinical Exercise Physiology

After completing this chapter you will be able to:

1. Describe the historical development of clinical exercise physiology.
2. Explain the duties and responsibilities of a clinical exercise physiologist.
3. List the physiologic data collected during a graded exercise test.
4. Describe the components of health-related physical fitness testing.
5. Identify the primary cardiovascular, respiratory, metabolic, and neuromuscular diseases.

Physical activity and exercise play an essential role in the prevention of, treatment of, and recovery from a variety of disease conditions and physical disabilities. Clinical exercise physiology involves the use of physical activity and exercise to prevent or delay the onset of chronic disease in healthy individuals or provide **therapeutic** or **functional** benefits to individuals with disease conditions or physical disabilities. Individuals trained in exercise science and possessing certification to work in clinical environments are called clinical exercise physiologists. Assisting other healthcare specialists in diagnostic and functional capacity testing; prescribing individual exercise based on needs, desires, and abilities; and instructing, supervising, and monitoring exercise programs in clinical settings are the primary responsibilities of clinical exercise physiologists (25). Employment as a clinical exercise physiologist can occur in a variety of medical settings such as hospitals, rehabilitation centers, outpatient clinics, weight management clinics, in community, corporate, commercial, and university fitness and wellness centers, nursing homes, and retirement communities. The range of practice includes apparently healthy individuals with no known medical problems and individuals with diagnosed cardiovascular, pulmonary, metabolic, rheumatologic, orthopedic, and/or neuromuscular diseases and conditions (25).

Clinical exercise physiologists must have a solid educational background in exercise physiology, including the understanding of how the body responds to acute and chronic physical activity and exercise in both a healthy and diseased condition. Advanced knowledge of the **pathophysiology** of chronic diseases, pharmacology of drugs and medicines, medical terminology, medical record keeping and charting, electrocardiographic interpretation, exercise testing for special populations, and nutrition is also valuable to the clinical exercise physiologist. Undergraduate students interested in clinical exercise physiology should complete a clinical internship, which allows work with patients in a medical setting, interactions with a variety of healthcare professionals, and opportunities to prescribe and monitor exercise in a variety of locations (25). Individuals desiring to become clinical exercise physiologists should obtain a certification from a professional organization such as the ACSM (see Chapter 11).

HISTORY OF CLINICAL EXERCISE PHYSIOLOGY

Although clinical exercise physiology is relatively new as a defined body of knowledge, individuals have been interested in how physical activity and exercise influence health and recovery from illness and diseases since the time of the early Greeks (11). Early historic events in medicine, physiology, and exercise that helped define many of the disciplines in exercise science have also influenced the development of clinical exercise physiology. Many of those important historic events are described in Chapters 1 and 3. The material contained in this section should be considered a supplement to these chapters and will contain only information specific to the development of clinical exercise physiology.

Early Influences

The use of physical activity and exercise in cardiovascular disease recovery can be traced to the eighteenth and nineteenth centuries (43). William Heberden

(1710–1801) was the first to describe the condition of **angina pectoris** (chest pain) during physical exertion (21) and the use of physical activity with patients who experienced angina pectoris (22). Heberden and William Stokes (1804–78) are credited with being the first physicians to recommend the use of physical activity and exercise to promote the recovery from heart disease (41,43). Unfortunately, prior to the middle of the twentieth century, there was little written about the role of physical activity and exercise in the prevention of chronic disease development or in the recovery process from diseases conditions (25).

Recent Influences

One of the most significant events in the development of clinical exercise physiology was a renowned study of coronary heart disease in London bus drivers and conductors performed by Jeremy N. Morris and his colleagues and published in 1953 (33). This study is considered the first to demonstrate the relationship between physical activity and the reduced risk of developing heart disease and it helped initiate interest in disease risk reduction and public health epidemiology. The foundation for **cardiac rehabilitation** began to take shape in the 1950s with the major focus on the restoration of functional capacity after a cardiovascular event. Around this time, Samuel A. Levine and Bernard Lown were the first to recommend armchair exercises for patients with heart disease (30) and H. K. Hellerstein provided a step-by-step plan for the rehabilitation of the cardiac patients (23). Although the use of physical activity and exercise in heart disease patients was not common prior to 1960 (19), the work of Hellerstein, Levine, Lown, and Morris and colleagues created a foundation for using physical activity and exercise to promote the prevention of and recovery from various diseases. Throughout the 1960s and 1970s, experiments in both animals and humans led to using physical activity and exercise in the recovery process for patients with acute heart attacks (19). For example, several prospective studies supported the use of a structured physical activity and exercise program for reducing morbidity and mortality and improving the various clinical, medical, and psychological factors in patients with heart disease (14,28). The development of cardiac rehabilitation programs advanced significantly during the 1970s when professional organizations such as the American Heart Association and the American College of Sports Medicine released textbooks addressing the proper procedures for the testing and training of healthy and diseased individuals (5–7). These books were very popular and remain in wide use today.

The use of physical activity and exercise to promote recovery in patients with pulmonary disease is credited to Alvin L. Barach (43). Considered by many

---

Therapeutic Of or relating to the treatment of disease or disorders by remedial agents or methods.

Functional Performing or being able to perform a regular function.

Pathophysiology Functional changes that accompany a disease condition.

Angina pectoris Severe chest pain caused by an insufficient supply of blood to the heart.

Cardiac rehabilitation A medically supervised program to help heart patients recover quickly and improve their overall physical and mental functioning.

experts to be the "Father of modern day pulmonology," Barach used a variety of procedures and strategies to improve the conditions of individuals with congestive heart failure, pneumonia, and other pulmonary disorders (10). Beginning in 1958, William F. Miller and Thomas Petty published a series of papers promoting the use of physical activity and exercise for treating individuals with chronic pulmonary disorders including airway obstruction and emphysema (31,32,36). The development of **pulmonary rehabilitation** as an appropriate part of the treatment for diseased individuals was further advanced when, in 1981, the American Thoracic Society released a statement supporting pulmonary rehabilitation as a necessary procedure for enhancing functional status in pulmonary patients (9,43).

In 1974, the *Journal of Cardiac Rehabilitation* began publication, providing practitioners access to a scientific, peer-reviewed journal devoted to the dissemination of information vital to the rehabilitation of individuals with various forms of heart disease (43). In 1986, the content of the journal was expanded to include pulmonary rehabilitation and the journal was renamed the *Journal of Cardiopulmonary Rehabilitation* (43). The development of a professional association for practicing cardiopulmonary rehabilitation specialists occurred in 1985, when the American Association of Cardiovascular and Pulmonary Rehabilitation (AACVPR) was established (43). The mission of the AACVPR is to reduce morbidity, mortality, and disability from cardiovascular and pulmonary diseases through education, prevention, rehabilitation, research, and aggressive disease management (43). The knowledge base in cardiac and pulmonary rehabilitation was expanded through research and the publication of guidelines and position statements by the AACVPR. Table 4.1 lists some important publications that helped further the development of cardiopulmonary rehabilitation. The AACVPR further enhanced the profession of cardiopulmonary rehabilitation with the establishment of certification for cardiac and pulmonary rehabilitation programs in 1996 (43).

The development of individual certification programs by a number of other professional organizations has led to further professional growth of cardiopulmonary rehabilitation. Major professional organizations such as the ACSM and the National Strength and Conditioning Association offer professional certifications to individuals

Table 4.1	Important Publications in Cardiopulmonary Rehabilitation	
PUBLICATION		**DATE**
Guidelines for Cardiac Rehabilitation and Secondary Prevention Programs, 4th Edition (2)		2004
Guidelines for Pulmonary Rehabilitation Programs, 3rd Edition (3)		2004
Clinical Competency Guidelines for Pulmonary Rehabilitation Professionals (40)		1995
Outcome Measurement in Cardiac Rehabilitation (16)		2002
Pulmonary Rehabilitation: Joint ACCP/AACVPR Evidence-Based Clinical Practice Guidelines (37)		2007

desiring to work with healthy and diseased populations. Additional information about certification and licensure opportunities can be found in Chapter 11.

The endorsement of the health benefits obtained from physical activity and exercise by the United States Surgeon General in 1996 was a significant milestone in the promotion of physical activity and exercise for healthy and diseased individuals. The Surgeon General's report highlighted the positive health effects of physical activity and exercise on the musculoskeletal, cardiovascular, respiratory, and endocrine systems including a reduced risk of premature mortality and reduced risks of coronary heart disease, hypertension, colon cancer, and diabetes mellitus. Recommendations for the appropriate amount of physical activity and exercise helped establish the standards for using exercise to assist in the treatment of diseased individuals (35).

> ➤ *Thinking Critically*
>
> *In what ways could the historic development of cardiopulmonary rehabilitation and the 1996 Surgeon General's report be used to promote participation in physical activity and exercise for the prevention and treatment of disease conditions?*

Throughout the 1990s and early into the twenty first century, government agencies such as the Department of Health and Human Services and the Centers for Disease Control and Prevention established health promotion programs designed to reduce the risk of disease development in healthy individuals and improve the health of those with disease conditions. The National Institutes of Health and other professional organizations such as the American Heart Association and the American Diabetes Association continue to promote research activities and public health programs designed to improve health and reduce disease risk. As we move further into the twenty first century, additional education and health promotion programs will be instrumental in promoting the use of physical activity and exercise for ensurin g good health

> ➤ *Thinking Critically*
>
> *In what ways does the professional organization, AACVPR, contribute to the development of clinical exercise physiology as both a profession and a discipline?*

and promoting recovery from disease conditions. Table 4.2 provides a list of the significant events in the historic development of clinical exercise physiology.

DUTIES AND RESPONSIBILITIES

Clinical exercise physiologists take part in a number of significant duties and responsibilities to evaluate the health status of and prescribe physical activity and exercise to both healthy individuals and individuals with disease conditions. The primary duties of clinical exercise physiologists include conducting pre-exercise screening, performing exercise testing and evaluation, developing exercise prescriptions, instructing individuals in proper training techniques, and supervising safe and effective exercise programs in various healthcare, community, and employment settings. Clinical exercise physiologists must understand the normal physiologic responses of the body to acute and chronic physical activity and

Pulmonary rehabilitation A medically supervised program to help patients with chronic respiratory disease stabilize or reverse systemic manifestations.

Table 4.2	Significant Events in the Historic Development of Clinical Exercise Physiology
DATE	**HISTORIC EVENT**
1802	Heberden describes using physical exertion to treat angina pectoris
1854	Stokes recommends using physical activity and exercise during the recovery from heart disease
1948	Barach promotes the use of physical activity and exercise to promote recovery in individuals with pulmonary disease
1952	Levine and Lown recommend armchair exercises for patients with heart disease
1953	Morris demonstrates a relationship between physical activity and a reduced risk of developing heart disease
1957	Hellerstein and Ford outline a plan for rehabilitation of cardiac patients
1958	Miller and Petty publish a series of papers promoting the use of physical activity and exercise for treating individuals with chronic pulmonary disorders
1972 and 1975	American Heart Association and the American College of Sports Medicine release textbooks addressing the proper testing and training of healthy and diseased individuals
1974	Publication of the *Journal of Cardiac Rehabilitation*
1985	American Association of Cardiovascular and Pulmonary Rehabilitation is established
1996	Surgeon General's report highlights the positive health effects that physical activity has on the physiologic systems and the reduction of chronic disease risk

exercise to maximize the use of physical activity and exercise for the prevention, management, or rehabilitation of disease. It is also important to understand how different diseases and the medical management of the disease conditions affect the physiologic responses during rest and exercise (25).

Exercise Testing and Evaluation

Exercise testing is an important component of clinical exercise physiology as it is used to clear individuals for safe participation in physical activity and exercise and as a basis for developing an exercise prescription. Diagnostic testing and functional capacity testing are the two broad classifications of exercise testing and evaluation.

Diagnostic testing is commonly used to assess the presence of cardiovascular or pulmonary disease. Figure 4.1 illustrates the type of diagnostic exercise testing performed by clinical exercise physiologists. If an individual has symptoms of

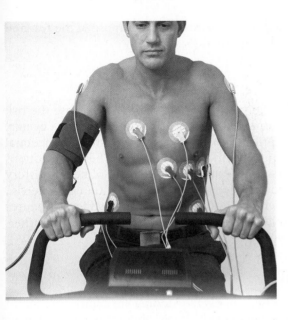

FIGURE 4.1 ▼ A diagnostic exercise test.

heart or lung disease, a history of a possible abnormal cardiac incident, abnormal electric activity of the heart, or a high probability of an underlying disease condition, then diagnostic testing is performed. Exercise tests also help diagnose the presence of heart disease, primarily on the basis of abnormal changes during the test. During exercise, the demands placed on the heart allow abnormal responses and disease conditions to become more readily apparent. Although the clinical exercise physiologist plays an important role in administering the test, only a medical doctor can provide a medical diagnosis of disease (5).

Functional capacity testing provides information about an individual's capacity to participate in physical activity and exercise. The information obtained from testing can be used to prescribe an appropriate physical activity and exercise program to improve fitness. Functional capacity is usually determined by a submaximal or maximal exercise test that progressively increases in intensity. Functional capacity testing may also be used to determine if an individual has normal cardiovascular and pulmonary responses to physical activity and exercise (5).

Both diagnostic and functional capacity testing are used to evaluate the cardiopulmonary response to a standard exercise workload. Diagnostic and functional capacity tests use workloads that are incremental and are referred to as graded exercise tests (GXT). During a GXT the intensity progresses in stages from light to maximal exertion or to a previously determined ending point. There are general guidelines to be followed when performing a GXT, which is typically conducted on a treadmill or a cycle ergometer. Several standard exercise protocols are

Diagnostic testing Used to determine a specific disease condition or possible illness.
Functional capacity testing Used to provide an objective measure of an individual's safe functional abilities.

available for use and the protocol selected depends on the purpose of the test and the characteristics of the individual being tested (5).

Pretesting Procedures

Physical activity and exercise stress the systems of the body and increase the risk of musculoskeletal injury and abnormal cardiovascular and pulmonary events. Certain precautions must be taken prior to conducting a diagnostic or functional capacity GXT to reduce the risk of injury or an abnormal event. These precautions include pretesting screening, a physical examination, collection of health history information, and obtaining individual informed consent (5). Clinical exercise physiologists are instrumental in performing some of the pretesting procedures including pretest screening for health risk, collection of health history information, and acquiring informed consent.

Pretest Screening for Health Risk

Determining if physical activity, exercise, and exercise testing are appropriate for an individual is very important. For most healthy individuals, physical activity and exercise do not pose a safety risk if proper exercise techniques and principles are observed. However, physical activity and exercise may not be safe for everyone, especially if a preexisting medical condition such as cardiovascular, pulmonary, or metabolic disease exists. Some individuals may not be able to participate in exercise testing for specific medical reasons. A list of contraindications can be found in the *ACSM's Guidelines for Exercise Testing and Prescription Manual* (5). The level of risk for an individual participating in physical activity and exercise must be determined before administering a diagnostic or functional capacity test and the start of an exercise program.

Physical Examination

Certain individuals who are physically inactive and have multiple risk factors for disease require a physician's referral before they can undergo exercise testing or begin an exercise program. In this situation, the physical examination is designed to assess the risk of an abnormal event while participating in exercise or exercise testing. The *ACSM's Guidelines for Exercise Testing and Prescription Manual* can be used to assist clinical exercise physiologists and healthcare professionals in determining the safety of exercise for individuals (5).

Health History

The assessment of an individual's personal health history and risk factors for cardiovascular disease is an important component of the pretesting screening phase of exercise testing and prescription. The assessment of individual health history is designed to

- identify individuals with **medical contraindications** to exercise
- identify individuals with clinically significant disease conditions who should be referred to a medically supervised exercise program

- identify individuals with symptoms and risk factors for a disease who should receive further medical evaluation before starting an exercise program
- identify individuals with special needs for safe exercise participation (e.g., elderly, pregnant women) (5)

A number of instruments are available for recording and evaluating an individual's health history. The American Heart Association/ACSM Health/Fitness Preparticipation Screening Questionnaire and the Physical Activity Readiness Questionnaire are examples of instruments that can be used in the pretesting screening phase of exercise testing and prescription. Questionnaires should be designed to collect health history information about the individual and his or her family. Figure 4.2 shows an example of a comprehensive health history questionnaire (5).

Informed Consent

Informed consent is a process whereby the individual participating in the exercise test is made aware of and understands the purposes, risks, and benefits associated with the test or exercise program. A signed informed consent should be obtained from an individual prior to diagnostic or functional capacity testing. All of the procedures involved in the exercise test and the potential risks and benefits should be thoroughly explained before any testing is done. During the collection of informed consent, participants should be encouraged to ask questions to clarify and resolve uncertainties about the testing procedures. Figure 4.3 shows an example of a comprehensive informed consent document (5).

Performing the Test

After the collection and evaluation of the health history information and the informed consent, the GXT can begin if the individual being tested meets the accepted level of health and disease risk for participation in exercise testing. Figure 4.4 provides a chart that can be used to identify those individuals who can participate in submaximal or maximal GXT and whether a physician needs to be present during testing. During the GXT, physiologic measures such as resting and exercise heart rate and blood pressure are collected. Additional measures collected often include the **rating of perceived exertion** (RPE), electric activity of the heart using an **electrocardiograph** (ECG), oxygen consumption (VO_2) to determine **maximal oxygen consumption** (VO_{2max}), and physical work capacity. A GXT can be either submaximal or maximal depending on the prescreening information and whether the test is for diagnostic or functional capacity assessment (5).

Medical contraindication A condition which makes a particular treatment or procedure inadvisable.

Rating of perceived exertion A subjective assessment of how hard an individual feels he/she is working.

Electrocardiograph An instrument that measures electric potentials on the body surface and generates a record of the electric currents associated with heart muscle activity.

Maximal oxygen consumption The maximal amount of oxygen used by the body during maximal effort exercise.

Assess your health status by marking all *true* statements

History
You have had:
_____ a heart attack
_____ heart surgery
_____ cardiac catheterization
_____ coronary angioplasty (PTCA)
_____ pacemaker/implantable cardiac
_____ defibrillator/rhythm disturbance
_____ heart valve disease
_____ heart failure
_____ heart transplantation
_____ congenital heart disease

Symptoms
_____ You experience chest discomfort with exertion.
_____ You experience unreasonable breathlessness.
_____ You experience dizziness, fainting, or blackouts.
_____ You take heart medications.

*If you marked any of these statements in this section, consult your physician or other appropriate health care provider before engaging in exercise. You may need to use a facility with a **medically qualified staff.***

Other health issues
_____ You have diabetes.
_____ You have asthma or other lung disease.
_____ You have burning or cramping sensation in your lower legs when walking short distances.
_____ You have musculoskeletal problems that limit your physical activity.
_____ You have concerns about the safety of exercise.
_____ You take prescription medication(s).
_____ You are pregnant.

Cardiovascular risk factors
_____ You are a man older than 45 years.
_____ You are a woman older than 55 years, have had a hysterectomy, or are postmenopausal.
_____ You smoke, or quit smoking within the previous 6 months.
_____ Your blood pressure is >140/90 mm Hg.
_____ You do not know your blood pressure.
_____ You take blood pressure medication.
_____ Your blood cholesterol level is >200 mg/dL.
_____ You do not know your cholesterol level.
_____ You have a close blood relative who had a heart attack or heart surgery before age 55 (father or brother) or age 65 (mother or sister).
_____ You are physically inactive (i.e., you get <30 minutes of physical activity on at least 3 days per week).
_____ You are >20 pounds overweight.

*If you marked two or more of the statements in this section you should consult your physician or other appropriate health care provider before engaging in exercise. You might benefit from using a facility with a **professionally qualified exercise staff**[†] to guide your exercise program.*

_____ None of the above

You should be able to exercise safely without consulting your physician or other appropriate health care provider in a self-guided program or almost any facility that meets your exercise program needs.

*Modified from American College of Sports Medicine and American Heart Association. ACSM/AHA Joint Position Statement: Recommendations for cardiovascular screening, staffing, and emergency policies at health/fitness facilities. *Med Sci Sports Exerc.* 1998:1018.

[†]Professionally qualified exercise staff refers to appropriately trained individuals who possess academic training, practical and clinical knowledge, skills, and abilities commensurate with the credentials defined in Appendix F.

FIGURE 4.2 ▼ Comprehensive health history questionnaire (5). (From *ACSM's Guidelines for Exercise Testing and Prescription.* 8th ed. Philadelphia (PA): Lippincott, Williams & Wilkins; 2009.)

Informed Consent for an Exercise Test

1. **Purpose and Explanation of the Test**

   You will perform an exercise test on a cycle ergometer or a motor-driven treadmill. The exercise intensity will begin at a low level and will be advanced in stages depending on your fitness level. We may stop the test at any time because of signs of fatigue or changes in your heart rate, ECG, or blood pressure, or symptoms you may experience. It is important for you to realize that you may stop when you wish because of feelings of fatigue or any other discomfort.

2. **Attendant Risks and Discomforts**

   There exists the possibility of certain changes occurring during the test. These include abnormal blood pressure, fainting irregular, fast or slow heart rhythm, and in rare instances, heart attack, stroke, or death. Every effort will be made to minimize these risks by evaluation of preliminary information relating to your health and fitness and by careful observations during testing. Emergency equipment and trained personnel are available to deal with unusual situations that may arise.

3. **Responsibilities of the Participant**

   Information you possess about your health status or previous experiences of heart-related symptoms (e.g. shortness of breath with low-level activity, pain, pressure, tightness, heaviness in the chest, neck, jaw, back, and/or arms) with physical effort may affect the safety of your exercise test. Your prompt reporting of these and any other unusual feelings with effort during the exercise test itself is very important. You are responsible for fully disclosing your medical history, as well as symptoms that may occur during the test. You are also expected to report all medications (including nonprescription) taken recently and, in particular, those taken today, to the testing staff.

4. **Benefits to Be Expected**

   The results obtained from the exercise test may assist in the diagnosis of your illness, in evaluating the effect of your medications or in evaluating what type of physical activities you might do with low risk.

5. **Inquiries**

   Any questions about the procedures used in the exercise test or the results of your test are encouraged. If you have any concerns or questions, please ask us for further explanations.

6. **Use of Medical records**

   The information that is obtained during exercise testing will be treated as privileged and confidential as described in the Health Insurance Portability and Accountability Act of 1996. It is not to be released or revealed to any person except your referring physician without your written consent. However, the information obtained may be used for statistical analysis or scientific purposes with your right to privacy retained.

7. **Freedom of Consent**

   I hereby consent to voluntarily engage in an exercise test to determine my exercise capacity and state of cardiovascular health. My permission to perform this exercise test is given voluntarily. I understand the I am free to stop the test at any point if I so desire. I have read this form, and I understand the test procedures that I will perform and the attendant risks and discomforts. Knowing these risks and discomforts, and having had an opportunity to ask questions that have been answered to my satisfaction, I consent to participate in this test.

_____   _____
Date   Signature of Patient

_____   _____
Date   Signature of Witness

_____   _____
Date   Signature of Physician or Authorized Delegate

FIGURE 4.3 ▼ A comprehensive informed consent document. (From *ACSM's Guidelines for Exercise Testing and Prescription*. 8th ed. Philadelphia (PA): Lippincott, Williams & Wilkins; 2009.)

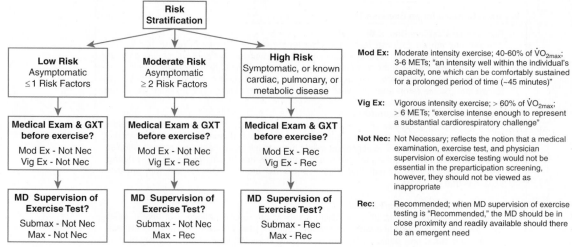

FIGURE 4.4 ▼ Exercise testing and testing supervision recommendations based on risk factor stratification. (From *ACSM's Guidelines for Exercise Testing and Prescription*. 8th ed. Philadelphia (PA): Lippincott, Williams & Wilkins; 2009.)

Heart Rate

Resting heart rate is usually measured after the individual has been sitting quietly for 5 minutes or longer. An electronic heart rate monitor is often used to obtain heart rate in healthy individuals. In all clinical settings, however, the heart rate is determined from the ECG recordings or directly off the digital display of the **oscilloscope**. Many factors can influence the resting and exercise heart rate including smoking, caffeine ingestion, fever, high humidity, stress, food digestion, certain medications, and prior physical activity or exercise. That is why pretesting instructions to individuals often prohibit the use of caffeine, food consumption, or activity prior to exercise testing. During exercise, the heart rate is recorded periodically to ensure an appropriate cardiovascular response to exercise and for later use in developing an exercise prescription (5).

Blood Pressure

Blood pressure is measured after a period of quiet sitting and often at the same time as the resting heart rate. Blood pressure is the force exerting pressure against the walls of the blood vessels in the circulatory system. The highest pressure recorded during a **cardiac cycle** (one heart beat to the next heart beat) occurs during the contraction phase (systole) of the left ventricle and is called the systolic blood pressure. A measurement of systolic blood pressure provides an estimation of the work of the heart, as well as the pressure exerted against the walls of the blood vessels. The period between heart beats is called the relaxation phase of the heart (diastole) and the pressure recorded during this period is called the diastolic blood pressure. During diastole, the blood pressure is decreased and this measurement gives an indirect indication of the ease with which blood flows through the circulatory system (5).

Blood pressure is an important indicator of overall health. When resting blood pressure is chronically elevated, a disease condition called hypertension

Table 4.3	Categories of Normal and Elevated Blood Pressure	
BLOOD PRESSURE CLASSIFICATION	SYSTOLIC BLOOD PRESSURE (mm Hg)	DIASTOLIC BLOOD PRESSURE (mm Hg)
Normal	<120	And <80
Prehypertension	120–139	Or 80–89
Stage 1 hypertension	140–159	90–99
Stage 2 hypertension	≥160	Or ≥100

exists. Individuals with hypertension have an increased risk of stroke and cardiovascular disease (27). In clinical exercise settings, blood pressure can be measured manually or by an automated analyzer. The manual method uses a sphygmomanometer (blood pressure cuff) and a stethoscope and is often performed by a clinical exercise physiologist. The automated analyzer eliminates much of the individual variability associated with the manual method assessment. Table 4.3 provides the categories and values of normal and elevated blood pressure (27).

Physical activity and exercise cause an increase in blood pressure. A GXT is used to evaluate the blood pressure response to increasing workloads and to help identify any abnormal responses that may occur. During testing, blood pressure is normally measured every 1 to 3 minutes. Systolic blood pressure can increase to approximately 200 mm Hg in healthy, fit men and women during maximal exercise. Diastolic pressure should remain the same or decrease slightly during a GXT. Abnormal blood pressure responses typically indicate a problem with the cardiovascular system (5).

Rating of Perceived Exertion

During a GXT, an assessment of the psychological perception of the intensity of exercise is often made. The Borg RPE scale is commonly used to assess the subjective level of difficulty the individual is experiencing during exercise (13). This RPE scale provides a moderately accurate measure of how the individual feels in relation to the level of physical exertion. The RPE scale also allows the technician conducting the test to know when the individual being tested is nearing exhaustion. Figure 4.5 illustrates the Borg 14 point RPE scale. The 6–20 point numerical RPE scale relates closely to the heart rates from rest to maximal exercise when multiplied by a factor of 10 (60 to 200 beats · min^{-1}). A revised RPE scale attempts to provide a category-ratio scale of the RPE values (ranging from 0 to 11) that are anchored with the terms "nothing at all" and "absolute maximum" (12). An additional perceived exertion scale called the Omni scale has been developed that uses pictures to help individuals identify the level of difficulty associated with exercise (38,39).

Oscilloscope An electronic instrument that produces an instantaneous trace on the screen that corresponds to oscillations of voltage and current.
Cardiac cycle A complete beat of the heart, including systole and diastole and the intervals between.

Category Scale	Category-Ratio Scale†	
6	0 Nothing at all	"No I"
7 Very, very light	0.3	
8	0.5 Extremely weak	Just noticeable
9 Very light	0.7	
10	1 Very weak	
11 Fairly light	1.5	
12	2 Weak	Light
13 Somewhat hard	2.5	
14	3 Moderate	
15 Hard	4	
16	5 Strong	Heavy
17 Very Hard	6	
18	7 Very strong	
19 Very, very hard	8	
20	9	
	10 Extremely strong	"Strongest I"
	11	
	• Absolute maximum	Highest possible

* Copyright Gunnar Borg. Reproduced with permission. For correct usage of the Borg scales, it is necessary to follow the administration and instructions given in Borg G. Borg's Perceived Exertion and Pain Scales. Champaign, IL: Human Kinetics, 1998.

†Note: ON the Category-Ratio Scale, "I" represents intensity.

FIGURE 4.5 ▼ Borg 14 point RPE Scale (12). (From *ACSM's Guidelines for Exercise Testing and Prescription*. 7th ed. Baltimore (MD): Lippincott, Williams & Wilkins; 2006.)

An added benefit to collecting the RPE is that the information can be used in the development of an exercise prescription, because individuals can easily learn to exercise at a particular RPE that corresponds to a given exercise intensity (5).

Electrocardiogram

The electrical activity of the heart is usually recorded using an ECG during a diagnostic test. This information helps in the overall evaluation of health and disease status. The electrical activity of the heart can be recorded from electrodes placed on the surface of the chest. The ECG is a valuable component of the exercise test because of its use in determining the presence of cardiovascular disease. The diagnosis of these conditions is made easier during exercise because many of these problems do not become apparent until the heart is required to beat faster and generate more force than when at rest (5). Some of the more common cardiovascular abnormalities include ST segment depression and atrial and ventricular arrhythmia. Figure 4.6 illustrates the assessments made during a GXT.

Echocardiography

The functional condition and disease status of the heart can also be assessed using **echocardiography**. An echocardiogram is an instrument that uses sound waves

Echocardiography The use of sound waves to create a moving picture of the heart.

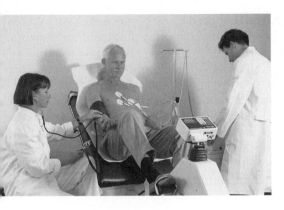

FIGURE 4.6 ▼ Assessments made during a GXT.

to create a moving picture of the heart that is much more detailed than an X-ray image, and it involves no radiation exposure. An echocardiogram allows health-care professionals to see the beating heart and to visualize many of the structures of the heart. Occasionally, a body structure such as the lungs or ribs may prevent the sound waves and echoes from providing a clear picture of heart function. In this instance, a small amount of contrast material (i.e., dye) may be injected into a vein to provide a clearer picture of the inside of the heart. An echocardiogram can also be combined with a GXT (called a stress echocardiogram). This type of test allows healthcare professionals to learn how the heart functions when it is made to work harder. The echocardiogram combined with the GXT is especially useful in diagnosing coronary artery disease (18).

Oxygen Consumption and Functional Capacity

Functional capacity testing measures the degree to which a person can increase physical activity and exercise intensity and maintain this increased level. It is related to the ability of the body to change carbohydrates, fats, and proteins into energy for exercise. An individual's functional capacity is strongly influenced by the health and fitness level of the cardiovascular, respiratory, and muscular systems. The measurement of VO_{2max} is the best assessment of cardiovascular fitness and a good measure of overall physical fitness. The VO_{2max} is defined as the maximal rate at which oxygen can be taken up, distributed, and used by the body during exer-cise that involves a large muscle mass (26). During a maximal GXT, the workload is gradually increased until the individual being tested can no longer exercise. The oxygen consumption measured at this point is considered the VO_{2max}. Specific test criteria have been established to ensure that a true maximal level of exercise and oxygen consumption has been achieved by individuals during the GXT (26).

Submaximal Graded Exercise Tests

A submaximal GXT can be used to evaluate the cardiovascular, respiratory, and muscular systems' responses to a standard submaximal exercise bout. The submaxi-mal GXT is conducted to an intensity that elicits between 70% and 85% of the age-predicted maximal heart rate. Information obtained during this test can be used to calculate an estimate of an individual's maximal fitness level. Cardiovascular fitness can be estimated from equations that predict VO_{2max} from the last workload achieved during the test, from the oxygen consumption requirement for horizontal and graded walking on a treadmill, or from the individual's heart rate response to a series of submaximal workloads (typically used during a cycle ergometer test). Heart rate and blood pressure are normally recorded at each stage of the test, with an ECG tracing obtained, if necessary. Abnormal responses in heart rate, blood pressure, or the ECG indicate a cessation of testing and referral for further medical evaluation. A submaximal test is usually easier to administer, less costly, and safer than a maximal GXT because the individual is not required to exercise to maximal effort. In some exercise settings, an estimate of VO_{2max} is sufficient for approving exercise participation and in developing an individualized exercise prescription (5).

Maximal Graded Exercise Testing

A maximal GXT is often employed when a direct assessment of cardiovascular, respiratory, and muscular function is needed. A maximal GXT does not stop at a predetermined workload (e.g., 70% to 85% of age-predicted maximum) but is continued to the point of exhaustion or to the point at which abnormal physiologic responses occur. If the test is diagnostic in nature, it may be conducted until abnormal responses in blood pressure and/or ECG activity as well as chest pain (angina pectoris), shortness of breath (**dyspnea**), or lightheadedness are observed. This type of test is often called a symptom-limited stress test. It is often important to be able to take individuals to maximal effort exercise because many abnormal signs and symptoms of disease do not occur until the exercise workload is at a high intensity. The major concern associated with a maximal GXT is the level of physical stress placed on the participants, especially those who are not physically active, as this may increase the risk for an abnormal cardiovascular event (5).

> ➤ **Thinking Critically**
> *Why is it important for a clinical exercise physiologist to collect information on heart rate, blood pressure, perceived exertion, and ECG activity during a graded exercise test in both healthy and diseased individuals?*

Health-Related Physical Fitness Testing and Interpretation

The assessment of health-related physical fitness is a common and appropriate practice in preventive and rehabilitative physical activity and exercise programs. Health-related physical fitness testing can

- provide information to individuals about their current health-related fitness relative to standards and age- and gender-matched norms
- provide information that is helpful in developing exercise prescriptions
- allow the evaluation of progress by individuals in an exercise program
- enhance motivation by establishing fitness goals
- identify the level of risk for certain cardiovascular diseases (5)

Dyspnea A feeling of difficult or labored breathing.
Normative data Data generated that allows comparison of an individual to a group.

Table 4.4	Assessments Used to Determine Health-Related Physical Fitness (5)	
HEALTH-RELATED PHYSICAL FITNESS COMPONENT	**EXAMPLES OF ASSESSMENT**	
Body composition	Body mass index, waist and hip circumference measurements, skinfold measurements, bioelectric impedance	
Cardiovascular-respiratory fitness	Maximal and submaximal GXT using treadmill, cycle ergometer, or box stepping	
Muscular strength	One repetition maximum in the bench press or leg press	
Muscular endurance	Maximum number of repetitions performed with a set amount of weight in the bench press or leg press	
Flexibility	Sit and reach test	

Information obtained during health-related physical fitness testing can be combined with an individual's health and medical information to assess the level of risk for certain disease conditions and to develop appropriate exercise prescriptions. The tests selected should provide results that are indicative of the current state of physical fitness, sensitive enough to reflect changes from physical activity or exercise, and be directly comparable to **normative data** so that the level of fitness can be determined. Table 4.4 provides examples of assessments used to determine health-related physical fitness (5).

Exercise Prescription

Increased levels of physical activity and regular exercise are useful for improving health and reducing the level of risk for a variety of disease conditions. After the completion of testing, clinical exercise physiologists play an important role in developing an exercise prescription specific for the individual. An exercise prescription is a plan for physical activity and exercise developed to achieve specific outcomes such as improvement in fitness, reduction in cardiovascular disease risk, or weight loss. For individuals with diagnosed disease, the exercise prescription should be individualized to optimize the probability of safe and effective exercise. Advances in basic and applied exercise physiology and clinical exercise physiology have led to a better understanding of the process of prescribing physical activity and exercise to healthy individuals and those with chronic diseases. Formulating a prescription that meets the interests, goals, health needs, and clinical condition of an individual must be based on sound principles and innovative programming. Exercise prescriptions should specify the type

> ▶ *Thinking Critically*
> *What information should be used by a clinical exercise physiologist when developing a safe and effective exercise program for promoting health and reducing the risk of chronic disease conditions in a middle-aged adult?*

of activity and the intensity, duration, and frequency of training. The results of the exercise testing, clinical evaluations, and individual goals should be used to develop the exercise program (5).

SPECIFIC DISEASE CONDITIONS

Clinical exercise physiologists design physical activity and exercise programs to improve health, prevent complications associated with disease conditions, compensate for loss of anatomic or physiologic function, and optimize functional capacity (25). Increased levels of physical activity and exercise are appropriate intervention strategies to achieve these goals because nearly 70% of disabling conditions limit mobility and function by interfering with the function of the cardiovascular, pulmonary, and musculoskeletal systems. Therefore, clinical exercise physiologists must have a comprehensive knowledge of the physiology of exercise and its application in the clinical environment. Clinical exercise physiologists must also be familiar with the drugs commonly used in the pharmacologic treatment of disease conditions (29). Treatment interventions for many health conditions include medical surgery, pharmacologic interventions, dietary alterations and therapy, lifestyle modifications (e.g., stress reduction), weight loss, and exercise. Most disease conditions can be classified into the following groups: cardiovascular disease, respiratory disease, metabolic disease, and neuromuscular disease (25). The following sections will provide a short overview of disease conditions and how clinical exercise physiologists can use exercise to improve health and reduce disease risk.

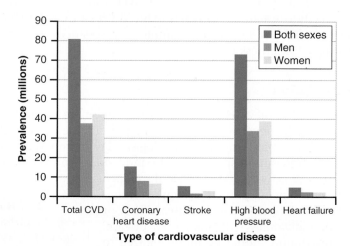

FIGURE 4.7 ▼ Prevalence of cardiovascular diseases in 2005 in the United States (8).

Ischemia A decrease in the blood supply to a bodily organ, tissue, or part caused by constriction or obstruction of the blood vessels.

Cardiovascular Disease

Cardiovascular disease is the leading cause of death in the United States and contributes to considerable morbidity (17). Figure 4.7 shows the prevalence of cardiovascular diseases for the year 2005 in the United States (8). For many of the cardiovascular disease conditions, increased levels of physical activity and exercise can play a beneficial role in restoring normal physical and physiologic function. Table 4.5 illustrates the potential benefits of exercise for the primary cardiovascular disease conditions.

Myocardial Infarction

A myocardial infarction, also commonly referred to as a heart attack, occurs when an area of heart muscle is deprived of oxygen. The cause is usually due to a blockage of a diseased coronary artery that results in a decreased blood flow (called **ischemia**) to an area of the heart supplied by those blood vessels (Figure 4.8). A myocardial infarction is typically accompanied by chest pain (angina pectoris) radiating down one or both arms. There is usually damage to

Table 4.5	Potential Benefits of Exercise for Cardiovascular Disease Conditions (4)
DISEASE CONDITION	**PRIMARY BENEFITS OF EXERCISE**
Myocardial infarction	Increased VO_{2max}; reduction in heart rate, blood pressure, and myocardial oxygen requirements; improvements in blood lipid profile; improved well-being and self-efficacy; protection against triggers of a myocardial infarction
Coronary artery disease	Increased VO_{2max}; reduction in heart rate, blood pressure, and myocardial oxygen requirements; improvements in blood lipid profile; improved well-being and self-efficacy; protection against triggers of a myocardial infarction
Angina pectoris	Reduction in myocardial oxygen demand
Cardiac arrhythmia	Reduction in heart rate at rest and submaximal workloads
Valvular heart disease	Improved working capacity of skeletal muscle improves ability to perform activities of daily living
Chronic heart failure	Improved in skeletal muscle metabolism and distribution of blood to the tissues of the body
Peripheral vascular disease	Increased limb blood flow; better redistribution of blood flow; improvement of muscle function
Hypertension	Reduction in the rise of blood pressure over time; reduction in resting systolic and diastolic blood pressure

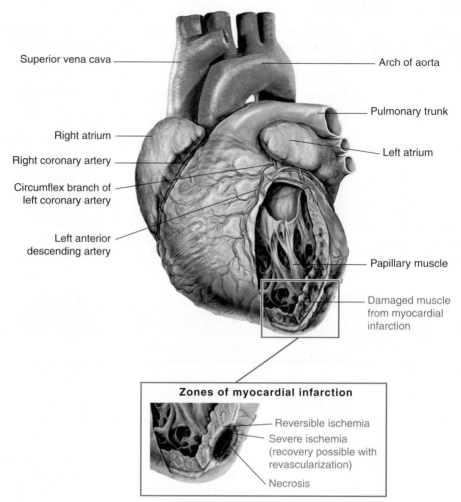

Superior vena cava

Arch of aorta

Pulmonary trunk

Right atrium

Left atrium

Right coronary artery

Circumflex branch of
left coronary artery

Left anterior
descending artery

Papillary muscle

Damaged muscle
from myocardial
infarction

Zones of myocardial infarction

Reversible ischemia
Severe ischemia
(recovery possible with
revascularization)
Necrosis

FIGURE 4.8 ▼ Myocardial ischemia and infarction. (Asset provided by Anatomical
Chart Co.)

the cardiac muscle, the severity of which varies with the extent and location of
the damage (4).

Coronary Artery Disease

Coronary artery disease involves a localized accumulation of fibrous tissue and, to
a lesser extent, lipid matter within the coronary artery. The resultant narrowing of
the opening of the vessel is often referred to as coronary **atherosclerosis**. This condition reduces the blood flow through the coronary arteries to the cardiac muscle.
The reduced blood flow usually results in ventricular dysfunction, angina pectoris,
and frequently a myocardial infarction. Coronary artery disease becomes clinically
significant when approximately 75% of the blood vessel is obstructed (4).

Angina Pectoris

Angina pectoris is a feeling of pain or discomfort in the chest that originates behind the sternum and radiates to the shoulders, arms, neck, or jaw. Some individuals experience shortness of breath, nausea, or excessive sweating (called **diaphoresis**). These symptoms usually last for 10 to 20 seconds at a time but can occur for as long as 30 minutes or longer. Angina pectoris is usually a response to reduced blood flow to cardiac muscle, brought about by coronary artery disease. There are two types of ischemia: symptomatic and silent. Symptomatic ischemia results in the development of the symptoms described above. Silent ischemia is a reduced blood flow without any accompanying symptoms (4).

Cardiac Arrhythmia

In the heart, nervous tissue in the right atrium is responsible for initiating contraction of the heart muscle and for setting the heart rate. In a normal healthy heart, the rhythm and rate are set to meet the demands of the body for blood and oxygen. An arrhythmia is when the normal rate and rhythm are affected. For example, an abnormal heart rhythm called atrial fibrillation is characterized by chaotic, rapid, and irregular electric activity of the atria. Atrial fibrillation is a common **arrhythmia** and it occurs more frequently with advancing age. The irregular contractions result in a reduced filling of the ventricles with blood and a decreased delivery of blood to the tissues of the body (4).

Valvular Heart Disease

The anatomic structure of the heart is designed so that one-way valves of fibrous tissue separate the ventricles (lower chambers) from the atria (upper chambers). These valves allow for coordinated and regulated blood flow through the heart and to the tissues of the body. Valvular heart disease can result from rheumatic fever, congenital abnormalities, infection, and aging. Valvular heart disease can result in a significant reduction of **cardiac output** leading to health complications, thereby affecting the ability to perform physical activity and exercise. The symptoms, limitations, and recommendations for physical activity and exercise in an individual with valvular heart disease depend on the heart valve which is affected, the condition of the valve, and the presence of any other disease condition (4).

Chronic Heart Failure

Chronic heart failure is characterized by the inability of the heart to deliver adequate amounts of blood to the tissues of the body. Chronic heart failure results in a depressed systolic function, depressed diastolic function, or a combination of

---

Atherosclerosis A condition characterized by a reduced opening in the blood vessels.

Diaphoresis A condition of excessive sweating.

Arrhythmia Irregular electric activity of the heart.

Cardiac output The volume of blood ejected from the ventricles of the heart in minute.

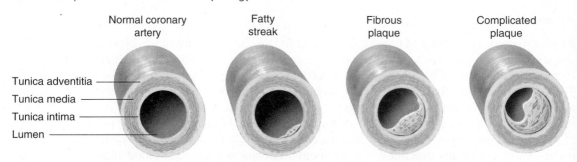

Tunica adventitia
Tunica media
Tunica intima
Lumen

FIGURE 4.9 ▼ Progression of peripheral artery disease. (Asset provided by Anatomical Chart Co.)

both. Depressed systolic function occurs when the heart loses muscle (usually due to a myocardial infarction) or there is a reduction in the contractile force generated by the cardiac muscle. Depressed diastolic function is characterized by an increased resistance to filling of the ventricles. Chronic heart failure is associated with changes to other tissues including alterations in skeletal muscle metabolism, impaired **vasodilation** of blood vessels, and an inability of the kidneys to remove waste products from the body (called **renal insufficiency**) (4).

Peripheral Vascular Disease

Peripheral vascular disease can affect the arteries, the veins, or the lymph vessels of the body tissues outside the heart. The most common and important type of peripheral vascular disease is peripheral artery disease, which is a condition similar to coronary artery disease. In peripheral artery disease, fatty deposits build up in the inner linings of the artery walls resulting in a blockage and restriction of blood flow, mainly in arteries leading to the kidneys, stomach, arms, legs, and feet (Figure 4.9). Peripheral vascular disease becomes more common with aging. Individuals with peripheral vascular disease have a four to five times higher risk of heart attack or stroke (4).

Hypertension

Hypertension is an abnormally high level of blood pressure. The high blood pressure results from an increased amount of blood pumped by the heart or from an increased resistance to the flow of blood through the arterial blood vessels of the body. Hypertension is generally defined as a blood pressure reading greater than 140 (systolic) over 90 (diastolic) mm Hg. Blood pressures of 120 to 139 (systolic) over 80 to 89 (diastolic) mm Hg are now considered prehypertensive and should create greater awareness for allied healthcare professionals (27). In primary or essential hypertension, the cause of the condition is unknown. When the cause of the hypertension is known, (e.g., a disorder of the adrenal glands, kidneys, or

Vasodilation The dilation of a blood vessel.

Renal insufficiency An inability of the kidneys to remove waste products from the body.

Table 4.6	Potential Benefits of Exercise for Various Respiratory Disease Conditions
DISEASE CONDITION	**BENEFITS OF EXERCISE**
Obstructive pulmonary disease	Improved cardiovascular and ventilatory function; increased muscular strength and flexibility; improved body composition
Restrictive pulmonary disease	Improved cardiovascular and ventilatory function; improved oxygen extraction in the lungs
Asthma	Improved overall fitness
Cystic fibrosis	Increased work capacity; improved ventilatory function; greater mucus clearance; delayed deterioration of pulmonary function

arteries), the condition is known as secondary hypertension. Several risk factors such as heredity, obesity, smoking, and emotional stress are believed to contribute to the development of hypertension (4).

Respiratory Disease

Respiratory disease contributes to considerable morbidity and mortality in Americans. For many respiratory disease conditions, increased levels of physical activity and exercise can play a beneficial role in restoring normal air flow into and out of the lungs. Table 4.6 illustrates the potential benefits of exercise for various respiratory disease conditions.

Obstructive Pulmonary Disease

Chronic obstructive pulmonary disease (COPD) affects more than 30 million Americans and is a leading cause of death in the United States. Individuals with COPD typically have symptoms of both chronic bronchitis and emphysema (Figure 4.10). The majority of COPD is a result of tobacco abuse, although cystic fibrosis and other forms of lung diseases may also contribute to the development of COPD. Individuals with COPD are susceptible to many problems that can quickly lead to the development of other disease conditions. Ventilatory and gas exchange impairments in the lungs occur with COPD, but there can also be impairments of normal cardiovascular and muscular functions. Individuals with COPD also experience chronic anxiety and often depression that arises from the difficulty with breathing and performing physical activity and exercise (4).

Restrictive Pulmonary Disease

Restrictive lung diseases are characterized by reduced lung volume, caused by an alteration in the lung tissue or because of a disease associated with the lung tissue, chest wall, or neuromuscular breathing process. Restrictive lung diseases

Emphysema

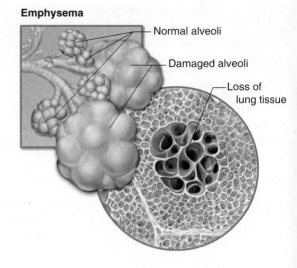

Normal alveoli

Damaged alveoli

Loss of lung tissue

FIGURE 4.10 ▼ Chronic obstructive pulmonary disease as a result of emphysema.

are distinguished by a decreased total lung capacity, vital capacity, or resting lung volume. If caused by **parenchymal lung disease**, restrictive lung disease is accompanied by reduced oxygen and carbon dioxide transfer between the lungs and the blood. The numerous disorders that cause a reduction or restriction of lung volumes may be divided into two groups based on anatomic structures. Intrinsic lung diseases (diseases of the lung tissue) cause inflammation or scarring of the lung tissue or result in filling of the air spaces with fluid and debris. Intrinsic lung diseases can be characterized according to causal factors and include lung diseases with no known cause, connective tissue diseases, drug-induced lung disease, and primary diseases of the lungs. Extrinsic lung diseases (diseases caused by factors outside of the lung) are the result of abnormal functioning of the chest wall, pleura, and respiratory muscles. Diseases of these structures result in lung restriction, impaired ventilatory function, and respiratory failure (4).

Asthma

Asthma is a lung condition characterized by reversible obstruction to airflow and increased bronchial airway responsiveness to a variety of stimuli, both **allergenic** and environmental. An acute worsening of asthma is called an asthma attack, which is characterized by shortness of breath, coughing, wheezing, and chest discomfort. Individuals with asthma experience a wide range of severity during an asthma attack, ranging from very mild, provoked by an allergen or exercise, to very severe, which is largely irreversible despite optimal medication administration.

Parenchymal lung disease A disease affecting the tissue of the lungs.

Allergenic A substance that causes an allergy.

Fibrosis The development of stiff cartilaginous tissue.

Exercise-induced asthma is characterized by brief airway obstruction that usually occurs 5 to 15 minutes after the start of exercise. The symptoms may last up to 30 minutes following the completion of exercise (4).

Cystic Fibrosis

Cystic fibrosis is an inherited disorder that causes the mucous secretions in many parts of the body to become thick and viscous. One in every 25 Whites carries the cystic fibrosis gene, and a child will be afflicted if he or she inherits the gene from both parents. The thick mucus primarily affects the respiratory and digestive systems. Mucus accumulates in the respiratory airways, creating a reduced airflow and difficulty in getting air into the lungs. Lung tissue is extremely susceptible to infection, inflammation, and eventually **fibrosis** and irreversible loss of pulmonary function. The mucus also prevents the pancreatic enzymes from reaching the digestive tract, thereby causing difficulties with digestion and absorption of the macronutrients and micronutrients. Individuals with cystic fibrosis can be treated with daily therapy that can assist in the removal of mucus from the lungs and with oral supplements to replace the pancreatic enzymes. Despite aggressive treatment programs, individuals with cystic fibrosis usually die prematurely (4).

Metabolic Disease

Various metabolic diseases contribute both directly and indirectly to considerable morbidity and mortality. Figure 4.11 shows the prevalence of the three most common metabolic disease conditions: high blood cholesterol, diabetes mellitus, and overweight and obesity (8). These disease conditions can arise from a variety of sources and treatment often includes lifestyle modification and pharmacologic interventions. Table 4.7 illustrates the potential benefits of exercise for each metabolic disease condition.

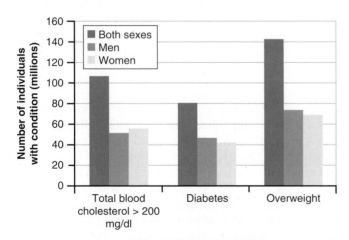

Metabolic disease condition

FIGURE 4.11 ▼ Prevalence of the three most common metabolic disease conditions: high blood cholesterol, diabetes mellitus, and overweight and obesity (8).

Table 4.7	Potential Benefits of Exercise for Various Metabolic Disease Conditions	
DISEASE CONDITION	**BENEFITS OF EXERCISE**	
Diabetes	Improved blood glucose control; improved fitness; reduction in body fat; reduction in stress	
Hyperlipidemia	Improvement in blood lipid profile	
Obesity	Reduction in body weight and percent body fat; improvement in fitness	
Metabolic syndrome	Reduction in body weight and percent body fat; improvement in fitness; improvement in blood lipid profile; improved blood glucose control	

Diabetes Mellitus

Diabetes mellitus is a condition characterized by disordered metabolism and blood glucose levels consistently above normal. There are three types of diabetes: type 1, type 2, and gestational. Type 1 diabetes mellitus is characterized by an insufficient amount of insulin produced by the beta cells of the pancreas. Type 2 diabetes is characterized by insulin resistance in tissues, but there may also be some impairment of normal beta cell function. Gestational diabetes also involves insulin resistance, as some of the hormones secreted during pregnancy can impair normal glucose metabolism. Diabetes can cause many medical complications including the acute complications of **hypoglycemia** and **ketoacidosis**. Long-term complications include an increased risk of cardiovascular disease, chronic kidney failure, retinal damage of the eye, nerve tissue damage, and damage to the small blood vessels in the body. Inadequate blood flow to tissues may result in poor wound healing, particularly in the feet, which can often lead to amputation (4).

Hyperlipidemia

Hyperlipidemia is the presence of elevated levels of lipids and/or lipoproteins in the blood. Lipids are not water soluble and therefore must be transported in the body attached to a protein capsule in the blood. The density of the lipids and the type of protein determine the fate of the lipoprotein and its influence on metabolism. Hyperlipidemia is common in the general population and arises as a result of genetic influence, smoking, excess body fat, poor dietary choices, and physical inactivity. Hyperlipidemia is a strong risk factor for cardiovascular disease because it contributes to the development of atherosclerosis and coronary artery disease. The four classifications of lipoproteins include chylomicrons, very low density lipoproteins (VLDL), low-density lipoproteins (LDL), and high-density lipoproteins (HDL). Hypertriglyceridemia is a condition of elevated triglyceride concentration, whereas hypercholesterolemia is a condition of elevated cholesterol concentration (4).

Obesity

Obesity is an excess amount of body fat that can result in a significant impairment of health and physical function. Excess body weight and fat are the result of environmental, genetic, and metabolic disorders as well as increased calorie intake and low levels of physical activity and exercise. Obesity results in a variety of altered physiologic functions including increased fasting insulin, increased insulin response to glucose, and decreased insulin sensitivity (1). Obesity is associated with high morbidity and mortality rates and increases the risk for diabetes mellitus, cancer, hypertension, and coronary heart disease. Typical treatment for obesity includes behavior modification, lifestyle management, nutritional modification, and increased physical activity and exercise. Pharmacologic and surgical interventions are available to those individuals who have been unsuccessful in repeated attempts to lose weight (42). Individuals who are obese and lose weight display a high rate of recidivism, with a high percentage of those who lose weight regaining the weight within one year (4).

Metabolic Syndrome

The metabolic syndrome is characterized by a clustering of metabolic risk factors including abdominal obesity, **atherogenic dyslipidemia**, elevated blood pressure, insulin resistance or glucose intolerance, a **prothrombotic state** (e.g., high fibrinogen or plasminogen activator inhibitor–1 in the blood), and a proinflammatory state (e.g., elevated C-reactive protein in the blood) (15). Individuals with metabolic syndrome are at increased risk of coronary heart disease and other diseases related to atherosclerosis (e.g., stroke and peripheral vascular disease) and type 2 diabetes. Metabolic syndrome has become increasingly common in the United States with estimates of more than 50 million Americans having the condition (15). The dominant underlying risk factors for metabolic syndrome appear to be abdominal obesity and insulin resistance. Other conditions associated with the syndrome include physical inactivity, aging, hormonal imbalance, and genetic predisposition. There are no well-accepted criteria for diagnosing the metabolic syndrome, but many experts agree that the presence of three or more of the following indicates the presence of metabolic syndrome: elevated waist circumference, elevated triglycerides, reduced HDL cholesterol, elevated blood pressure, and elevated fasting glucose (20).

Orthopedic and Neuromuscular Disease

Orthopedic and neuromuscular disease can significantly affect participation in physical activity and exercise, contributing to considerable morbidity and mortality. Figure 4.12 shows the prevalence of the two most common orthopedic and neuromuscular diseases: arthritis and osteoporosis (24,34). The diseases provided

---

Hypoglycemia Below normal levels of blood glucose.

Ketoacidosis An acidotic condition caused by the increased production of ketone bodies.

Atherogenic dyslipidemia Abnormal levels of blood lipids that promote the development of atherosclerosis.

Prothrombotic state A condition of the body that favors the development of blood coagulation.

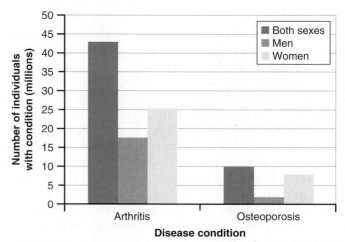

FIGURE 4.12 ▼ Prevalence of the two most common orthopedic and neuromuscular diseases: arthritis and osteoporosis (24,34).

in the following sections are some of the more common conditions experienced by clinical exercise physiologists in healthcare settings. Table 4.8 illustrates the potential benefits of exercise for each orthopedic and neuromuscular disease condition.

Arthritis

Arthritis is a painful condition affecting a joint or numerous joints in the body. About 46 million individuals have arthritis, and it is a leading cause of disability in individuals older than age 55 (24). The two most common arthritic conditions are osteoarthritis, which is a degenerative joint disease, and rheumatoid arthritis, which is an inflammatory joint disease. Osteoarthritis is localized to the affected joint or joints and first appears as a deficit in the soft cartilage around the ends of the bones that constitute the joint. Also known as degenerative joint disease, osteoarthritis typically occurs following trauma to the joint, following an infection of the joint, or simply as a result of aging. Rheumatoid arthritis occurs as a result of an inflammatory response of the immune system against the joint tissue. In this case, the inflammatory response may affect numerous joints and other organ systems as well. Treatment of arthritic conditions varies depending on the type of arthritis but typically includes physical and occupational therapy, lifestyle modification to include increased physical activity and exercise, weight loss, and pharmacologic treatment. Joint replacement surgery may be required in severe cases involving joint deterioration (4).

Osteoporosis

Osteoporosis, a condition of decreased bone mass, occurs when the normal replenishment of bone tissue is severely disrupted, resulting in weakened bones and an increased risk of fracture. **Osteopenia** is a condition that occurs when bone-mass loss is significant but not as severe as in osteoporosis. Although osteoporosis can occur in anyone, with more than 10 million individuals having the disease, it is

Table 4.8	Potential Benefits of Exercise for Various Orthopedic and Neuromuscular Diseases
DISEASE CONDITION	**BENEFITS OF EXERCISE**
Arthritis	Improvement in fitness; decreased joint swelling and pain
Osteoporosis	Improvement in fitness; slowing of the age-related decline in bone mass
Muscular dystrophy	Improvement in strength and functional capacity
Multiple sclerosis	Improvement in short-term physical fitness and functional performance
Cerebral palsy	Improved fitness; increased sense of well-being

most common in underweight postmenopausal White women (34). Bone mass is typically at its greatest during a person's third decade of life (Figure 4.13). Thereafter, a gradual reduction in bone mass occurs as bone is not replenished as quickly as it is lost. In postmenopausal women, the production of estrogen, which helps maintain the levels of calcium and other minerals necessary for normal bone regeneration, decreases substantially. This decreased level of estrogen contributes to an accelerated loss of bone mass of up to 3% per year over a period of 5 to 7 years. Other factors contributing to an increase in bone loss include smoking, excessive alcohol consumption, and a sedentary lifestyle. The development of osteoporosis also has a genetic component. A receptor gene that affects calcium uptake and bone density has been identified, and the different forms of this gene appear to correlate with differences in levels of bone density among individuals with osteoporosis (4).

Muscular Dystrophy

Muscular dystrophy is an umbrella term used to describe several inherited diseases characterized by the progressive wasting of skeletal muscles. There are five main forms of the disease. They are classified according to the age at onset of symptoms, the pattern of inheritance, and the part of the body primarily affected. Muscular dystrophy is characterized by a progressive degeneration of muscle fibers that are replaced by fibrous tissue. Muscular dystrophy appears early in life and causes **symmetric** weakness and wasting of groups of muscles such as those of the lower limbs, shoulder girdle, and face. The most common form of the disease (*Duchene* type) is due to a defect on the X chromosome and only affects boys. The muscle cell membrane lacks a specific protein called *dystrophin*, which normally prevents the muscle structure from being destroyed by its own contractions. There is no known treatment or

Osteopenia A condition of bone in which decreased calcification, decreased density, or reduced mass occurs.
Symmetric Affecting corresponding parts simultaneously and similarly.

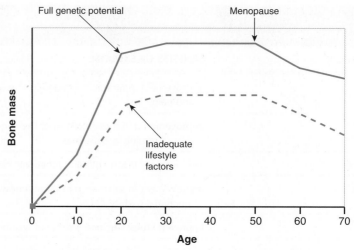

FIGURE 4.13 ▼ Acquisition and loss of bone mass during the lifespan. (Adapted from Heaney et al. Peak bone mass. Osteoporosis International. 2000;11:985–1009.)

cure for muscular dystrophy. Supportive measures and physical activity and exercise can improve the quality of life and preserve mobility for as long as possible (4).

Multiple Sclerosis

Multiple sclerosis is a chronic, slowly progressive **autoimmune** disease in which the immune system attacks the protective myelin sheaths that surround the nerve cells of the brain and spinal cord. This results in damaged areas of the nervous system that are unable to transmit nerve impulses. Multiple sclerosis also slowly damages the nerves themselves. The onset of multiple sclerosis is usually between the ages 20 and 40 years. The many symptoms associated with multiple sclerosis affect almost every system of the body and result in problems with vision, emotional disturbances, speech disorders, convulsions, paralysis or numbness of various regions of the body, bladder disturbances, and muscular weakness. The course of the disease varies considerably among individuals. In some individuals, the symptoms diminish and return, sometimes at frequent intervals and sometimes after several years. In other individuals the disease progresses steadily. There is a genetic predisposition to multiple sclerosis and environmental factors may also be involved in disease development. There is no cure for multiple sclerosis, but a number of drugs can slow its progression and reduce the frequency of attacks (4).

Cerebral Palsy

Cerebral palsy is a disability caused by brain damage before or during birth or in the first years of life, resulting in a loss of voluntary muscular control and

Autoimmune The immune response of body against its own tissues or organs.

coordination. Although the exact cause is unknown, several factors may predispose a child for developing cerebral palsy including diseases such as rubella or genital herpes simplex, very low infant birth weight, injury or physical abuse, maternal smoking, alcohol consumption, and ingestion of certain drugs. Most cases of cerebral palsy are associated with prenatal problems. The severity of the affliction depends on the extent of the brain damage. Individuals with mild cases of cerebral palsy may have only a few muscles affected, whereas severe cases can result in total loss of coordination or even paralysis. There are many different forms of the disability, each caused by damage to a different area of the brain. Spastic cerebral palsy accounts for more than half of all cases and results from damage to the motor areas of the cerebral cortex. This condition causes the affected muscles to be contracted and over responsive to stimuli. Other types of cerebral palsy include athetoid, choreic, and ataxic. The different types of cerebral palsy may occur singularly or in combination. Some individuals who are affected have a degree of mental retardation, but in many individuals, the intellect is unimpaired. There is no cure for the disorder and treatment usually includes physical, occupational, and speech therapy (4).

> ➤ **Thinking Critically**
> How might coursework in exercise science prepare an individual for a professional career as a clinical exercise physiologist and assist in the use of physical activity and exercise for the management of a chronic disease condition?

I N T E R V I E W

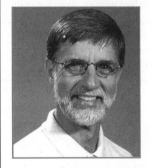

Jeffrey L. Roitman, EdD, Rockhurst University, Clinical Exercise Physiologist

Brief Introduction

I majored in physical education and English as an undergraduate student at the University of Missouri and obtained an EdD at the University of Northern Colorado where I majored in physical education with an emphasis in exercise physiology. I taught for 8 years at the college level, before taking a position as a clinical exercise physiologist in a cardiac rehabilitation program in Michigan. In 1981, I became the Director of Cardiac Rehabilitation at Research Medical Center in Kansas City, Missouri, where I remained for 26 years. Currently, I am the Director of Sports Science at Rockhurst University.

➤ **Why did you choose to become a clinical exercise physiologist?**

Initially, I moved from the academic environment to clinical exercise physiology because I thought it offered an increased intellectual challenge. In retrospect, I think the challenge is from within. The constant evolution of clinical practice and research literature is an ongoing challenge in which any professional can choose to participate.

➤ **What individuals or experiences were most influential in your career development?**

Dr Nancy Van Anne, one of my first graduate professors was a great teacher who demanded excellence. The team of exercise physiologists that I began my career with, Dr Gordon Schultz, Dr Richard Parr, and Dr Jon Pavlisko, were my original influences with respect to the clinical

(Continued)

and adult fitness and fitness programming. Dr Enrique Leguizamon, a cardiologist and my first medical director demanded that we all learn basic clinical cardiology and that we keep up with the literature. His presence required that we all be professionals of the highest caliber and his influence was deep and broad for me. Later in my career, Dr Larry Kenney, Dr Reed Humphrey, and Dr Mark Williams all provided me with professional association volunteer opportunities that were unlikely without them. I would be remiss if I did not mention the staff and patients who stimulated me to continue to learn so that our program would be current. The end result of this was that patients benefited from being exposed to our programs and classes throughout the years.

> ### What are your top professional accomplishments?

My work with ACSM's Certification Committee during its early years was certainly one of the most meaningful professional experiences of my career. I believe that the early efforts of that Committee have improved the credibility, quality, and the standing of exercise professionals over the past 25 years. As a member of the Publications Subcommittee of Certification, I helped establish the precursor to *ACSM's Health and Fitness Journal*. Though still a developing publication, I believe that the journal is (and will increasingly be) a

critical link between the practicing exercise professional and the research that drives our profession. Finally, I think I am most proud of having worked for more than 25 years with hundreds of patients and with many staff members who have passed through our program. I believe that their experiences helped them live better, healthier lives.

> ### What advice would you have for a student exploring a career in exercise science?

My first bit of advice would be not to choose your career too early. It is, perhaps, best to choose your passion (or maybe it chooses you) and follow it. Get as much varied experience as you can. Working with many clinical (and nonclinical) populations can only enhance your knowledge, understanding, and ability to work with people. I strongly recommend that young professionals become involved in volunteer work with their professional association early and work to make the profession better. You reflect your profession and your profession is a reflection of you. Finally, I think it is important to realize early in one's career that we cannot change other people. We can only present information and give them tools to change. Change comes from within. People do not change because we lecture, model, demonstrate, teach, inform, tell, or want a change to occur.

SUMMARY

- Physical activity and exercise that can prevent or delay the onset of chronic disease in healthy individuals or provide therapeutic or functional benefits to individuals with disease conditions is the hallmark of clinical exercise physiology.
- Clinical exercise physiologists play an important role in the complete healthcare team by providing expertise in the prevention, treatment, and rehabilitation of a numerous disease conditions and physical disabilities.
- Clinical exercise physiologists use physical activity and exercise as a means of evaluating functional capacity; assisting healthcare specialists in diagnostic testing; prescribing exercise based on individual needs, desires, and abilities; and instructing, supervising, and monitoring exercise programs in clinical settings.
- Cardiovascular, respiratory, metabolic, orthopedic, and neuromuscular disease conditions can be positively affected by the use of individualized physical activity and exercise program.

FOR REVIEW

1. What are the primary employment settings for a clinical exercise physiologist?

2. What significant events occurred during the 1950s that contributed to the understanding of the role of physical activity and exercise in the prevention of cardiovascular disease?

3. Define diagnostic and functional capacity testing.

4. What are primary functions of a graded exercise test?

5. What is the purpose of pre-exercise screening?

6. Why must an individual provide informed consent prior to participation in a graded exercise test?

7. Why is it important to collect the rating of perceived exertion, heart rate, and blood pressure during a graded exercise test?

8. What is the difference between a submaximal and maximal graded exercise test?

9. What are the components of health-related physical fitness testing?

10. Define the primary cardiovascular diseases:
    a. Myocardial infarction
    b. Coronary artery disease
    c. Angina pectoris
    d. Valvular heart disease
    e. Chronic heart failure
    f. Peripheral vascular disease
    g. Hypertension

11. Define the primary respiratory diseases:
    a. Obstructive pulmonary disease
    b. Restrictive pulmonary disease
    c. Asthma
    d. Cystic fibrosis

12. Define the primary metabolic diseases
    a. Diabetes
    b. Hyperlipidemia
    c. Obesity
    d. Metabolic syndrome

13. Define the primary orthopedic and neuromuscular diseases:
    a. Arthritis
    b. Osteoporosis
    c. Muscular dystrophy
    d. Multiple sclerosis
    e. Cerebral palsy

REFERENCES

1. Allison DB, Downey M, Atkinson RL, et al. Obesity as a disease: A white paper on evidence and arguments commissioned by the Council of The Obesity Society. *Obes Res.* 2008;16:1161–77.
2. American Association of Cardiovascular and Pulmonary Rehabilitation. *Guidelines for Cardiac Rehabilitation and Secondary Prevention Programs.* Champaign (IL): Human Kinetics; 2004.
3. American Association of Cardiovascular and Pulmonary Rehabilitation. *Guidelines for Pulmonary Rehabilitation Programs.* Champaign (IL): Human Kinetics; 2004.
4. American College of Sports Medicine. *ACSM's Exercise Management for Persons with Chronic Diseases and Disabilities.* Champaign (IL): Human Kinetics; 2003.
5. American College of Sports Medicine. *ACSM's Guidelines for Exercise Testing and Prescription.* 8th ed. Philadelphia (PA): Lippincott, Williams & Wilkins; 2009.
6. American Heart Association. *Exercise Testing and Training of Apparently Healthy Individuals: A Handbook for Physicians.* New York (NY): American Heart Association; 1972.
7. American Heart Association. *Exercise Testing and Training of Individuals with Heart Disease or at High Risk for its Development: A Handbook for Physicians.* Dallas (TX): American Heart Association; 1975.
8. American Heart Association. *Heart Disease and Stroke Statistics—2008 Update.* Dallas (TX): American Heart Association; 2008. p. 1–43.
9. American Thoracic Society. Pulmonary rehabilitation. *Am Rev Respir Dis.* 1981;24:663–6.
10. Barach AL. *Physiologic Therapy in Respiratory Disease.* Philadelphia (PA): J.B. Lippincott; 1948.
11. Berryman JW. Ancient and early influences. In: Tipton CM, editor. *Exercise Physiology: People and Ideas.* New York (NY): Oxford University Press; 2003. p. 1–38.
12. Borg GAV. *Borg's Perceived Exertion and Pain Scales.* Champaign (IL): Human Kinetics; 1998.
13. Borg GAV, Linderholm H. Perceived exertion and pulse rate during graded exercise in various age groups. *Acta Med Scand.* 1967;472:194–206.
14. Cain HD, Frasher WG, Stiuelman R. Graded activity program for safe return to self care following myocardial infarction. *JAMA.* 1961;177:111–5.
15. Churilla JR, Fitzhugh EC, Thompson DL. The metabolic syndrome: How definition impacts the prevalence and risk in U.S. adults: 1999–2004 NHANES. *Metab Syndr Relat Disord.* 2007;5:331–42.
16. Comoss P. The utility and viability of outcome measurement and monitoring in cardiac rehabilitation. *J Cardiopulm Rehab.* 2002;22:334–7.
17. Cooper R, Cutler J, svigne-Nickens P, et al. Trends and disparities in coronary heart disease, stroke, and other cardiovascular diseases in the United States: Findings of the National Conference on Cardiovascular Disease Prevention. *Circulation.* 2000;102: 3137–47.
18. Eisenmann JC, DuBose KD, Donnelly JE. Fatness, fitness, and insulin sensitivity among 7- to 9-year-old children. *Obes Res.* 2007;15:2135–44.
19. Froelicher VF. Cardiac rehabilitation. In: *Exercise and the Heart: Clinical Concepts.* Chicago (IL): Year Book Medical Publishers, Inc.; 1987. p. 423–86.
20. Hanse BC. The metabolic syndrome X. *Ann N Y Acad Sci.* 2000;1–24.
21. Heberden W. Some accounts of a disorder of the chest. *Med Trans Coll Phys.* 1772;2:59–66.
22. Heberden W. *Commentaries on The History and Care of Disease.* London: T. Payne; 1802.
23. Hellerstein HK, Ford AB. Rehabilitation of the cardiac patient. *JAMA.* 1957;164:225–31.
24. Helmich CG, Felson DT, Lawrence RC, et al. Estimates of the prevalence of arthritis and other rheumatic conditions in the United States. *Arthritis Rheum.* 2008;58:15–25.
25. Hornsby WG, Bryner RW. Clinical exercise physiology. In: Brown SP, editor. *Introduction to Exercise Science.* Philadelphia (PA): Lippincott, Williams & Wilkins; 2001. p. 212–34.
26. Howley ET, Bassett DR, Welch HG. Criteria for maximal oxygen uptake: Review and commentary. *Med Sci Sports Exerc.* 1995;27:1292–301.
27. Joint National Committee on Prevention DEaToHBP. The seventh report of the Joint National Committee on prevention, detection, evaluation, and treatment of high blood pressure (JNC VII). *Hypertension.* 2003; 157:2413–46.
28. Kallio V, Hamalainen H, Hakkila J, Luurila OJ. Reduction in sudden deaths by a multifactorial intervention programme after acute myocardial infarction. *Lancet.* 1979;2:1091–4.
29. Kostoff D. Parmacotherapy. In: Ehrman JK, Gordon PM, Visich PS, Keteyian SJ, editors. *Clinical Exercise Physiology.* Champaign (IL): Human Kinetics; 2009. p. 31–59.
30. Levine SA, Lown B. Armchair treatment of acute coronary thrombosis. *JAMA.* 1952;148:1365–7.
31. Miller WF. Physical therapeutic measures in the treatment of chronic bronchopulmonary disorders. *Am J Med.* 1958;24:929.
32. Miller WF. Rehabilitation of patients with chronic lung diseases. *Med Clin North Am.* 1967;349–56.
33. Morris JN, Heady JA, Raffle PAB, Roberts CG, Parks JW. Coronary heart disease and physical activity of work. *Lancet.* 1953;1053–7,1111–20.
34. National Osteoporosis Foundation. *Fast Facts on Osteoporosis.* Washington (DC): National Osteoporosis Foundation; 2008.
35. Pate RR, Pratt M, Blair SN, et al. A recommendation from the Centers for Disease Control and Prevention and the American College of Sports Medicine. *JAMA.* 1995;273:402–7.
36. Petty TL, Nett LM, Finigan NM, Brink GA, Corsello PR. A comprehensive care program for chronic airway obstruction. *Ann Intern Med.* 1969;70: 1109–20.
37. Ries AL, Bauldoff GS, Carlin BW, et al. Pulmonary rehabilitation: Joint ACCP/AACVPR evidence-based clinical practice guidelines. *Chest.* 2007;131:4S–42S.

38. Robertson RJ, Goss FL, Boer N, et al. OMNI scale perceived exertion at ventilatory breakpoint in children: Response normalized. *Med Sci Sports Exerc.* 2001; 33:1946–52.

39. Robertson RJ, Goss FL, Rutkowski J, et al. Concurrent validation of the OMNI perceived exertion scale for resistance exercise. *Med Sci Sports Exerc.* 2003; 35:333–41.

40. Southard DR, Cahalin LP, Carlin BW. Clinical competency guidelines for pulmonary rehabilitation professionals. *J Cardiopulm Rehab.* 1995;15:173–8.

41. Stokes W. *Disease of the Heart and Aorta.* Philadelphia (PA): Lindsay; 1854.

42. Sugerman HJ, Kral JG. Evidence-based medicine reports on obesity surgery: A critique. *Int J Obes.* 2005; 29:735–45.

43. Wilson PK. AACVPR: The first 20 years. *J Cardiopulm Rehab.* 2005;25:242–8.

CHAPTER

Athletic Training and Sports Medicine

At the completion of this chapter you will be able to do the following:

1. Describe the importance of athletic training and sports medicine as they relate to enhancing the understanding of physical activity, exercise, sport, and athletic performance.

2. Describe the key highlights in the historic development of athletic training and sports medicine.

3. Identify the primary responsibilities of an athletic trainer and a sports medicine team physician.

4. Describe some of the important knowledge areas for athletic trainers and sports medicine physicians.

Athletic training is an area of exercise science that is involved in the prevention, treatment, and rehabilitation of injuries to physically active individuals and athletes (Figure 5.1). Many individuals often think of athletic trainers as only working with athletes in a sport setting; however, athletic trainers also work closely with other allied health professionals to provide care to anyone who may have an injury caused by participation in physical activity or exercise. Certified athletic trainers perform professional practice in a variety of work environments including secondary schools, colleges and universities, sports medicine clinics, professional sports programs, and other healthcare settings. Athletic trainers work closely with sports medicine physicians to form the primary athletic medicine team (49).

Sports medicine is an umbrella term used to describe all of the various issues interrelated among medicine, physical activity, exercise, health promotion, and disease prevention (38). Sports medicine has four primary component areas:

- Medical supervision and care of recreational and competitive athletes
- Use of exercise and sports for people who are physically or mentally handicapped

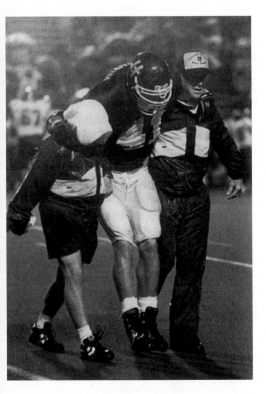

FIGURE 5.1 ▼ Athletic trainers assist with injury prevention, diagnosis, and rehabilitation. (From Brown SP. *Introduction to Exercise Science*. Baltimore (MD): Lippincott Williams & Wilkins; 2001.)

Athletic training An area of exercise science that helps with the prevention, treatment, and rehabilitation of injuries to physically active individuals and athletes.

Sports medicine An umbrella term used to describe all things related to medicine, physical activity, exercise, health promotion, and disease prevention.

• Helping people develop and maintain physical fitness
• Use of exercise to treat and rehabilitate people who have been ill or injured.

The profession of sports medicine has created a balance between caring for competitive athletes and treating general patients by promoting exercise for health and disease prevention. The sports medicine physician may be either an athlete's primary care physician or a physician hired by the school, university or college, or professional team to supervise all aspects of medical care to athletes. Sports medicine physicians, although at one time a group primarily comprised of orthopedic surgeons, now include those physicians who have successfully passed a subspecialty exam in sports medicine. The athletic trainer and sports medicine physician work together and often with other exercise science and healthcare professionals such as physical therapists to provide the best medical care and treatment possible to athletes and physically active individuals who have been injured (38).

Injuries are a common occurrence in individuals who are participating in physical activity and exercise programs, as well those actively involved in sport and athletic competition. Athletic trainers, sports medicine physicians, and other exercise science and allied healthcare professionals have a primary responsibility to help reduce the risk of injury among active individuals and also provide rehabilitation following the injury. Despite using many injury prevention precautions, individuals participating in sport and athletic competition are at risk for sport-related injuries. The following set of figures illustrates the incidence of injuries in certain high school and college sports and sport and recreational injuries treated at emergency rooms. Figure 5.2 provides information on the injury rates for the top five sports with the highest injury rate among high school athletes participating in sports during the 2005–06 school year (13). Figure 5.3 provides information on the injury rate during game competition and practice activities for 15 National Collegiate Athletic Association–sponsored sports during the period from 1988–89 through 2003–04 (31). Figure 5.4 provides information on all nonfatal sport and

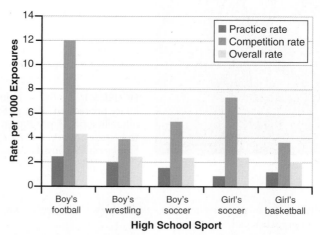

FIGURE 5.2 ▼ Overall injury rates for the top five sports with the highest injury rate among high school athletes participating in sports during the 2005–06 school year (13).

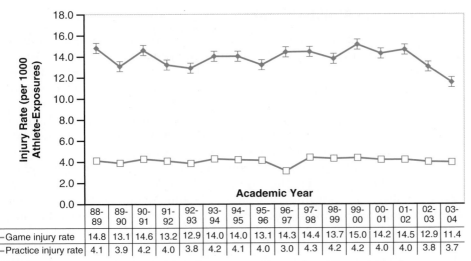

	88-89	89-90	90-91	91-92	92-93	93-94	94-95	95-96	96-97	97-98	98-99	99-00	00-01	01-02	02-03	03-04
Game injury rate	14.8	13.1	14.6	13.2	12.9	14.0	14.0	13.1	14.3	14.4	13.7	15.0	14.2	14.5	12.9	11.4
Practice injury rate	4.1	3.9	4.2	4.0	3.8	4.2	4.1	4.0	3.0	4.3	4.2	4.2	4.0	4.0	3.8	3.7

FIGURE 5.3 ▼ Overall injury rate during game competition and practice activities for 15 National Collegiate Athletic Association–sponsored sports during the period from 1988–89 through 2003–04 (31).

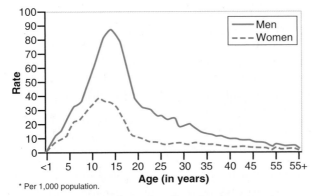

* Per 1,000 population.

FIGURE 5.4 ▼ Overall rate for all nonfatal sport and recreation injuries treated at emergency rooms during the period of July 2000 to June 2001 (12).

recreation injuries treated at emergency rooms during the period of July 2000 to June 2001 (12). From the figures, it is clear to see that participating in competitive sport and recreational activities carries an inherent risk of injury.

HISTORIC DEVELOPMENT OF ATHLETIC TRAINING AND SPORTS MEDICINE

The history of athletic training and sports medicine are intertwined because both professions grew primarily out of the professional service of providing care to injured athletes. This section begins with a brief history of athletic training and then concludes with an overview of the historic development of sports medicine.

Early History of Athletic Training

The formal development of athletic training as a profession occurred in the early 1900s, and its growth coincided with the emergence of the sport of American tackle football (46). In reality however, athletic training probably had its origin with primitive man. To survive, early man had to continuously develop physical skills and maintain fitness to meet the demands and dangers of the environment. These early hunters believed in a medicine man, called a "Shaman," who was a specialist in healing. The shaman used herbs and heat to keep the hunter healthy so that he could continue his search for food and survival (46).

The Greek and Roman civilizations played an important role in the development of athletic training. The Greeks had trainers called Paidotribes, Aleittes, and Gymnastes. The meaning of Paidotribes and Aleittes were boy-rubber and anointer, respectively. The use of these terms in Greek writings suggests that massage was an important part of the duties of the trainer (21). Herodicus of Megura, considered the greatest of all the Greek trainers, was also considered a physician as well. He was the advocate of modern gymnastics and was the teacher of Hippocrates, the father of modern medicine. The medical gymnastae were not responsible for training individuals in a particular skill or sport activity but to possess some idea of the effect of diet, rest, and exercise on the development of the body (46).

Claudius Galen (130–200 AD) is considered one of the first "athletic trainers" and team physicians. Galen wrote broadly about medicine and athletics and his writings frequently criticized other athletic trainers and coaches for their practices and training of athletes. He recommended that patients exercise in the gymnasia as a means to recover from sickness and fatigue. Unfortunately, from the time of Galen until early in the twentieth century there is little written record of the work of athletic trainers (46).

Recent History of Athletic Training

In the early twentieth century, athletic trainers began to understand the need for the development and advancement of athletic training as profession. A group of athletic trainers began to envision the development of a professional organization, which ultimately became the National Athletic Trainers Association (NATA). The NATA has had a profound impact on the professional development of athletic training. The first national association for athletic trainers was organized in 1938; however, the challenges of travel, communication, financial limitations, and the influence of World War II led to the dissolution of the first NATA in 1944 (46).

The reemergence of the NATA was the result of the development of regional associations of athletic trainers within various collegiate athletic conferences. These associations eventually came together to form the distinct regional organizational structure of the NATA and included the following conference associations: Southern, Eastern, Pacific Coast, Southwest, and Southeastern. This original regional structure remained in place when the conference associations were designated as districts in the NATA (46).

In 1950, the NATA was officially formed by representatives from the regional collegiate conference associations. A total of nine districts comprised the new organizational structure of the NATA. The organizational leaders at the time wanted the association to build and strengthen the profession of athletic training through the exchange of ideas, knowledge, and methods of athletic training. Central to the development of the NATA was the Cramer Chemical Company, a producer of athletic training and sports medicine equipment that covered all the expenses of the association for the first 5 years of its existence (46). In 1956, in an effort to disseminate information about the profession of athletic training, the NATA began publication of a journal titled *The Journal of the National Athletic Trainer's Association*. The NATA later changed the name to *Athletic Training: The Journal of the National Athletic Trainers Association* before finally settling on the name *Journal of Athletic Training* (46).

From 1950 to 1975, the NATA steadily expanded its professional influence and standing in the athletic communities through two major accomplishments. In 1969, the NATA Committee on Professional Advancement developed and implemented rules and regulations for the certification of athletic trainers. A national certification examination was developed and in 1970, the NATA began testing and certifying professional athletic trainers. Also during this time period, a curricular program was approved by the NATA Professional Education Committee for a program of study in athletic training. This educational program was adopted as part of the college and university curricula for the professional preparation of athletic trainers. The NATA Board of Certification, Inc. oversees the certification of all athletic trainers. Only graduates of an athletic training program accredited by the Commission on Accreditation for Athletic Training Education (CAATE) may become a certified athletic trainer. The NATA remains a key advocate for the development of athletic training as a profession. A summary of some of the key historic events in the development of athletic training is presented in Table 5.1.

Early History of Sports Medicine

Sports medicine, like many other disciplines related to health and medicine, had its origin in Greek and Roman times. For example, early writings have Claudius Galen serving as a physician to Greek gladiators (5). Much of the early written work, however, is centered more on the role of physicians in their dealings with

Table 5.1	Key Historic Events in Athletic Training	
DATE	**DEVELOPMENT**	
1938	First attempt at formation of the NATA	
1950	Formation of the NATA	
1956	First publication of the *Journal of Athletic Training*	
1969	Development of certification program for athletic trainers	
1970	Development of accreditation guidelines for college and university athletic training education programs	

health, physical activity, and exercise. During the period of enlightenment in the eighteenth century, there was a surge in the interest of orthopedic medicine. For example, in 1741, Nicolas Andry, a professor of medicine at the University of Paris published the first edition of *Orthpaedia*. Andry developed the concept of the splinted tree for practicing orthopedic medicine in children and thereby helping to correct and prevent deformaties. The concept for the splinted tree arises from the Greek meaning of the word orthopedic; ortho meaning straight and pais meaning child. From this origin, orthopedic sports medicine grew into the professional discipline that we know today (1).

Recent History of Sports Medicine

In the first half of the twentieth century, orthopedic medicine was a specialty area with a primary focus on children and only a limited role in the treatment of traumatic injuries. Following World War II, orthopedic surgeons expanded their medical treatment of fractures and severe trauma through the use of advanced surgery. For example, the development of the total joint replacement procedure allowed reconstructive surgery to grow as a specialty area throughout the 1950s and 1960s. In the early 1970s, the birth of modern day sports medicine occurred. Initially, sports medicine was described as "locker room medicine" (61). Much of the science behind sports medicine was anecdotal, and the papers were mostly testimonials and observations of physicians and surgeons who were working with athletes. The practice of sports medicine initially focused on competitive athletes but gradually expanded its scope to include recreational athletes. The acceptance of primary care sports medicine for athletes signaled a major change in the field. A team approach for sports medicine developed in the 1980s and 1990s and incorporated orthopedists, primary care physicians, athletic trainers, physical therapists, exercise physiologists, cardiologists, nutritionists, and others (1).

Another key historic development in sports medicine occurred in 1989 with the recognition of sports medicine as a subspecialty by the American Board of Medical Specialties. The development of several professional organizations such as the American Orthopaedic Society for Sports Medicine (AOSSM) and the ACSM have further facilitated the growth and maturation of sports medicine. The AOSSM was founded in 1972 and began publishing the *American Journal of Sports Medicine* in 1974. The ACSM serves sports medicine physicians as part of an overall organizational structure. The publication of the *Sports Medicine Bulletin* and the Team Physician Consensus Statements (22–29) has allowed the ACSM to distribute current information to physicians and help shape the care given to those individuals participating in competitive sports and athletics. The American Medical Society for Sports Medicine (AMSSM) was founded in 1991 and is a multidisciplinary organization that serves primary care physicians with fellowship training in sports medicine, nonsurgical sports medicine, and full time team physician programs (2).

Several advancements in the treatment of injured athletes and other preventative measures have helped further shape sports medicine. One of the key technologic advancements was the development of the arthroscopic surgery procedure. First used in the early 1930s, arthroscopy grew dramatically so that by the late 1990s approximately 700,000 knee and shoulder arthroscopic procedures were being performed each year (1). A diagnostic and treatment intervention called soft-tissue endoscopy decreases the time it takes for athletes who have had tendon injuries to return to play. Once considered revolutionary, anterior cruciate ligament (ACL) surgery and ulnar collateral ligament reconstruction are now considered common in the sports medicine field. Future advances in sports medicine care will likely include treatments such as chondrocyte implantation, bone morphogenic protein, and gene therapy (58).

Several prominent orthopedic surgeons were instrumental in promoting the development of sports medicine. Frank Jobe performed the first ulnar collateral ligament reconstruction procedure on a baseball pitcher named Tommy John in 1974. James Andrews is known for his pioneering work on the surgical correction of knee, elbow, and shoulder injuries. In 1984, Jack Hughston opened the Hughston Sports Medicine Hospital, the first facility of its kind in the country. Hughston is well known for his work in treating knee injuries and for being the first to establish postdoctoral fellowships in sports medicine. Hughston was also one of the founders of the AOSSM, and in 1972 he founded the *American Journal of Sports Medicine* (1).

Recently, sports medicine physicians and other exercise science professionals have continued to improve the care given to athletes by further refining the preparticipation physical examination (43) and providing guidelines for exercise during pregnancy (16). Sports medicine professionals have also advanced the understanding of the female athlete triad (22), the higher prevalence of ACL injuries in female athletes (3), and improved head concussion management and treatment (28). The generation of knowledge within the discipline has been enhanced by having sports medicine professionals embrace the scientific inquiry and evidence-based approach to the treatment and care of injured athletes (57). Table 5.2 provides some of the significant historic events in the development of sports medicine.

> ➤ *Thinking Critically*
> *How has the historic development of athletic training and sports medicine contributed to providing better medical care for individuals injured during participation in exercise or sport activities?*

Table 5.2	Key Historic Events in Sports Medicine
DATE	**DEVELOPMENT**
1741	Andry published the first edition of *Orthpaedia*
1934	Development of the arthroscopic surgery procedure
1972	Formation of the American Orthopaedic Society for Sports Medicine
1974	Jobe performed the first ulnar collateral ligament reconstruction procedure also called John surgery
1989	Recognition of sports medicine as a subspecialty by the American Board of Medical Specialties
1991	Formation of the American Medical Society for Sports Medicine

PRIMARY RESPONSIBILITY AREAS OF ATHLETIC TRAINING PROFESSIONALS

The core body of knowledge comprising athletic training has been divided into six domains by the Board of Certification, Inc. (49). Table 5.3 illustrates those six domains. Individuals studying in a CAATE-accredited program will develop knowledge, skills, and abilities in each of the domains. Only those individuals graduating from an accredited college or university athletic training program are eligible to take the certification examination to become a certified athletic trainer and only certified individuals are allowed to practice professionally as athletic trainers. The following sections contain information about the primary responsibilities of an athletic trainer.

Prevention of Athletic Injuries

Participation in exercise and sport activities comes with an inherent risk of injury. This level of risk depends on a variety of factors including the physical condition of the individual, the skill level of the individual, and the environment in which the individual is participating. One of the main responsibilities of an athletic trainer is to make sure that the level of risk of injury is as low as possible. One of the most important preventive measures that physically active individuals can do to ensure a reduced risk of injury is to have a preparticipation physical examination performed prior to engaging in training for any sport or athletic competition. Athletic trainers, working with other sports medicine personnel, are an integral part of the complete preparticipation physical examination assessment team (43,49).

Athletic trainers must also be aware of the physical and environmental conditions that may increase the risk of injury to an individual. Reducing the risk of injury may be as simple as making sure that equipment is in proper working order and meets health and safety guidelines for use. Performing a visual survey of the practice and playing areas for any equipment or conditions that can potentially increase the risk of injury is something that athletic trainers must be vigilant about. Athletic trainers should work with coaches to ensure that groups of athletes work in different areas of the practice facility to reduce the risk of unintended collisions. Athletic trainers can help reduce the risk of injury by making sure that individuals comply with safety equipment guidelines such as wearing mouthguards and using

Table 5.3	Domains of Athletic Training
Prevention of athletic injuries	
Recognition, evaluation, and assessment of athletic injury	
Immediate care of athletic injuries	
Treatment, rehabilitation, and reconditioning of athletic injuries	
Organization and administration	
Professional development and responsibility	

other equipment designed to enhance safety and reduce injury risk. If working in an industrial setting, athletic trainers may spend time with employees on job-specific training before a worker becomes part of the production community. Athletic trainers must also be aware of extreme environmental conditions such as hot temperatures, high relative humidity, cold temperatures with high wind velocity, and air pollution that can contribute to heat injury, hypothermia, and pulmonary disorders (49).

Recognition, Evaluation, and Assessment of Athletic Injuries

Recognizing, evaluating, and assessing injuries to athletes that occur during training and competition is a primary responsibility of athletic trainers. This is probably the most visible responsibility as an athletic trainer is most likely the first person to intervene when an injury occurs to an athlete (Figure 5.5). Athletic trainers are responsible for taking a systematic approach to injury evaluation so that a comprehensive written record can be generated for communication with physicians and other sports medicine personnel. The extensive preparation received in educational activities and field experiences provide the foundation by which athletic trainers can be successful in this role (49). A specific evaluation process is utilized when initially encountering an injured athlete. A primary survey is completed first, followed by a secondary survey. Both the primary and secondary surveys have specific steps to follow in the process (49). Figure 5.6 provides an example of the steps used by athletic trainers when evaluating an injury situation.

Athletic trainers must be fully prepared to deal with a variety of injury situations. This includes having knowledge of emergency care and personal care procedures. Athletic trainers are required to be certified in cardiopulmonary resuscitation (CPR) from an accredited certifying agency such as the American Red Cross, American Heart Association, or the National Safety Council. Although not required, it is strongly encouraged that athletic trainers be certified in basic first aid (50). This is such a critical component of the skill set that many athletic trainers also receive training and certification as emergency medical technicians. Athletic trainers should also be concerned about their own personal safety especially as it relates to exposure to bloodborne pathogens. Athletic trainers must take precautionary measures to avoid contact with blood and other bodily fluids when

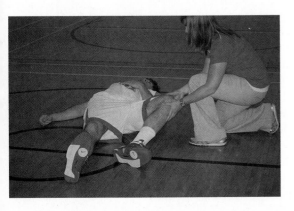

FIGURE 5.5 ▼ Evaluation of an acute injury by an athletic trainer.

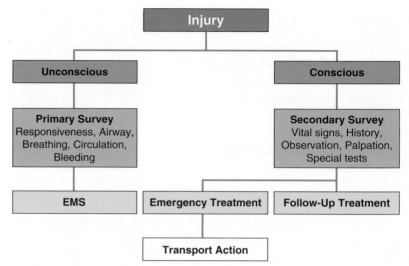

FIGURE 5.6 ▼ Steps involved in an injury evaluation process (53). (From Brown SP. *Introduction to Exercise Science*. Baltimore (MD): Lippincott Williams & Wilkins; 2001.)

performing an evaluation or first aid procedures. Athletic trainers are required to use latex gloves and proper disposal and cleanup procedures whenever blood or other fluids are present (47).

Primary Survey

Athletic trainers perform a primary survey when an athlete is injured. This includes assessing the ABCs (airway, breathing, and circulation) and activating the emergency medical service (EMS), if necessary. Unconscious patients are carefully monitored and if necessary, CPR or rescue breathing is initiated. Even if the injured athlete is conscious, a primary survey is still a required part of the evaluation and assessment processes. After completion of the primary survey, the secondary survey is performed (49).

Secondary Survey

Table 5.4 provides the steps involved in the secondary survey. This process includes an extensive assessment of the athlete and injured body area in an effort to provide a comprehensive evaluation and make a decision as to the most appropriate course of action. If during the secondary survey any of the information gathered would indicate an unfavorable outcome from further testing, the athletic trainer terminates the evaluation and the athlete is transported to an appropriate medical facility for further care. The secondary survey begins with an injury history. Information regarding when, how, and what happened to cause the injury is important for obtaining an accurate diagnosis from medical personnel. The athletic trainer must determine if any previous injuries occurred to the injured body part as this information has a bearing on any structural and functional testing done on the

Table 5.4	Secondary Survey of Injury Assessment
Collection of injury history and observation of body language	
Observation of any deformities, change in skin color, and/or change in the shape and size of structures	
Palpitation of the injured area, including both bone and soft tissue	
Assessment of ROM	
Administration of specific structure tests designed to identify the presence of injury	
Assessment of functional performance	
Decision on the course of action	

new injury site. During and after collection of injury history, the athletic trainer observes the athlete's body language as this can provide an indication of the level of pain or discomfort the athlete is experiencing and how much the athlete is favoring the injured body part. During a more formal observation of the injured area, the athletic trainer is looking for any deformities, change in skin color, and/or change in the shape and size of various structures. The next step is to **palpate** the injured area, including both bone and soft tissue. The injured athlete is asked to identify the most painful area. The athletic trainer then palpates the body part distal to the area of pain working toward the injury and finally arriving at the site of greatest discomfort (49).

If warranted, the athletic trainer can perform testing to establish the structural and functional integrities of an injured body area. The athletic trainer checks for circulation beyond the injury site, the injured athlete's response to touch, and the athlete's ability to activate the muscle of the injured area. If all of these are determined to be normal, the range of motion (ROM) of the body area is tested in three successive stages: active, passive, and resistive ROM. Active ROM requires the athlete to move the body part in response to the athletic trainer's instructions. Passive ROM involves a comparison of what ROM is achieved by the athlete compared to the ROM achieved by the athletic trainer when the muscles are relaxed. The third ROM assessment involves resistance applied by the athletic trainer as the athlete moves the injured body part through the normal ROM (49).

All of the information collected during the primary and secondary surveys is used to help determine which additional assessments will be made. If the assessments completed are normal, then functional testing involving activity-specific movements is used to determine if the athlete may safely return to full activity. During all testing and assessments, comparisons to the opposite side (bilateral) of the body are made to account for the variability found in individual people (49).

Palpate To examine by feeling and pressing with the palms of the hands and the fingers

Table 5.5	The SOAP Method for Record Keeping (49)	
S	Subjective information	What the athlete tells the athletic trainer
O	Objective information	Quantifiable information including signs, observations, palpation, and special tests performed by the athletic trainer
A	Assessment	Professional opinion of the athletic trainer or other healthcare professionals about the nature and extent of the injury
P	Plan	Includes all treatments rendered and disposition of the injury, whether referral or continued local intervention and rehabilitation

Course of Action

Upon completion of the injury evaluation, the athletic trainer must decide on the course of action. If the injury is mild, the athlete may be released to return to activity. If the injury is moderate to severe, the athlete is removed from the practice or competition and often referred to a physician for further evaluation and treatment. For some severe and all potentially catastrophic injuries, the EMS system is activated and the athlete is transported to the nearest appropriate facility for treatment (49).

Record Keeping

After completion of the injury evaluation, the athletic trainer completes a detailed written record. The results of all assessments and tests are recorded for later use by medical personnel performing a complete diagnosis and treatment of the injury. The injury evaluation and treatment report can be used by other athletic trainers, sports medicine physicians, and allied healthcare personnel to supervise the rehabilitation of the injured athlete. The SOAP method for recording the written record is probably the most commonly used method for recording information. SOAP is an acronym that stands for subjective, objective, assessment, and plan (36). Table 5.5 provides a detailed description of the SOAP record keeping format.

Immediate Care of Athletic Injuries

Athletic trainers are the most common healthcare professional to treat an acute injury. This means athletic trainers must be trained and ready to respond to any injury situation whether commonplace or life threatening. The primary and secondary surveys provide information that dictates the course of action an athletic trainer will follow when responding to an injury. All athletic training settings should have a written emergency action plan (49). A well-designed and executed emergency care plan will greatly limit secondary injury caused by inappropriate movement, treatment, or time spent activating the EMS. If the EMS is activated by the athletic trainer, the EMS personnel take responsibility for the athlete (49).

Acute musculoskeletal injuries are most commonly treated by using rest, ice, compression, and elevation (the acronym is RICE) (49). Rest of the injured body part may mean removal from practice or competition for a specific period of time.

If the injured body part requires immobilization, the sports medicine physician can employ crutches, a sling, or a cast to limit and restrict movement. Ice packs and compression wraps should be applied to the injured body part. The ice and compression helps limit the swelling of the injured area. The application of a compression wrap and cold treatment is usually 20 minutes in duration with removal of the cold treatment for a duration sufficient to allow the tissue to rewarm (37).

Treatment, Rehabilitation, and Reconditioning of Athletic Injuries

Pain, swelling, decreased ROM, and loss of normal function are the immediate effects of an acute injury to a body part. Following an acute injury, there is usually a period of inactivity that, depending on the length of inactivity, can lead to significant changes in the muscle including atrophy, and decreased strength, endurance, and neuromuscular coordination as well as reduced function of other body systems (49). A proper treatment, rehabilitation, and reconditioning program can reduce the amount of time required to return an athlete to practice and competition.

The various tissues (e.g., tendons, ligaments, and bone) and systems (e.g., muscular, cardiovascular, and respiratory) of the body all require regularly applied physical activity and exercise to maintain normal function and optimal performance (9,49). For example, the immobilization of a lower extremity can decrease various markers of cardiorespiratory function in a relatively short period of time (9,49). Muscle strength and performance will decrease as the number of days of inactivity increase (45). To reduce this loss of function, a systematic rehabilitation program must be followed. Active and passive exercises, as well as aerobic and resistance exercise should be used in a comprehensive rehabilitation program of an injured athlete. Exercises should be selected that minimize stress to the injured body part, yet provide a complete body workout.

Restoring a normal ROM to an injured body part is critical for preparing an injured athlete for returning to action. Completing physiologic and accessory movements is the key to increasing the ROM of a joint. Physiologic movements are those normally ascribed to a joint and include, for example, flexion and extension of the elbow joint. Accessory movements are small movements that reposition the bones for the maximum efficiency of physiologic movement and include additional movements. Normal function and ROM of a joint requires that both physiologic and accessory movements be properly coordinated. Large muscle activity through active, passive, and resistive ROM, performed throughout the entire ROM, is typically used to increase physiologic movements. Accessory movements of a joint are more commonly restored with joint mobilization techniques (35,49).

Exercise Activities

Athletic trainers can choose from a variety of muscle actions in the rehabilitation process, including isometric, isotonic, and isokinetic. **Isometric** muscle

---

Isometric The generation of force by a muscle without any movement of the joint.

action involves contracting a muscle but not moving the joint involved with the muscle through a ROM. Force is generated by the muscle, but there is no movement of the muscle during the contraction process. Isometric muscle actions can increase muscle strength but only for about a 15-degree ROM (angle) around the joint position at which the muscle is contracted (18). To improve muscle strength through the entire ROM, muscle contractions must be performed at several joint angles. Isometric contractions are performed against a machine or individual (e.g., athletic trainer) who provides resistance against the muscle contraction (35).

Isotonic muscle actions involve contracting a muscle against resistance and allowing the joint to move through the ROM. Force is generated by the muscle, and there is movement of the muscle during the contraction process. Isotonic muscle actions are performed using either free weights or a machine to provide resistance against the muscle movement. During isotonic exercises, the resistance provided by the external force stays constant, but the force generated by the muscle changes as the joint angle changes. When the joint angle changes, there are changes in the lever action of the joint and the force that must be generated by the muscle (18). Isotonic muscle actions are performed at variable speeds against a fixed resistance.

Isokinetic muscle actions consist of contracting a muscle against a resistance and moving the joint through the ROM at a constant velocity. Specific machines called isokinetic dynamometers allow the muscle to contract at a controlled speed, generally somewhere between 0 and 360 degrees per second. At the same time, resistance is provided against the muscle movement requiring the muscle to generate force (18). Isokinetic exercises are performed at a fixed speed with variable accommodating resistance.

Both isotonic and isokinetic exercises require the muscle to perform concentric and eccentric muscle actions. **Concentric muscle actions** occur when a muscle shortens in length and develops tension. **Eccentric muscle actions** occur when a muscle increases in length and develops tension.

Athletic trainers also use **closed kinetic chain** and **open kinetic chain** activities to facilitate the rehabilitation of injured athletes. The functional anatomic relationships that exist in the upper and lower extremities provide the basis for kinetic chain exercises. When an individual is in a weight bearing position, the lower extremity kinetic chain involves the transmission of forces among the foot, ankle, lower leg, knee, thigh, and hip. The hand as an upper extremity

---

Isotonic The generation of a constant force by a muscle and movement of the joint.

Isokinetic The generation of force by a muscle and movement of the joint at a constant speed or velocity.

Concentric muscle action When a muscle shortens in length and develops tension.

Eccentric muscle action When a muscle increases in length and develops tension.

Closed kinetic chain When forces along the body are transmitted to an adjacent structure, usually the floor or a piece of equipment.

Open kinetic chain When forces along the body are allowed to dissipate into the air.

Therapeutic modalities Machines, devices, or substances that are used to enhance recovery from an injury.

weight-bearing surface transmits forces to the wrist, forearm, elbow, upper arm, and shoulder girdle (48,49). In a closed kinetic chain, the foot or hand is weight bearing, whereas in an open kinetic chain there is no hand or foot contact with a surface (48,49). In a closed kinetic chain, the forces begin at the contact point between the foot or hand and the surface and then work their way along each joint. In a closed kinetic chain, forces must be absorbed by various tissues and anatomic structures rather than simply dissipating as would occur in an open chain (56). Closed kinetic chain strengthening techniques have become an extremely popular rehabilitation treatment by many athletic trainers in part because they are more functional than are open kinetic chain activities (49). Closed kinetic chain exercises are also more sport or activity specific because these exercises involve movement that more closely approximates the desired activity (49).

Therapeutic Modalities

Athletic trainers also use a variety of **therapeutic modalities** to assist in the rehabilitation process (Figure 5.7). Therapeutic modalities can provide effective support to the various techniques used in rehabilitation exercise (49). Appropriate rehabilitation protocols and proper progression of treatment must be based primarily on the physiologic responses of the tissues to injury and on an

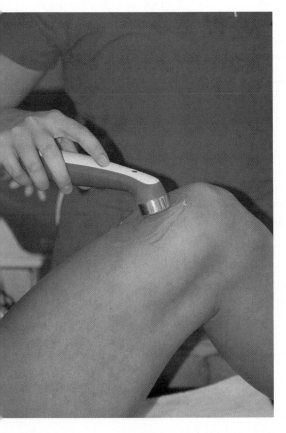

FIGURE 5.7 ▼ Treatment of an injury by an athletic trainer.

Table 5.6	Commonly used Therapeutic Modalities (49)	
MODALITY	PRINCIPLE	EXAMPLES
Cryotherapy	Cooling decreases physiologic function	Ice massage, cold or ice water immersion, ice packs, vapocoolant sprays
Cryokinetics	Cool the body part to analgesia and then work to increase the ROM	Ice immersion, cold packs, ice massage
Thermotherapy	Heating increases physiologic function	Moist heat packs, whirlpool baths, paraffin bath, contrast bath, fluidotherapy
Ultrasound	Deep heats tissues to increase tissue temperatures	High frequency generator transmits continuous or pulsed ultrasound waves, phonophoresis
Electrotherapy	Increases the excitability of nerve tissue	Transcutaneous electric stimulators deliver biphasic, monophasic, or polyphasic currents
Massage	Manipulation of soft tissue causes mechanical, physiologic, and psychological responses	Effleurage, petrissage, friction, tapotement, vibration, deep friction massage, acupressure massage
Traction	Produces separation of vertebral bodies to reduce pressure on spinal column and associated tissues and joints	Manual, mechanical, positional, wall-mounted, and inverted traction
Intermittent compression	Increased pressure controls or reduces swelling and reduces edema	Pneumatic inflatable sleeve and cryo-cuff

understanding of how various tissues progress through the healing process. An athletic trainer must consider the signs, symptoms, and various phases of the healing process when making a decision on which therapeutic modalities may be best used to treat an injured athletic (49). The common therapeutic modalities used by an athletic trainer are contained in Table 5.6. There are specific governmental laws regarding the use of therapeutic modalities, and athletic trainers must be aware of and follow those laws that dictate the use of the modalities. When used inappropriately, the therapeutic modalities may cause significant harm and injury and therefore athletic trainers must use great care when employing a therapeutic modality in the rehabilitation of an injured athlete (49).

Organization and Administration

Many athletic trainers often work in a position of autonomy. This requires the athletic trainer to be responsible for a variety of issues related to the organization and administration of an athletic training program including personnel management, professional development, facility management and design, budgeting, preparticipation physical examinations, medical record keeping, insurance, and public relations (51). It is important for athletic trainers to be responsive to these issues so that the best possible care can be provided to the athletes. The following sections provide an overview of some of the areas of responsibility.

Professional Development and Responsibility

Individuals who belong to a profession have a responsibility to maintain knowledge and skills at the current standard of care and practice. Athletic trainers must continue to advance their content knowledge and treatment skills through various continuing education activities and programs. For example, athletic trainers must maintain certification in emergency first aid and CPR to remain certified as an athletic trainer. Furthermore, athletic trainers must continue to obtain continuing education credits (CUEs) to satisfy the requirement of professional development established by the Board of Certification, Inc. Athletic trainers also have a responsibility to promote the profession to the general public. Because of the close relationship established with athletes, athletic trainers must often serve as a counselor to the athlete and his or her family members. These responsibilities are important in providing effective total care to the athlete (49).

Providing Coverage

Athletic trainers are responsible for providing coverage at the athletic training facility and at practices and competitions. The athletic training facility is generally a place where treatment and rehabilitation, preparation for competition, and injury management occurs. In college and university settings and often in commercial sports medicine facilities, the facility may be open all day. In a high school setting, the facility may be open only for a limited time. To provide the best care and protection to athletes, a certified athletic trainer should be in attendance at all practices and home and away competitions. Colleges and universities typically have sufficient personnel to provide concurrent coverage to several sports. In a high school setting, there are usually only one or two athletic trainers who must decide what sport practices or competitions will be covered during a specific time. In this situation, a schedule should be developed so that the athletic trainer is in attendance for part of the practice time (49).

Legal and Insurance Issues

Athletic trainers must keep current and accurate records as part of the comprehensive athletic training program. The essential components of the records to be kept include medical records and injury reports, treatment logs, personal information, injury evaluations and progress rates, supply and inventories, and annual program reports. A solid understanding of the laws governing confidentiality is critical to the effective functioning of the athletic trainer and athletic training program. The Health Insurance Portability and Accountability Act (HIPPA) and the Family Educational Rights and Privacy Act (FERPA) are responsible for protecting the medical and educational information of individuals, respectively. HIPPA regulates how anyone who has private health information about an individual (e.g., athlete) can share that information with others (33). HIPPA ensures that all individuals have certain rights over the control and use of their medical records, and provides a clear path of recourse if their medical privacy is compromised (49). FERPA is a law that protects the privacy of student's educational records. FERPA gives parents certain rights to their children's educational records until the child reaches 18 years of age or attends a postsecondary school. To release any information from a student's educational record, a school must have written permission from the parent or eligible student (49).

Given the significant changes in our healthcare system, it is becoming increasing important for athletic trainers and other exercise science professionals to understand a variety of issues related to healthcare delivery. All athletes should have a general health insurance policy, usually a family health insurance plan that covers illness, hospitalization, and emergency care (49). It is important for the school or university to ensure that personal health insurance is arranged for or purchased by athletes not covered under family policies (52). Accident insurance is available to student athletes and this covers accidents on school grounds while the student is in attendance. Professional liability insurance protects athletic trainers against damages that may arise from injuries occurring on school property and often covers claims of negligence on the part of individuals (15). Catastrophic insurance is often available to athletes through sports-governing agencies to assist with the costs associated with a permanent disability. Although catastrophic injuries are extremely rare, the extensive medical and rehabilitation care associated with these types of injuries can create a financial burden on the athlete and his/her family (49).

Athletic trainers may also acquire third-party payment for services rendered while working in a variety of settings, including hospitals, physician's offices, sports rehabilitation clinics, and colleges and university settings (32). In many states, certified athletic trainers are viewed as licensed healthcare professionals and therefore eligible for reimbursement for services by most third-party payers (i.e., health insurance companies). To facilitate this process, the athletic trainer must file insurance claims immediately and correctly (54). It is important that the athletic trainer keep accurate and up-to-date records when billing for and receiving reimbursement for treating an injury sustained to an athlete.

Working with the Team Physician

In most high school, college, and professional sports settings, the athletic trainer works primarily under the supervision of the team physician, usually a sports medicine physician (Figure 5.8). A working environment of mutual respect and cooperation between the athletic trainer and the team physician ensures that athletes receive the best care possible. Athletic trainers are often the first person to initiate contact with an injured athlete. They must be clear and concise in relaying information about the nature of the injury to the athlete to the sports medicine or primary care physician. The team physician, who is ultimately responsible for directing the total healthcare of the athlete will diagnose the extent of the injury and recommend follow-up care. Physicians in charge of sports teams should be aware of the progress of rehabilitation of

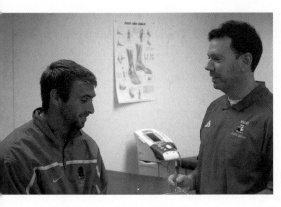

FIGURE 5.8 ▼ A team physician interviewing an athlete about an injury.

the athlete through the recovery period and make the final determination as to when an athlete can return to practice and competition (49). There are several roles and responsibilities that a team physician should assume with regard to injury prevention and the healthcare of the athlete that are presented in the next section of this chapter.

> ➤ *Thinking Critically*
> *What personal qualities and professional characteristics do you believe are important for athletic trainers to possess to fulfill their primary responsibilities?*

SPORTS MEDICINE

The professional practice of sports medicine has increased dramatically since the early 1980s, mostly in response to the demand for high quality healthcare for athletes. The number of sport-related injuries has increased, and many factors have contributed to this increase (41). Figures 5.1 and 5.2 provide the prevalence rates for injuries in high school and intercollegiate sports. Table 5.7 provides some suggested reasons for the increased number of sport-related injuries. Sports medicine physicians contribute to total athlete care by being an integral component of the primary athletic medicine team and working with other healthcare providers from orthopedics, physical medicine and rehabilitation, athletic training, biomechanics, cardiology, nutrition, optometry, pharmacology, physical therapy, exercise physiology, psychology, and podiatry (41).

Guidelines for Sports Medicine Physicians

Often the sports medicine physician serves as the leader of the primary athletic medicine team through his or her role as the team physician. The importance of this role has resulted in several organizations working together to provide several Team Physician Consensus Statements. These statements are used to guide the activities and responsibilities of the team physician (22–29). A list of the current Team Physician Consensus Statements written in collaboration through numerous professional organizations is provided in Table 5.8.

The first Team Physician Consensus Statement published in 2000 provides physicians, school administrators, team owners, the general public, and individuals who are responsible for making decisions regarding the medical care of

Table 5.7	Reasons for Increased Sports-related Injuries (41)
Increased participation in sports	
Increased numbers of previously sedentary individuals becoming active	
Increased variety of sports available	
Increased opportunities for participation	
Increased sophistication of participants in sports	
Increased participation intensity which often leads to increased risk of injury	
Athlete specialization at a young age leading to overuse injury	
Poor coaching and training methods leading to increased sport injuries	

Table 5.8	Team Physician Consensus Statements	
TOPIC		**YEAR PUBLISHED**
Team Physician Consensus Statement		2000
Sideline Preparedness for the Team Physician: A Consensus Statement		2001
The Team Physician and Conditioning of Athletes for Sports: A Consensus Statement		2001
The Team Physician and Return-To-Play Issues: A Consensus Statement		2002
Female Athlete Issues for the Team Physician: A Consensus Statement		2003
Mass Participation Event Management for the Team Physician: A Consensus Statement		2004
Psychological Issues Related to Injury in Athletes and the Team Physician: A Consensus Statement		2006
Concussion (Mild Traumatic Brain Injury) and the Team Physician: A Consensus Statement		2006

athletes and teams with guidelines for choosing a qualified team physician and an outline of the duties expected of a team physician (26). This consensus statement provides clear and concise information about the definition, qualifications, and duties of a team physician. Each of the subsequent consensus statements has identified important topics relevant to providing the best medical care for athletes at all levels of participation. Table 5.9 provides a summary of the responsibilities of the sports medicine team physician.

Advances in the Treatment of Sport-related Injuries

The primary responsibility of sports medicine professionals is to provide the best care possible to physically active individuals and athletes. There are several

Table 5.9	Responsibilities of the Team Physician (26,51)
RESPONSIBILITY	**PHYSICIAN ACTIONS**
Work with the athletic trainer	Supervise and advise athletic training staff; share philosophy regarding injury management and rehabilitation
Work with other sports medicine personnel	Provide the best possible care using the expertise of the primary sports medicine team
Compiling medical history	Oversee medical history; conduct physical examinations for each athlete
Diagnosing injury	Assume responsibility for diagnosing an injury; make recommendations for treatment to the athletic trainer and other sports medicine personnel
Deciding on disqualification and return to play	Determine when an athlete should be disqualified from competition and when that injured athlete may return to play
Attending practice and games	Attend as many practices, scrimmages, and competitions as possible; be available to other sports medicine personnel for consultation or advice
Commitment to sports and athletes	Demonstrate a strong affection and dedication to the athlete and sports
Academic Program Medical Director	Be responsible for the coordination and guidance of the medical aspects of an accredited athletic training education program

advances in the medical treatment of orthopedic injuries that have accomplished that aim. In most cases, these advancements have resulted in the development of minimally invasive procedures and a shorter recovery time for the athlete. In some instances, the careers of athletes have been saved or extended as a result of these advancements. Examples of these procedures include arthroscopy, ACL reconstruction, ulnar collateral ligament reconstruction, and chondrocyte implantation. Each is discussed in the following sections. The examples provided are not meant to be an inclusive list of significant developments in athlete care, but a sampling of advancements made over the years.

Arthroscopy

Arthroscopy or arthroscopic surgery is a minimally invasive procedure used to examine and treat damage to the interior of a joint. The procedure is performed by a sports medicine physician using an arthroscope and is shown in Figure 5.9. Arthroscopic surgery is used to evaluate and treat many orthopedic conditions such as torn floating cartilage, torn surface cartilage, and the ACL of the knee

Arthroscopy A minimally invasive surgical procedure used to repair damaged tissue.

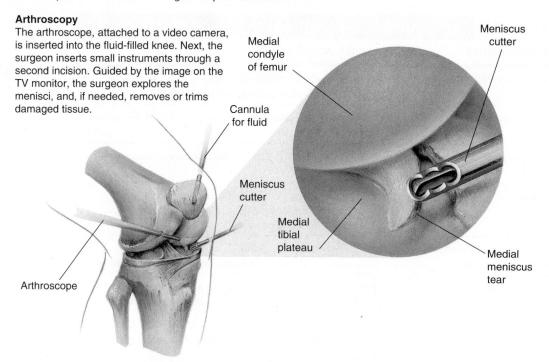

Arthroscopy
The arthroscope, attached to a video camera, is inserted into the fluid-filled knee. Next, the surgeon inserts small instruments through a second incision. Guided by the image on the TV monitor, the surgeon explores the menisci, and, if needed, removes or trims damaged tissue.

FIGURE 5.9 ▼ Arthroscopic surgery of the knee joint. (Asset provided by Anatomical Chart Co.)

joint. Arthroscopic surgery does not require the treated joint to be surgically opened. Only two small incisions are made, one for the arthroscope and one for the surgical instruments. The physician views the joint area on a video monitor and can diagnose and repair torn joint tissue including ligaments and cartilage. The postoperative recovery time is reduced and the surgery success rate is usually increased because there is reduced trauma to the connective tissue of the joint. This procedure is especially useful for athletes who require a rapid recovery time following surgery. Arthroscopic surgery is commonly used for joints of the knee, shoulder, elbow, wrist, ankle, and hip (10).

Anterior Cruciate Ligament Reconstruction

Anterior cruciate ligament reconstruction (ACL reconstruction) is a surgical procedure that uses a graft replacement of a torn ACL in the knee (Figure 5.10). A torn ACL dramatically decreases the stability and functional ability of the knee

Anterior cruciate ligament reconstruction A surgical procedure that uses a graft to replace a torn anterior cruciate ligament in the knee

Ulnar collateral ligament reconstruction A surgical procedure in which a ligament in the medial elbow is replaced with a tendon from elsewhere in the body.

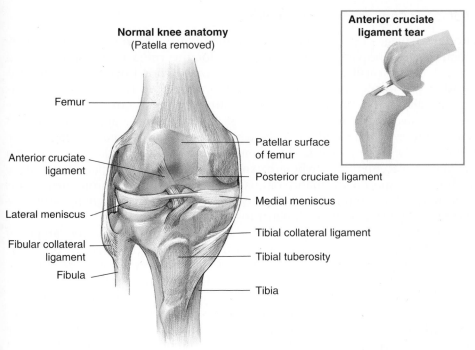

Normal knee anatomy
(Patella removed)

Anterior cruciate ligament tear

Femur

Anterior cruciate ligament

Lateral meniscus

Fibular collateral ligament

Fibula

Patellar surface of femur

Posterior cruciate ligament

Medial meniscus

Tibial collateral ligament

Tibial tuberosity

Tibia

FIGURE 5.10 ▼ Anterior cruciate ligament tear. (Asset provided by Anatomical Chart Co.)

joint and is usually treated medically. Torn ligaments do not heal, so surgery is often required to medically treat the injury. An ACL reconstruction requires a tissue graft from another part of the body. The torn ligament is removed from the knee before the graft is inserted, and attachment is made to the tibia and the femur. The types of surgery differ mainly in the type of graft that is used. Part or all of the ACL reconstruction is performed using arthroscopic surgery (10).

Ulnar Collateral Ligament Reconstruction

Ulnar collateral ligament reconstruction is a surgical procedure in which a ligament in the medial elbow is replaced with a tendon from elsewhere in the body, usually from the forearm, hamstring, knee, or foot. Damage to the ulnar collateral ligament usually occurs in response to the stress of the throwing motion. In the procedure, the replacement tendon is woven in a figure-eight pattern through tunnels that have been drilled in the ulna and humerus bones that are part of the elbow joint. Ulnar collateral ligament reconstruction is also known as Tommy John surgery. John was a pitcher for the Los Angeles Dodgers who was the first professional athlete to undergo the surgery, which was performed by Dr Jobe. Following surgery, an extensive rehabilitation process is undertaken by the athlete. ROM and resistance training exercises are performed for about 6 months. Thereafter, the athlete can begin a throwing program.

Autologous Chondrocyte Implantation

Articular cartilage covers the ends of the long bones of the body, is essentially frictionless, and provides a smooth surface for the contact and movement of bones. Articular cartilage is formed by cells called chondrocytes. **Autologous chondrocyte implantation** (ACI) is used to repair defects in the articular cartilage, usually in the knee. Patients eligible for treatment with ACI usually have joint pain, swelling, catching, or grinding. ACI is generally applied to patients between the ages of 15 and 55 years, with little or no additional damage to the knee joint. These are patients who do not have enough knee damage to need a total knee replacement, but who are experiencing considerable pain that may be impairing their sport performance or quality of life. Clinically appropriate patients are identified through traditional diagnostic methods, such as magnetic resonance imaging, X-ray evaluation, and an arthroscopic examination (8).

Once a patient is determined to be eligible for ACI, a **biopsy** sample of between 200 and 300 mg of the patient's articular cartilage is collected. The tissue sample is then sent to a laboratory, where the chondrocytes are separated from their surrounding cartilage and cultured for 4 to 5 weeks, generating between 5 and 10 million cells. The implantation of the cells is a surgical procedure in which the patient's joint is exposed by the orthopedic surgeon. The defect area is prepared by removing dead cartilage and smoothing the surrounding living cartilage. A piece of periosteum, the membrane that covers bone, is taken from the patient's tibia and attached over the prepared area. The cultured cells are injected by the surgeon under the periosteum, where they will grow and mature over time. In about 10 and 12 weeks, the patient can put full weight on the knee but complete recovery may take up to 1 year (8).

> ➤ *Thinking Critically*
>
> *Why is it important for sports medicine physicians to be knowledgeable of current research activities in medicine in general and in sports medicine in particular?*

CURRENT ISSUES IN ATHLETIC TRAINING AND SPORTS MEDICINE

With the rapid advances in the identification and treatment of sports-related injuries athletic trainers, sports medicine physicians, and other allied healthcare professionals must maintain current knowledge to provide the best possible healthcare to the athletes they work with. To remain certified, an athletic trainer must accumulate 75 CEUs over a 3-year period. Sports medicine physicians must accumulate continuing medical education (CME) credits to remain licensed. The number of CMEs required varies by state licensing boards. The CEUs and CMEs can be obtained by participating in several educational activities. Many of these activities focus on issues currently being addressed by researchers,

---

Autologous chondrocyte implantation A medical procedure used to repair damaged cartilage in joints of the body.

Biopsy The collection of body tissue using a special needle.

scholars, athletic trainers, and sports medicine professionals. Issues of particular importance to both athletic trainers and sports medicine physicians are wide ranging and include maintaining hydration status (11), preventing exertional heat illness (6), managing sudden cardiac arrest (17) and asthma (42) in athletes, and injury surveillance and prevention (31). The management of concussions sustained in sport competition and the increased incidence of ACL injures in female athletes are particularly important and discussed in greater detail in the following section.

Concussion Management

One of the most potentially severe injuries that can be sustained by an athlete is a concussion to the brain. Athletic trainers and sports medicine physicians must use the most recent scientific and clinic-based evidence for managing sport-related concussion. From 1968 to 1990, there was a significant reduction in brain and cervical spine fatalities in high school and college football players (20,44). The decrease was attributed to a variety of factors including rule changes, enhanced player education, improvements in equipment safety, and enhanced evaluation techniques by athletic trainers and sports medicine personnel (20). Science- and clinic-based information has been used to develop guidelines for reducing the incidence and severity of sport-related concussion and improving return-to-play decisions (20). The NATA and the ACSM have position and consensus statements on the medical management of sport-related concussions (20,28).

The most common sport-related concussion is the diffuse brain injury. This type of injury occurs when a linear acceleration–deceleration motion (side-to-side or front-to-back) causes the brain to be shaken within the skull (Figure 5.11). A sudden momentum change by the brain can result in tissue damage. Cerebral concussion can best be classified as a mild, diffuse injury that results in one or more of the following conditions: headache, nausea, vomiting, dizziness, balance problems, feeling "slowed down," fatigue, trouble sleeping, drowsiness, sensitivity to light or noise, blurred vision, difficulty remembering, or difficulty concentrating (55). Even though the purpose of bone is to protect the brain mass, it is in contact with the cranium that results in a concussion. Athletic trainers and sports medicine personnel are responsible for making on-site evaluations and often use a grading scale for assistance when making the decision on when to return to play (20).

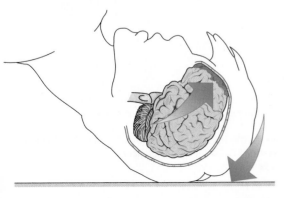

FIGURE 5.11 ▼ Example of how a concussion of the brain occurs.

Anterior Cruciate Ligament Injuries in Females

Since the passage of Title IX of the Educational Assistance Act more women are participating in sports. Unfortunately, an increased number of ACL injuries have accompanied the increased participation (3). Female athletes experience 4 to 10 times more ACL injuries than male athletes (14,19,34), and ACL injuries in female athletes are considerably higher than male athletes performing the same sports (3). The reasons for the different rates of injury in men and women are unclear, but may be related to differences in structure and knee alignment (60), ligament laxity (4,7,62), and muscle strength (40).

In the knee joint, an intercondylar notch (compartment) lies between the two rounded ends of the thigh bone (femoral condyles). The ACL moves within this notch, connecting the femur (thigh bone) and tibia (shin bone) and providing stability to the knee. It prevents the tibia from moving too far forward and from rotating too far inward under the femur (Figure 5.12). Women have a narrower

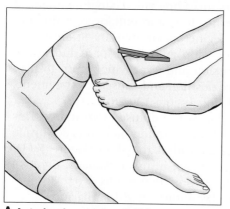

A Anterior drawer sign (ACL)

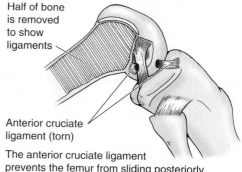

Half of bone is removed to show ligaments

Anterior cruciate ligament (torn)

The anterior cruciate ligament prevents the femur from sliding posteriorly on the tibia and hyperextension of the knee and limits medial rotation of the femur when the foot is on the ground, and the leg is flexed.

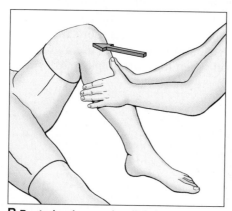

B Posterior drawer sign (PCL)

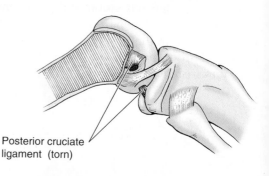

Posterior cruciate ligament (torn)

The posterior cruciate ligament prevents the femur from sliding anteriorly on the tibia, particularly when the knee is flexed.

FIGURE 5.12 ▼ Mechanism for an ACL injury in the knee. Anterior drawer sign (ACL) (**A**) and posterior drawer sign (**B**). (Modified from Moore KL, Dalley AF, II. *Clinical Oriented Anatomy.* 4th ed. Baltimore (MD): Lippincott Williams & Wilkins; 1999.)

notch than men have; therefore, the space for ACL movement is more limited in women than in men (59,60). Within this restricted space, the femoral condyles can more easily pinch the ACL as the knee bends and straightens out, especially during twisting and hyperextension movements. The pinching of the ACL in the joint can lead to its rupture or tear (59).

In the knee, the femur meets the tibia at an angle (called the quadriceps, or Q angle). The width of the pelvis determines the size of the Q angle. Females have a wider pelvis than males; therefore, the Q angle is greater in females compared to males. At this greater angle, forces are concentrated on the ligament each time the knee twists, increasing the risk for an ACL tear. A twisting injury in the knee of a male may only stretch the ACL; however, because of the greater Q angle, the same type of twisting injury in the knee of a female may cause a complete ACL tear (59,60).

Female hormones such as estrogen and progesterone allow for greater flexibility and looseness of muscles, tendons, and ligaments. This looseness may help prevent injuries because it enables certain muscles and joints to absorb more impact before being damaged. This looseness however, may contribute to ACL injuries in females. If the ligaments and muscles around the knee are too loose, they cannot absorb the stresses placed on them. In this situation, normal loads or forces may be transferred directly to the ACL, making it prone to tearing or rupture. In this situation, the ACL must maintain stability of the knee, and also compensate for the instability in a generally loose knee. During the menstrual cycle, hormone levels vary and may affect knee stability. Recent studies have shown that, at specific points within the menstrual cycle, the knee becomes looser than normal, and ACL rupture is more common (4,7,62).

When males and females compete in the same sporting events and at the same level of competition, they have nearly equal twisting and loading forces placed across their knee joints. Females, however, have less muscle strength in proportion to bone size than males have, and the muscles that help hold the knee stable are stronger in males than in females (40). Therefore, females rely less on the muscles and more on the ACL to hold the knee in place. In this situation, the ACL may have to absorb more forces making it more prone to rupture (40).

> ### ➤ *Thinking Critically*
> *In what ways have athletic training and sports medicine contributed to the understanding of how injuries occur during physical activity, exercise, sport, and athletic performances?*

> ### ➤ *Thinking Critically*
> *In what ways have athletic training and sports medicine professionals improved the rehabilitation management of individuals and athletes injured during exercise and sport competition?*

Developing an understanding of the best way to prevent ACL injuries in females is particularly important given the potentially debilitating nature of the injury and poor long-term prognosis following surgical reconstruction (30,39). Athletic trainers and sports medicine personnel are focusing efforts on identifying those factors that make females more susceptible than males to ACL injuries and on developing interventions to aid in the prevention of ACL injuries.

INTERVIEW

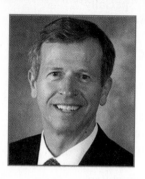

David H. Perrin, PhD, ATC, FACSM, Professor Department
of Exercise and Sport Science, University of North Carolina, Greensboro

Brief Introduction

I was an undergraduate physical education major at Castleton State College and a combination of courses (and great professors) in exercise physiology, kinesiology, and care/prevention of athletic injuries fostered my interested in athletic training. I attended graduate school at Indiana State University where I was able to study athletic training and become eligible to sit for the NATA certification examination. Although I was serving as director of the undergraduate athletic training education program at the University of Pittsburgh, I earned a PhD in exercise physiology, with a research focus on isokinetic muscle performance.

➤ **Why did you choose to become an athletic trainer?**

An undergraduate course in care and prevention of athletic injuries provided my first exposure to athletic training. The summer before my senior year in college, I attended an athletic training workshop in Buzzards Bay, Massachusetts directed by Koko Kassabian from Northeastern University. I knew at that point I wanted to pursue a career in athletic training.

➤ **Which individuals or experiences were most influential in your career development?**

Dr Charles Ash, my college basketball coach and exercise physiology and kinesiology professor, provided the spark for life-long learning. Kip Smith and Dr James McMaster provided the opportunity to launch my athletic training career at the University of Pittsburgh. Joe Gieck recruited me to the University of Virginia and provided the opportunity to direct an accredited master's degree program in athletic training and participate in the development of a fledgling doctoral program in sports medicine.

➤ **What are your most significance professional accomplishments?**

At the University of Pittsburgh, I had the opportunity to direct an undergraduate athletic training education program that became an academic major. At the University of Virginia, I advised nearly 200 master's degree students in athletic training. I helped to develop a doctoral program in sports medicine, founded the Sports Medicine/Athletic Training Research Laboratory, and mentored about 50 doctoral students, most of whom were certified athletic trainers. To watch these former students make their mark on the profession is what it is all about for me.

➤ **What advice would you have for an undergraduate student beginning to explore a career in athletic training?**

The allied health profession of athletic training is a terrific way to combine one's interest in sports, physical activity, health, and medicine. The curriculum is rigorous, and the clinical experiences are time consuming. As such, athletic training students must dedicate themselves beyond what is required for many other academic majors. Students should always be good ambassadors for the profession, and conduct themselves at the highest level of professional and ethical behaviors.

I N T E R V I E W

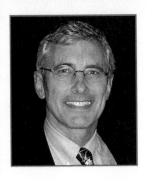

William Roberts, MS, MD, FACSM, Professor,
Department of Family Medicine and Community Health at the University of Minnesota Medical School; Program Director at Phalen Village Residency Clinic in St Paul, Minnesota; and past president of the American College of Sports Medicine.

Brief Introduction
I graduated from Rensselaer Polytechnic Institute in Troy, New York, with a degree in biology and the University of Minnesota Medical School with a Doctor of Medicine degree followed by a Master of Science in family medicine and community health. My special medical interests are in sports medicine and I have a subspecialty certificate in Sports Medicine. I am a charter member of the American Medical Society of Sports Medicine; a founding member and past president of the American Road Race Medical Society; an editorial board member of *Medicine and Science in Sports and Exercise, British Journal of Sports Medicine*, and *Clinical Journal of Sport Medicine*; a section editor for *Current Sports Medicine Reports*; the medical director for the Twin Cities Marathon; and the chair of the Sports Medicine Advisory Committee for the Minnesota State High School League and a member of the USA Soccer Cup Tournament Sports Medicine Advisory Committee. My research interests are in ice hockey and marathon injury.

➤ Why did you choose to become a sports medicine physician?

I enjoy taking care of athletes on the sidelines and in the office as a part of my family medicine practice, and that was my original intent. With time, I have come to realize that exercise is a critical component of a healthy lifestyle and I have integrated the philosophy that every patient is an athlete into my routine practice. This fits with current initiatives to promote exercise as medicine.

➤ Which individuals or experiences were most influential in your career development?

It would be nearly impossible to list all the physicians, scientists, and athletes who helped shaped my career. Three organizations deserve mention however, the American College of Sports Medicine, the Twin Cities Marathon, and the Minnesota State High School League each shaped my career with educational, administrative, and practice opportunities.

➤ What are your most significance professional accomplishments?

As the medical director of the Twin Cities Marathon, I have been able to develop care protocols for collapsed runners that are now used worldwide, to promote runner safety in hot and cold conditions, and to publish the outcomes of our care protocols to help runners in other races. As a member and now chair of the Minnesota State High School League Sports Medicine Advisory Committee, I have been able to promote on field measures to improve athlete safety with regard to environmental, nutrition, concussion, weight control and minimum wrestling certification, and skin issues. I became a fellow of the American College of Sports Medicine early in my career and was the first family physician elected to the office of President of ACSM.

➤ What advice would you have for an undergraduate student beginning to explore a career in exercise science or possibly as a sports medicine physician?

Find something you are passionate about and put your energy into developing a career around that

(Continued)

interest. Exercise science and sports medicine are very broad fields with great opportunities for those with interest. To become a sports medicine physician, you will have to enter one of the medical schools and complete a residency that will allow you to do a fellowship in the area. That is an 8 to 10 year commitment after college. I think that exercise science is a fantastic background for medical training and a career in sports medicine because it emphasizes the systems that are critical to life and health. I have been more than satisfied with my career choices of family medicine and sports medicine as I am constantly challenged by the changes in the field and the daily interactions with patients.

SUMMARY

- Athletic trainers have an important role to play in keeping an athlete safe and injury free during training and competition.
- As part of the primary care sports medicine team, athletic trainers are often the first to diagnose and respond to an injury.
- Working in close conjunction with other sports medicine personnel, the athletic trainer develops an individual rehabilitation program to help an injured athlete return to practice and competition.
- Sports medicine physicians work closely with other allied healthcare professionals to ensure that athletes are provided with the best medical care possible.
- Numerous advancements in the identification, treatment, and rehabilitation of injuries have enhanced the overall care provide to individuals who are injured during physical activity, exercise, sport, and athletic competition.

FOR REVIEW

1. Describe the difference between athletic training and sports medicine.
2. Describe how the NATA was formed.
3. How has the development of the certification program by the NATA enhanced the profession of athletic training?
4. Name three prominent associations in the area of Sports Medicine.
5. What are the six domains of athletic training?
6. What is the difference between a primary and a secondary survey of an injured athlete?
7. Why is detailed record keeping an important aspect of an athletic training program?

(Continued)

8. What does RICE stand for?

9. Define the following muscle actions:
   a. Isometric
   b. Isotonic
   c. Isokinetic
   d. Concentric
   e. Eccentric

10. What is the difference between open and closed chain kinetic exercises?

11. What are therapeutic modalities used for?

12. What recent medical advances have allowed sports medicine to improve the opportunity for athletes to return to play quickly from an injury to the knee joint?

13. Discuss the key issues related to the higher incidence rate of ACL injuries to women.

REFERENCES

1. Twentieth century orthopaedics. *AAOS Bulletin*. 1999;47:35–41.
2. American Medical Society for Sports Medicine. American Medical Society for Sports Medicine, 2007. Website retrieved from: http://www.newamssm.org/.
3. Arendt E, Dick RW. Knee injury patterns among men and women in collegiate basketball and soccer: NCAA data and review of literature. *Am J Sports Med*. 1995;23:694–701.
4. Arendt EA, Bershadsky B, Agel J. Periodicity of noncontact anterior cruciate ligament injuries during the menstrual cycle. *J Gend Specif Med*. 2002;5:19–26.
5. Berryman JW. Ancient and early influences. In: Tipton CM, editor. *Exercise Physiology: People and Ideas*. New York (NY): Oxford University Press; 2003. p. 1–38.
6. Binkley HM, Beckett J, Casa DJ, Kleiner DM, Plummer PE. National Athletic Trainers Association position statement: Exertional heat illness. *J Athl Train*. 2002;37:329.
7. Boden BP, Griffin LY, Garrett WE, Jr. Etiology and prevention of noncontact ACL injury. *Physician Sports Med*. 2000;28:53–60.
8. Brittberg M. Autologous chondrocyte implantation—technique and long-term follow-up. *Injury*. 2008;39:40–9.
9. Brooks GA, Fahey TD, White TP, Baldwin KM. *Exercise Physiology: Human Bioenergetics and Its Applications*. Mountain View (CA): Mayfield; 2000.
10. Brukner P, Khan K. *Clinical Sports Medicine*. Sydney, Australia: McGraw-Hill; 2007.
11. Casa DJ, Armstrong LE, Hillman S. National Athletic Trainer's Association position statement: Fluid replacement for athletes. *J Athl Train*. 2007;35:212.
12. Centers for Disease Control and Prevention. Nonfatal sports and recreation related injuries treated in emergency departments—United States, July 2000 to June 2001. *Morb Mortal*. 2002;51:736–40.
13. Centers for Disease Control and Prevention. Sports related injuries among high school athletes—United States, 2005–06 school year. *Morb Mortal*. 2006;55:1037–40.
14. Chandy TA, Grana WA. Secondary school athletic injury in boys and girls: A 3-year comparison. *Physician Sports Med*. 1985;13:106–11.
15. Cotton DJ. What is covered by your liability insurance policy? A risk management essential. *Exerc Stand Malpract Rep*. 2001;15:54.
16. Davies GAL, Wolfe LA, Mottola MF, MacKinnon C. Joint SOGC/CSEP clinical practice guideline: Exercise in pregnancy and the postpartum period. *Can J Appl Physiol*. 2003;28:329–41.
17. Drezner JA, Courson RW, Roberts WO, Mosesso VN, Link MS, Maron BJ. Inter-association task force recommendations on emergency preparedness and management of sudden cardiac arrest in high school and college athletic programs: A consensus statement. *J Athl Train*. 2007;42: 143–58.

18. Fleck SJ, Kraemer WJ. *Designing Resistance Training Programs*. Champaign: Human Kinetics Books; 2004.

19. Grindstaff TL, Hammill RR, Tuzson AE, Hertel J. Neuromuscular control training programs and noncontact anterior cruciate ligament injury rates in female athletes: A numbers-needed-to-treat analysis. *J Athl Train*. 2006;41:450–6.

20. Guskiewicz KM, Bruce SL, Cantu RC, et al. National Athletic Trainers' Association position statement: Management of sport-related concussion. *J Athl Train*. 2004;39:280–97.

21. Harris HA. *Greek Athletes and Athletics*. London: Hutchinson of London; 1964.

22. Herring SA, Bergfeld JA, Boyajian-O'Neill L, et al. Female Athlete Issues for the Team Physician: A Consensus Statement. *Med Sci Sports Exerc*. 2003;35:1785–93.

23. Herring SA, Bergfeld JA, Boyajian-O'Neill L, et al. Mass Participation Event Management for the Team Physician: A Consensus Statement. *Med Sci Sports Exerc*. 2004;36:2004–8.

24. Herring SA, Bergfeld JA, Boyd J, et al. The Team Physician and Conditioning of Athletes for Sports: A Consensus Statement. *Med Sci Sports Exerc*. 2001; 33:1789–93.

25. Herring SA, Bergfeld JA, Boyd J, et al. Sideline Preparedness for the Team Physician: A Consensus Statement. *Med Sci Sport Exerc*. 2001;33:846–9.

26. Herring SA, Bergfeld JA, Boyd J, et al. Team Physician Consensus Statement. *Med Sci Sports Exerc*. 2000;32:877–8.

27. Herring SA, Bergfeld JA, Boyd J, et al. The Team Physician and Return-To-Play Issues: A Consensus Statement. *Med Sci Sports Exerc*. 2002;34:1212–4.

28. Herring SA, Bergfeld JA, Boyland A, et al. Concussion (Mild Traumatic Brain Injury) and the Team Physician: A Consensus Statement. *Med Sci Sports Exerc*. 2006;38:395–9.

29. Herring SA, Boyajian-O'Neill L, Coppel DB, et al. Psychological Issues Related to Injury in Athletes and the Team Physician: A Consensus Statement. *Med Sci Sports Exerc*. 2006;38:2030–4.

30. Hewett TE, Myer GD. Reducing knee and anterior cruciate ligament injuries among female athletes. *J Knee Surg*. 2005;18:82–8.

31. Hootman JM, Dick RW, Agel J. Epidemiology of collegiate injuries for 15 sports: Summary and recommendations for injury prevention initiatives. *J Athl Train*. 2007;42:311–9.

32. Hunt V. Reimbursement efforts continue steady progress. *NATA News*. October 2002:10–2.

33. Hunt V. Meeting clarifies HIPPA restrictions. *NATA News*. February 2003:10.

34. Hutchinson MR, Ireland ML. Knee injuries in female athletes. *Sports Med*. 1995;19:288–302.

35. Jackson MD. Rehabilitation. In: McKeag DB, Moeller JL, editors. *ACSM's Primary Care Sports Medicine*. Philadelphia: Lippincott, Williams & Wilkins; 2007. p. 563–93.

36. Kettenbach G. *Writing SOAP Notes*. Philadelphia (PA): Davis; 1995.

37. Knight KL. *Cryotherapy in Sports Injury Management*. Champaign (IL): Human Kinetics; 1995.

38. Matheson GO. Reflecting on 30 years of moving forward. *Physician Sports Med*. 2003;31:1–2.

39. McAlindon R. 1999 ACL injuries in women [Online]. Hughston Sports Medicine Foundation; 1999.

40. McClay-Davis I. Ireland ML. ACL research retreat: The gender bias. *Clin Biomech*. 2001;16:937–59.

41. McKeag DB. Moeller JL. Primary care perspective. In: McKeag DB, Moeller JL, editors. *ACSM's Primary Care Sports Medicine*. Philadelphia (PA): Lippincott, Williams & Wilkins; 2007. p. 3–9.

42. Miller MG, Weiler JM, Baker R, Collins J, D'Alonzo G. National Athletic Trainers' Association Position Statement: Management of Asthma in Athletes. *J Athl Train*. 2005;40:224–45.

43. Moeller JL, McKeag DB. Preparticipation screening. In: McKeag DB, Moeller JL, editors. *ACSM's Primary Care Sports Medicine*. Philadelphia (PA): Lippincott, Williams & Wilkins; 2007. p. 55–79.

44. Mueller FO, Cantu RC. Nineteenth Annual Report of the National Center for Catastrophic Sports Injury Research: Fall 1982-Spring 2001. Chapel Hill (NC): National Center for Catasrophic Sports Injury Research; 2002.

45. Mujika I, Padilla S. Detraining: Loss of training-induced physiological and performance adaptations. Part II. *Sports Med*. 2000;30:145–54.

46. O'Shea ME. *A History of the National Athletic Trainers Association*. Greenville (NC): National Athletic Trainers Association; 1980.

47. OSHA. The OSHA bloodborne pathogens standards. *Fed Regist*. 1991;55:64175.

48. Prentice WE. Mobilization and traction techniques in rehabilitation. In: Prentice WE, editor. *Rehabilitation Techniques in Sports Medicine and Athletic Training*. St. Louis: McGraw-Hill; 2004.

49. Prentice WE. *Arnheim's Principles of Athletic Training: A Competency-based Approach*. New York (NY): McGraw-Hill Companies; 2006.

50. Prentice WE. On-the-field acute care and emergency procedures. In: *Arnheim's Principles of Athletic Training: A Competency Based Approach*. New York (NY): McGraw-Hill; 2006. p. 319–59.

51. Prentice WE. The athletic trainer and the sports medicine team. In: *Arnheim's Principles of Athletic Training*. New York (NY): McGraw-Hill; 2006. p. 1–43.

52. Rankin J, Ingersoll C. *Athletic Training Management: Concepts and Applications*. New York (NY): McGraw-Hill; 2000.

53. Rankin JM. Athletic training. In: Brown SP, editor. *Introduction to Exercise Science*. Philadelphia (PA): Lippincott, Williams & Wilkins; 2001. p. 289–308.

54. Ray R. *Management Strategies in Athletic Training*. Champaign (IL): Human Kinetics; 2000.

55. Report of the Quality Standards Subcommittee of the American Academy of Neurology. Practice parameter: The management of concussion in sports (summary statement). *Neurology*. 1997;48:581–5.

56. Rivera J. Open vs. closed kinetic chain rehabilitation of the lower extremity. *J Sport Rehabil*. 1994;3:154.

57. Roberts WO. Sports medicine's primary focus: Health for all. *Physician Sports Med*. 2003;31:1–2.

58. Schnirring L. Mending injured athletes: A track record of orthopedic advances. *Physician Sports Med*. 2003;31:1–3.

59. Swenson EJ, Jr. Knee injuries. In: McKeag DB, Moeller JL, editors. *ACSM's Primary Care Sports Medicine*. Philadelphia (PA): Lippincott, Williams & Wilkins; 2007. p. 461–90.

60. Uhorchak JM, Scoville CR, Williams GN, Arciero RA, St Pierre P, Taylor DC. Risk factors associated with noncontact injury of the anterior cruciate ligament: A prospective four-year evaluation. *Am J Sports Med*. 2003;31:831–42.

61. Wappes JR. 30 years of sports medicine and *sports-medicine*. *Phys Sports Med*. 2003;31:1–4.

62. Wojtys EM, Huston LJ, Boynton MD, Spindler KP, Lindenfeld TN. The effect of the menstrual cycle on anterior cruciate ligament injuries in women as determined by hormone levels. *Am J Sports Med*. 2002;30:182–8.

Exercise and Sport Nutrition

After completing this chapter you will be able to:

1. Describe the importance of proper nutrition as it relates to enhancing health, physical activity, exercise, sport, and athletic performance.

2. Describe the key highlights in the historic development of nutrition and sport nutrition.

3. Identify the basic nutrients for healthy nutritional intake.

4. Explain the key issues in measuring nutritional intake.

5. Identify the key nutritional issues for an active individual.

6. Identify the key nutritional issues for a competitive athlete.

Proper nutrition is important for optimal health and successful performance in sport and athletic competition. As a society, we are becoming increasingly aware of the role of good nutrition for decreasing the risk of various disease conditions and improving the overall health of individuals across the lifespan. Athletes, coaches, and sport nutritionists are also paying closer attention to the influence of proper nutrition for enhancing training and improving performance during all types of sport and athletic competitions.

Nutrition is defined as the science that interprets the connection between food and the function of the living organism (35). Exercise and sport nutrition exist under the umbrella of exercise science. Nutrition as a profession consists of a number of subspecialty areas including clinical nutrition, nutritional biochemistry, community nutrition, food science nutrition, nutritional management, and nutritional counseling (83).

The terms diet and nutrition are often used interchangeably in today's society, although they have different meanings. In general, diet and nutrition are used to convey a description of the foods and beverages we consume (Figure 6.1). However, the word "diet" for many individuals means a restriction of food or calorie intake, which often results in one of the most commonly used phrases in today's society "I will start my diet tomorrow." Nutrition is a widely used term to describe all aspects related to food consumption (79). Nutrition is used in medicine and biologic sciences and by politicians, economists, social and behavioral scientists, and consumers (73).

Good health and a reduced risk for numerous diseases depend largely on proper nutrition (35). Nutritional intake (i.e., food consumption) strongly influences the development and progression of chronic diseases and poor health conditions such as coronary heart disease, hypertension, osteoporosis, a variety of cancers, and obesity (62,63). Research evidence supports relationships between elevated serum cholesterol levels and coronary heart disease (31,87), reduced calcium intake and osteoporosis (38), consumption of dietary fats and certain cancers (73), and excess calorie intake and obesity (11). Figure 6.2 shows the relationship between nutritional intake and several common disease conditions.

Proper nutrition is also important for successful sport and athletic performance. Athletes and coaches are becoming increasingly aware of how the macronutrients, vitamins, minerals, and fluid intake can improve sport and athletic performance during both training and competition. Proper nutritional intake

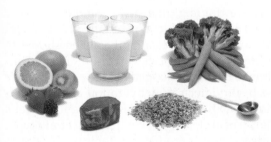

FIGURE 6.1 ▼ Optimal nutrition requires eating a variety of items from the food groups. (Photo by Photodisc/ Nicholas Eveleigh/Getty Images.)

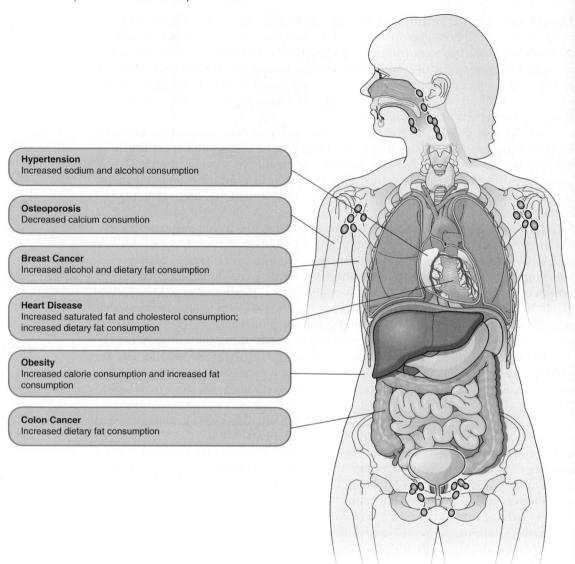

Hypertension
Increased sodium and alcohol consumption

Osteoporosis
Decreased calcium consumtion

Breast Cancer
Increased alcohol and dietary fat consumption

Heart Disease
Increased saturated fat and cholesterol consumption;
increased dietary fat consumption

Obesity
Increased calorie consumption and increased fat
consumption

Colon Cancer
Increased dietary fat consumption

FIGURE 6.2 ▼ The relationship between nutritional intake and several disease conditions.

allows for the maintenance of appropriate training intensity, promotes recovery from training and competition, enhanced energy production, and the development of skeletal muscle tissue. For example, carbohydrate loading has been shown to increase muscle glycogen levels and improve certain types of endurance performance (43). Fluid and carbohydrate intake during prolonged exercise can enhance performance and prevent the adverse health effects of dehydration and carbohydrate depletion (23). Adequate protein intake has the potential to enhance skeletal muscle development and the performance of athletes who compete in certain types of events that rely on muscular strength and power production. Table 6.1 illustrates how certain nutritional strategies can enhance sport and athletic performance.

Table 6.1	Nutritional Strategies for Enhancing Sport and Athletic Performance	
NUTRITIONAL STRATEGY	**EFFECTS ON PHYSIOLOGIC FUNCTION AND PERFORMANCE**
Increased carbohydrate consumption prior to prolonged exercise	Maximizes muscle glycogen prior to exercise, which delays glycogen depletion and fatigue
Carbohydrate and fluid ingestion during exercise	Spares muscle glycogen, maintains blood glucose concentration, maintains plasma volume, and prevents dehydration and fatigue
Adequate protein intake when combined with a resistance exercise training program	Maximizes lean mass development

Optimal nutritional intake consists of consuming the appropriate nutrients for tissue maintenance, repair, and growth and for providing the body with sufficient energy without an excess energy intake (61). There is no optimal nutritional intake for everyone as daily nutritional requirements will vary based on age, physical activity levels, gender, body size, and various health conditions such as diabetes or **hypercholesterolemia** (61). Exercise science professionals can play an important role in promoting proper nutrition for improving health and enhancing sport and athletic performance.

HISTORY OF NUTRITION

Though much has been realized about individual nutritional requirements in the last several decades, interest in diet and nutrition can be traced back in history for thousands of years. Awareness of the importance of nutrition and diet in human health can be observed in the recordings of the ancient Greeks and Romans (79). Many Greek writings in this era refer to energy requirements and a balanced diet for health, and that certain diseases can be treated with diet. For example, Hippocrates in the fourth century BC, formed a theory about the relationship between food and health that was followed for centuries (17). These early writings in nutrition laid the foundation for the expansion of our understanding of how food intake affects health, sport, and athletic performance.

Early History of Nutrition for Health

The word "nutrition" in its various forms of the English language appears to have originated somewhere between the fifteenth and sixteenth century. Throughout the seventeenth and eighteenth centuries, physicians and scientists used nutritional

Hypercholesterolemia The presence of high levels of cholesterol in the blood.

interventions as part of experiments on diseased individuals. For example, it was observed during this time period that increased iron intake could improve anemia and citrus fruit consumption could cure scurvy. During the early nineteenth century, François Magendie noted that dogs fed on only carbohydrate and fat lost body protein and died within a few weeks but dogs fed on a diet of carbohydrate, fat, and protein survived. This experiment demonstrated the importance of protein in the diet of animals (79).

In the early twentieth century, "diet" and "dietetics" were terms used widely when referring to problems relating to food (79) and several important advancements were made. In 1903, W.O. Atwater and Francis Gano Benedict invented a respiration chamber (Figure 6.3) and performed very accurate **direct calorimetry** and **indirect calorimetry** measurements of food metabolism and energy balance (67). These experiments formed the foundation for future work in the areas of energy intake and energy expenditure. In 1936, Eugene Du Bois coined the term **basal metabolic rate** and examined the relationship between age, gender, and weight (74). In 1937, Clive McCay demonstrated that restricting energy intake of rats by 33% led to increased longevity (by 25%), especially if simple carbohydrates were restricted (67). Ancel Keys from the University of Minnesota studied the influence of diet on health, in particular, the effects of different kinds of dietary fat on health. Keys was closely associated with two famous diets: Keys rations (more commonly known as K-rations), formulated as balanced meals for combat soldiers in World War II, and the "Mediterranean diet," which he popularized. Keys was also involved in the Minnesota Starvation Experiment, that provided considerable insight into the physiologic and psychological effects of severe and prolonged dietary restriction and the effectiveness of dietary rehabilitation strategies (46).

The recognition of nutrition as an academic discipline occurred in 1933 with the founding of the American Institute of Nutrition (AIN), which was instrumental in promoting nutrition as a science. The founding members of the AIN identified their disciplinary fields as nutrition, animal nutrition, chemistry, agricultural chemistry, biochemistry, physiologic chemistry, physiology, and anatomy. This diversity of background remains evident today with individuals from a wide variety of disciplines working in the field of nutrition and nutrition science. Although AIN has changed

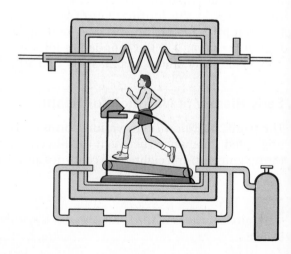

FIGURE 6.3 ▼ A human calorimeter.

its name to the American Society for Nutrition, it remains a premier research society dedicated to improving the quality of life through the science of nutrition (79).

During the early twentieth century, several laboratories were established to advance the understanding of nutrition. In 1904, The Nutrition Laboratory at the Carnegie Institute was created to study nutrition and energy metabolism. Established in 1927, the Harvard Fatigue Laboratory allowed for the further expansion of scientific research in the area of exercise and sport nutrition (78). Early scientific research in nutrition aimed to identify all the essential nutrients and the dietary requirements for each nutrient. Additional work was done to determine the distribution of each nutrient in various foods in an effort to define a nutritionally adequate diet or analyze a diet and determine whether it was nutritionally balanced for good health. This early research provided the foundation for the various computer databases that exist to provide both diet analysis and nutritional prescription (79).

Recent History of Nutrition for Health

The role of nutrition, particularly as it relates to chronic disease development, has received considerable attention over the last 50 years. **Epidemiologic studies** have provided us with much understanding of how various nutritional patterns influence the development of cardiovascular disease, cancer, and other diseases affected by individual's food intake (39). The Framington Heart Study (44), the Harvard Alumni Study (69), and the National Cholesterol Education Program (87) have helped identify specific dietary factors that are associated with cardiovascular disease including the consumption of high levels of saturated fat and cholesterol (62,63).

One of the most significant long-term epidemiologic studies about nutrition and health is the National Health and Nutrition Examination Survey (NHANES). NHANES began as a result of the National Health Survey Act of 1956, which was intended to establish a continuing National Health Survey to obtain information about the health status of U.S. citizens, including the services received for or because of health conditions. The first three National Health Examination Surveys (NHES I, II, and III) were conducted between 1959 and 1970. In response to numerous nutrition-related studies, the U.S. Department of Health, Education, and Welfare established a continuing National Nutrition Surveillance System in 1969 in an effort to measure the nutritional status of the U.S. population and monitor changes over time. The National Nutrition Surveillance System was merged with the National Health Examination Survey creating NHANES (64). Table 6.2 provides the dates and specific target groups and foci of the various surveys. Data from NHANES have

Direct calorimetry The measurement of heat produced by a chemical reaction or by the body.

Indirect calorimetry The measurement of energy production by the body using the amount of oxygen consumed and carbon dioxide produced.

Basal metabolic rate The level of metabolism, as measured by energy expenditure, required to maintain the normal physiologic functions of the body.

Epidemiologic studies The study of factors affecting the health and disease of large groups of individuals.

Table 6.2	Overview of NHANES Surveys from 1959 to the Present
SURVEY AND YEARS	**SPECIFIC FOCUS**
NHES I (1959–1962)	Selected chronic diseases of adults between 18 and 79 years of age
NHES II (1963–1965)	Growth and development of children between 6 and 11 years of age
NHES III (1966–1970)	Growth and development of adolescents between 12 and 17 years of age
NHANES I, (1971–1975)	Extensive dietary intake and nutritional status were collected by interview, physical examination, and a battery of clinical tests and measurements
NHANES II (1976–1980)	Expanded the age of the first NHANES sample by including individuals as young as 6 months of age; children and adults living at or below the poverty level were sampled at higher rates than their proportions in the general population ("oversampled") because these individuals were thought to be at particular nutritional risk
NHANES III (1988–1994)	Included infants as young as 2 months of age, with no upper age limit on adults; African Americans, Mexican Americans, infants, children, and those over 60 years old were oversampled; NHANES III also placed a greater emphasis on the effects of environment on health
1999, NHANES became a continuous survey	Surveys are conducted over a period of approximately 4 years with a break of at least 1 year between survey periods

provided considerable insight into how dietary patterns have changed during the past 50 years and how these changes have contributed to the development of disease conditions.

The American Dietetic Association (ADA) has been instrumental in promoting the dietetics profession, the enhanced understanding of nutrition, and the education of nutritional professionals. The ADA was founded in 1917 during a meeting of approximately 100 dieticians in Cleveland, Ohio. The first president, Lulu Grace Graves, helped establish the initial areas of practice: (a) dieto-therapy, (b) teaching, (c) social welfare, and (d) administration. These areas of practice remain at the heart of the mission of the ADA, which is to serve the public by promoting optimal nutrition, health, and well-being (17). Federal, state, and many private foundations continue to support nutritional science research in an effort to help better understand the role of nutrition intake in disease development and disease risk reduction.

> ➤ *Thinking Critically*
> *In what ways has our knowledge about nutrition contributed to a broader understanding of how individuals can improve physical fitness and promote good health?*

Sport Nutrition

The role of nutrition for enhancing sport and athletic performance has a rich history. The areas that have received the greatest attention and contributed most significantly to the development of sport nutrition have been carbohydrate and protein consumption, and vitamin and mineral supplementation. For example, historic recordings (ca. 500–400 BC) indicate that consumption of deer liver and lion heart would enhance bravery, speed, and strength in the athlete and warrior (5,60,81). Although early writings demonstrate people's awareness of the role of nutrition in promoting physical development, most of what we know about the role of nutrition for enhancing sport and athletic performance comes from more recent times. Early in the twentieth century, scholars described the importance of carbohydrate during prolonged exercise and the role of carbohydrates in maintaining adequate stores of muscle and liver glycogen (22,50). During the 1924 Boston Marathon, measures of blood glucose were made of the first 20 runners to cross the finish line. Many of the runners displayed hypoglycemia, symptoms of fatigue, stupor, and poor concentration (55). During the following year, runners were given large amounts of carbohydrate the day before the race and sugar candy during the race. The result of this nutritional strategy was a normalization of blood glucose levels and the alleviation of the symptoms of nervous system fatigue and poor concentration (34). The development and use of the **muscle biopsy** procedure by Swedish researchers in the 1960s allowed for the determination of how fast muscle glycogen was depleted during exercise (2). This information eventually led to the development of the carbohydrate loading procedure for improving endurance performance and the influence of carbohydrate consumption on muscle glycogen replenishment (9). Continued research in this area led to the use of sports drinks for delaying muscle fatigue and improving performance during prolonged exercise (86).

Experiments conducted in the 1940s demonstrated that increased protein consumption could enhance the development of skeletal muscle mass in individuals involved in resistance exercise training (5,49). Throughout the 1950s and 1960s, the increased consumption of milk and beef products led to greater protein consumption (5). The development of isolated protein powders and amino acids in the 1970s and early 1980s resulted in athletes using these products for increasing dietary protein intake. Additional research in the 1990s led to many athletes closely matching amino acid intake and resistance exercise training in an effort to secure the greatest enhancement of lean muscle mass development (5). The use of amino acid supplements by all types of athletes continues into the twenty first century, with athletes mixing various amino acids and growth-promoting agents in an effort to maximize protein synthesis and skeletal muscle mass during training.

Many water- and fat-soluble vitamins were discovered during the 1930s. The use of these compounds quickly spread through the sporting world so that by 1939, cyclists in the Tour de France reported performing better after taking vitamin supplements (60). Early scientific research did not support the use of vitamin supplements for enhancing athletic performance, but athletes remained committed to heavy vitamin supplementation. For example, during the 1972 Olympic Games athletes reported consuming large quantities of vitamins in an effort to enhance performance during competition (24). Athletes continue to use high doses of

Muscle biopsy A procedure whereby a small sample of muscle tissue is collected using a special needle.

vitamin supplementation in an effort to improve performance or at the very least as an insurance mechanism to ensure adequate levels of vitamins in the body (61).

Within the ADA, a dietary practice group called the Sports, Cardiovascular, and Wellness Nutritionists (SCAN) was established in 1981. The SCAN Dietetic Practice Group works to promote healthy, active lifestyles through excellence in dietetics practice in sports, cardiovascular, and wellness nutrition, and the prevention and treatment of disordered eating. Registered dieticians can also acquire board certification as a Specialist in Sports Dietetics indicating they are specialty trained to work with high school, collegiate, Olympic, and professional athletes to enhance sport performance (http://www.scandpg.org/).

Exercise and sport nutritionists working with other exercise science and allied health professionals continue to explore ways that nutrition can be used to promote good health and improve sport and athletic performance. Future research work and advancements in policy initiatives and educational program development will be a central focus as nutrition is used to address diet-related health problems, and individuals try and meet the dietary guidelines for good nutritional practices. Table 6.3 provides a list of significant recent events in the historic development of nutrition for health, sport, and athletic competition.

➤ *Thinking Critically*

In what ways has our knowledge about nutrition contributed to a broader understanding of how to enhance sport and athletic performance?

Table 6.3	Significant Events in the Historic Development of Nutrition for Health and Sport
YEAR	**EVENT**
1903	W.O. Atwater and Francis Gano Benedict invented a respiration chamber
1904	The Nutrition Laboratory at the Carnegie Institute was created to study nutrition and energy metabolism
1917	American Dietetic Association was founded
1925	First experiment on carbohydrate supplementation during exercise was conducted at the Boston Marathon
1927	Harvard Fatigue Laboratory was established
1933	American Society for Nutrition was founded
1937	Clive McCay demonstrated that restricting energy intake of rats by 33% led to increased longevity
1939	First report of vitamin supplementation improving performance in cyclists in the Tour de France
1956	First NHANES was administered
1981	The SCAN group of the ADA was formed
1999	NHANES became a continuous survey

BASIC NUTRIENTS

Each of us needs to consume adequate amounts of the **macronutrients** and micronutrients in our diet to ensure proper physiologic and structural function and good health. Although individual circumstances and preferences will dictate food intake, many individuals will meet the **recommended dietary intake** (RDI) for carbohydrate, fat, protein, vitamins, and minerals by consuming a diet that is consistent with general nutrition guidelines. Proper nutritional intake promotes optimal growth and development, appropriate energy balance and body composition, health and longevity, and normal physiologic function. Table 6.4 provides a list of the macro- and micronutrients and their primary functions related to physical activity, exercise, sport and athletic competition. The information contained in the following sections is designed to provide an overview of macro- and micronutrient function.

Carbohydrate

Carbohydrate is a macronutrient that provides energy to the body. Dietary carbohydrates exist in two forms: simple and complex. **Simple carbohydrates**, sometimes called simple sugars, come from the carbohydrates found in milk and

Table 6.4	The Macronutrients and Micronutrients and their Primary Functions Related to Physical Activity, Exercise, Sport, and Athletic Performance	
NUTRIENT	**PRIMARY FUNCTION RELATED TO PHYSICAL ACTIVITY, EXERCISE, SPORT, AND ATHLETIC PERFORMANCE**
Carbohydrates	• Provide energy during moderate to high intensity physical activity or exercise
Fats	• Provide energy during low to moderate intensity exercise
Protein	• Important component of skeletal muscle • Part of various compounds that regulate metabolism during rest and exercise
Vitamins	• Important for controlling metabolic pathways that produce energy during rest and exercise
Minerals	• Part of the structure of bone • Part of various compounds that regulate metabolism during rest and exercise

Macronutrient A chemical substance (such as protein, carbohydrate, or fat) required in relatively large quantities in an individual's daily nutritional intake.

Recommended dietary intake The recommended intake level of a nutrient that is considered to meet the daily needs of nearly all healthy individuals.

Simple carbohydrate A carbohydrate, such as glucose, that consists of a single monosaccharide unit.

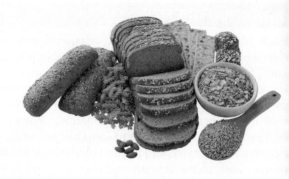

FIGURE 6.4 ▼ Complex carbohydrates.
(Photo by Tetra Images/Getty Images.)

fruit. A large percentage of the simple sugars consumed in the diet of individuals living in the United States are added to processed foods during the manufacturing process. These refined sugars, with sucrose and high fructose corn syrup being most popular, are frequently added to soft drinks, fruit drinks, candies, and desert items. **Complex carbohydrates**, also called starches, are found in whole grains (Figure 6.4) and certain vegetables such as potatoes, beans, and peas. Complex carbohydrates are generally considered healthier and more beneficial when performing exercise and participating in sport and athletic activities. Complex carbohydrates also contain large amounts of vitamins and minerals and result in a slower release into the body (35).

When carbohydrates are consumed in the diet, they are broken down in the gastrointestinal tract and absorbed in the small intestine as small six-carbon molecules such as glucose and fructose. Glucose is the most common and useful form of carbohydrates in the body. Glucose provides energy to the various tissues of the body in one of two forms; blood glucose or liver and muscle glycogen. Although almost all cells can use carbohydrate, fat, or protein for energy, the brain and nervous tissue depend almost exclusively on glucose to provide energy (35).

The storage form of glucose in the body is called glycogen. The liver and the skeletal muscle are the primary tissues for glycogen synthesis and storage. Normal fasting blood glucose levels are between 70 and 100 mg·dL^{-1}. When blood glucose decreases below 70 mg·dL^{-1} the condition of **hypoglycemia** occurs and symptoms such as drowsiness, irritability, and fatigue may appear. The body responds to hypoglycemia primarily by breaking down liver glycogen into glucose and releasing it into the blood. At the same time, various signals from the brain stimulate hunger and the desire for the individual to eat. Combined, these two actions serve to elevate blood glucose levels (35).

When blood glucose levels increase after food consumption, the body releases insulin from the beta cells of the pancreas. Insulin works with protein receptors (called glucose transport proteins) in the tissues of the body to promote glucose uptake for immediate energy use or conversion to glycogen for storage. This process results in a return of blood glucose to normal levels. A disease condition called diabetes mellitus occurs when either the pancreas does not produce sufficient amounts of insulin (**Type 1 diabetes mellitus**) or the insulin does not facilitate glucose uptake into the tissues of the body (**Type 2 diabetes mellitus**).

f the fasting blood glucose level is $100\,mg\cdot dL^{-1}$ to $125\,mg\cdot dL^{-1}$, the individual may have impaired fasting glucose, commonly known as prediabetes. A fasting blood glucose level of $126\,mg\cdot dL^{-1}$ or higher is consistent with either type 1 or type 2 diabetes when accompanied by classic signs and symptoms of diabetes, including increased thirst or hunger, frequent urination, weight loss or blurred vision (35).

Fat

Dietary fat and cholesterol are critical to the normal functioning of body tissues and overall good health of the body. Dietary fat is vital for the absorption of the fat-soluble vitamins (A, D, E, and K) and to provide key biochemical precursors that can be transformed into essential cellular products. Dietary fat also contributes to the flavor and texture of foods, and it is believed that fat maintains **satiety** and helps to keep us from being hungry. Fat also provides a concentrated form of energy for our body. Cholesterol is important in the formation of cell membranes and some hormones in the body (35).

Most consumed fats are broken down in the gastrointestinal tract into free fatty acids and **monoglycerides** for absorption in the small intestine. Dietary fat and cholesterol enter the blood stream and travel to the liver for further processing by the body. The fat absorbed from the small intestine is largely stored in the liver and **adipose tissue** and is later used in the body to provide energy at rest and during physical activity and exercise. Cholesterol travels through the circulatory system for use by various tissues of the body (35).

Excessive intake of dietary fat can result in the development of assorted disease conditions, including atherosclerosis, hyperlipidemia, and obesity. The consumption of a high fat diet, which often results in high total calorie intake, has been shown to be related to excessive weight gain and the development of obesity (6). Individuals who are obese have a higher risk of developing cardiovascular disease, type 2 diabetes, and certain types of cancer (16,28). The consumption of a high fat diet can also lead to excessive levels of blood lipids. The conditions of **hyperlipidemia** and **hypercholesterolemia** can increase an individual's risk of cardiovascular disease and stroke (26,87).

Complex carbohydrate A carbohydrate, such as sucrose or starch, that consists of two or more monosaccharide units.

Hypoglycemia An abnormally low level of sugar in the blood.

Type 1 diabetes mellitus Condition characterized by elevated blood glucose levels that are the result of a lack of insulin production by the pancreas.

Type 2 diabetes mellitus A metabolic disorder that is primarily characterized by insulin resistance, relative insulin deficiency, and hyperglycemia.

Satiety The feeling of fullness after eating.

Monoglycerides A chemical structure containing one glycerol molecule and one fatty acid molecule.

Adipose tissue The cells of the body that store fat derived from excess calorie intake.

Hyperlipidemia The presence of high levels of fat in the blood.

Hypercholesterolemia The presence of high levels of cholesterol in the blood.

Protein

Like carbohydrate and fat, protein is important for normal health and functioning of the body. Proteins are made from individual amino acids that are connected together to form chains. There are at least 20 individual amino acids that can be combined to form several proteins for use by the body. Proteins are primarily used for tissue growth and repair. As all tissues of the body contain proteins, this is an extremely important function. Proteins also form hormones and protein receptors that work to control a range of physiologic functions of the body. Proteins can also be broken down into amino acids, which can be further metabolized to provide energy for the body (35).

Dietary proteins come from animal and certain vegetable sources (Figure 6.5). During the digestion process, these proteins break down into individual amino acids and small chain proteins (3 to 6 amino acids in length). Once in the circulatory system, these amino acids and small proteins can be delivered to the tissues of the body. The defining characteristic of amino acids is the chemical amino group (NH_3) that exists on the compound. Our bodies are able to chemically transfer the amino group from one amino acid to another compound and create new amino acids, a process called **transamination**. Transamination allows for the formation of **nonessential amino acids** in the body. **Essential amino acids** cannot be made in the body and must be consumed in the diet on a daily basis (35).

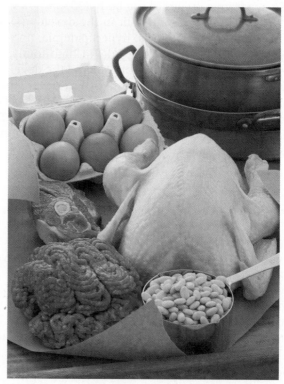

FIGURE 6.5 ▼ Different sources of dietary protein.
(Photo by Tetra Images/Getty Images.)

Normal physiologic function and growth and development require the consumption of about 0.8 g of protein per kg body mass per day. Insufficient dietary consumption of protein can result in **catabolism**. During catabolism, the body breaks down tissue proteins, typically skeletal muscle, to ensure the formation of the essential proteins of the body (e.g., hormones and neurotransmitters). Higher levels of protein consumption (>0.8 g per kg body weight per day) can lead the body into a state of **anabolism**, especially of the individual who participates in a regular resistance exercise training program. In an anabolic state, the body uses the amino acids to form proteins, including enzymes, hormones, and skeletal muscle (35,53).

Vitamins

Vitamins are organic substances required by the body in very small amounts to perform vital functions. Vitamins have no common chemical structure, do not supply energy, and do not contribute to the total mass of the body. The body cannot produce vitamins with the exception of vitamin D, and therefore vitamins must be supplied in the foods we consume or through dietary supplementation. There are 13 different vitamins and they are classified as either fat soluble or water soluble.

Fat-soluble vitamins are contained in dietary fat and are dissolved and stored in the fat tissues of the body. This storage process means that it may take years for a deficiency to develop, although this could be accelerated by consuming an extremely low fat or fat-free diet. Conversely, excessive intake of fat-soluble vitamins can be dangerous and lead to toxic effects. The consumption of fat-soluble vitamins (especially vitamins E and K) above the recommended level is believed to be of no additional health or athletic performance benefit (61).

Water-soluble vitamins are typically grouped together as the B-complex vitamins and vitamin C. Many water-soluble vitamins work with large protein compounds to form active enzymes that help regulate the chemical reactions in the body (35). Water-soluble vitamins are not stored in the body and therefore must be consumed in the diet on a regular basis. Excessive intake of vitamins, as is often the case with supplementation, leads to the excretion of the excess vitamins in the urine (61).

Transamination The transfer of an amino group from one chemical compound to another.

Non-essential amino acids An amino acid that can be synthesized by the body from other amino acids.

Essential amino acids An amino acid that cannot be synthesized by the body and must be consumed in the diet.

Catabolism Metabolic breakdown of complex molecules into simpler ones, often resulting in a release of energy.

Anabolism Phase of metabolism in which complex molecules, such as the proteins and fats that make up body tissues, are formed from simpler ones.

Fat-soluble vitamins Vitamins that dissolve and are stored in fat.

Water-soluble vitamins Vitamins that are easily dissolved in water.

Minerals

Minerals are a group of 22 mostly metallic inorganic elements required for normal physiologic function and used to form enzymes, hormones, and vitamins (61). Minerals appear either in combination with organic compounds or as free minerals in body fluids. Minerals present in large quantities with known biologic function are classified as major minerals; those present in very small quantities (<0.05% of body mass) are referred to as trace minerals. Excess minerals in the body provide no known biologic function and in some instances may even be harmful (35). Most minerals are found in water, topsoil of the ground, the root systems of plants and trees, and the tissues of animals that consume plants and water containing the minerals (35). Minerals play key roles in the function of the body because they provide for structure (e.g., bones and teeth), function (e.g., cardiac rhythm, muscle contraction), and regulation (e.g., energy metabolism) within the body. Minerals are also important for the synthesis of biologic nutrients; including glycogen, triglycerides, proteins, and hormones (35).

Water

Water plays an important part in maintaining health and proper physiologic function. Water does not contribute to the nutrient value of food, but the energy content of a specific food is generally inversely related to its water content. An individual's body weight is comprised of 40% to 60% water (36). Water content in tissue ranges from approximately 25% in adipose tissue to 75% in lean tissue such as skeletal muscle (36). Total body water content is therefore a function of the body composition (i.e., amount of adipose tissue vs. muscle tissue). The intracellular and extracellular compartments of the body contain water. Intracellular water comprises the fluid matrix that is the interior of the cell. The extracellular compartment comprises all the fluid that is external or outside the cell membrane and includes, for example, the blood plasma, lymph fluid, saliva, fluids of the eyes, and fluids secreted by glands and the intestines (35).

MEASURING NUTRITIONAL INTAKE

An accurate assessment of energy and nutrient intake is critically important for assuring the optimal health and fitness of individuals and the best performance of athletes during training and competition. Measuring habitual food consumption in humans, however, is one of the most difficult aspects of assessing nutritional intake (84). Two primary challenges for determining an accurate assessment that researchers, clinicians, and exercise science professionals face are the following: (a) obtaining a precise determination of an individual's normal food intake and

Dietary recall A process that requires individuals to recall from memory food items consumed during a prior period of time.

Dietary record A process that requires individuals to record food items consumed during a designated period of time.

(b) converting the information to nutrient and energy intake (84). When assessing dietary intake, it is important to verify that the technique used does not interfere with the individual's normal nutritional habits and thus influence the factor being measured. The two most common methods of measuring food intake at the individual level are the dietary recall and the dietary record (29).

Dietary Recall and Dietary Record

The **dietary recall** method requires an individual to report intake over the previous 24 hour period (called a 24-hour recall) or report the customary intake over the previous time period up to the past year (called a diet record). Food models, volume and size models, and pictures of food items can increase the accuracy of dietary recall. The **dietary record** method requires individuals to record the types and amounts of all foods consumed over a period of time (e.g., 3 days or 7 days). Figure 6.6 provides an example of a dietary record form. The

FOOD INTAKE RECORD		Date:_____	

Name:_____

Day/Time	Activity While Eating	Place of Eating	Food - Quality - Brand

FIGURE 6.6 ▼ A dietary record form.

Table 6.5	Advantages and Disadvantages of the Dietary Recall and Dietary Record Food Measurement Techniques (29)		
TYPE OF MEASUREMENT	**ADVANTAGES**		**DISADVANTAGES**
Dietary recall—24 h • Trained interviewer elicits food, portion size, place, and timing of meals eaten within past 24 h	• Easy to complete • Interview in person or by phone		• Relies on short-term memory • May not reflect typical intake • Data entry may be time-intensive
Dietary record • Trained interviewer instructs person to make detailed list of foods consumed, including preparation methods and brand names	• Does not rely on short-term memory • Accurate estimate of portion sizes with use of food models • Can include culture-specific foods		• Requires motivation for prolonged period of record keeping • Person may alter typical diet • Cost of carefully training participants is high

foods and fluids consumed by the individual are weighed or recorded in available household measures like spoons, cups, bowls, plates, serving size, or product size. The recorded information is converted to a weight or volume by measuring the actual devices used or adopting standard values from reference tables (84). Less used alternatives to the dietary recall and dietary record methods include the direct observation with weighted food records, food frequency questionnaire, double-portion technique, and the food supply technique (84). Table 6.5 illustrates important advantages and disadvantages of the dietary recall and dietary record food measurement techniques (29).

It is unclear how long food intake should be measured to determine customary nutritional consumption. If individuals live by a regular activity pattern (5 days of work or school and 2 days of nonwork or nonschool), it seems reasonable to suppose that their social and dietary habits are determined in part by this pattern of activity. The measurement of food intake should include samples of both workday/school day and nonwork/nonschool day intake. If possible, food intake is measured for the whole week. The length of the measurement period is determined by the level of day-to-day variability and the level of accuracy desired in the assessment. Generally, longer periods of measurement lead to a more accurate assessment of habitual food intake (84).

Once dietary intake data have been collected, conversion of this information to nutrient and energy intake occurs, typically using computer databases that contain the nutritional information of food samples. Several commercially available databases assess nutrient intake. The MyPyramid Tracker supplied by the Unites States Department of Agriculture (http://www.mypyramidtracker.gov/) is a very good Web-based tool for assessing nutritional intake. Other commercially available computer data–based programs are available for use. A primary challenge for obtaining accurate nutritional information lies in the interpretation of the item from the dietary record or recall and the selection of the matching food item from the database. Verifying specific information of the food item (size, volume, weight, brand, etc.) on the food intake record prior to entering the food into the database can improve accuracy. Additional accuracy can be obtained by using a database product that has several individual food items and also provides nutritional information on foods available in restaurants or prepackaged items from grocery stores. The information obtained from the nutritional assessment is then used to make recommendations for enhancing the nutritional intake of the individual (84).

NUTRITION FOR HEALTH

Habitual nutritional intake plays an important role in health promotion and disease prevention. Data from NHANES and other epidemiologic studies have demonstrated relationships between diet and increased risk for cardiovascular disease, hypertension, obesity, diabetes mellitus, osteoporosis, and certain forms of cancer (1,30,41,48,56,57,77). A primary treatment intervention for these lifestyle diseases and conditions is changing an individual's nutritional intake. Table 6.6 illustrates the potential beneficial effects of changing dietary intake on common disease conditions (35,66).

The importance of proper nutrition for optimal health cannot be underestimated. The federal government and private organizations and foundations have developed numerous promotional campaigns and programs aimed at improving nutritional intake in both the general population and in specific groups (e.g., those with high blood pressure or diabetes mellitus). Examples of some of these programs include the following:

- The **DASH Diet**, which stands for **D**ietary **A**pproaches to **S**top **H**ypertension, is designed to help individuals modify their diets in an effort to reduce blood pressure.
- **Fruits & Veggies-More Matters** is a public health initiative designed to increase the consumption of fruits and vegetables.

Table 6.6	Dietary Changes and Risk for Common Disease Conditions	
DIETARY CHANGE	**DISEASE CONDITION CHANGE**
Decreased sodium intake	Decreased blood pressure in hypertensive individuals
Taking a daily multivitamin that includes folic acid and limiting their intake of alcohol	Decreases excess risk of colon cancer associated with a family history of the disease
Decreased saturated fat and cholesterol intake	Decreased cardiovascular disease
Decreased calcium intake	Increased risk of osteoporosis
Decreased simple carbohydrate intake	Decreased risk of type II diabetes
Increased fruit and vegetable intake	Decreased risk of colon cancer

- **We Can!**, which stands for **W**ays to **E**nhance **C**hildren's **A**ctivity & **N**utrition is a national program designed for families and communities to help children maintain a healthy weight.
- The **FRESH START** program uses sequentially tailored materials to improve cancer survivors' diet and exercise behaviors.

Further support for the role that nutrition plays in optimizing health can be obtained by consulting the abundance of credible dietary self-help books, Internet Web sites, and commercial products for improving nutritional intake and improving health.

Dietary Guidelines for Health

The Dietary Guidelines for Americans, first published in 1980, provide science-based evidence to promote health and to reduce risk for chronic diseases through changing nutritional intake and physical activity patterns. The U.S. Department of Health and Human Services (HHS) and the U.S. Department of Agriculture (USDA) are responsible for developing and establishing the Dietary Guidelines of Americans. The process has evolved to include three stages for guideline development that are illustrated below (80):

- Stage 1 – An expert panel conducts an analysis of new scientific information on nutritional intake and health and issues a detailed report.
- Stage 2 – Key dietary recommendations are formed based on the report and from public and agency comments.
- Stage 3 – Communication of the recommendations (i.e., Dietary Guidelines) is made to the general public.

Every five years, the Dietary Guidelines Advisory Committee (DGAC) analyzes new scientific information during the revision of the Dietary Guidelines. This analysis is published in the DGAC Report (e.g., www.health.gov/dietary guide-lines/dga2005/report/) and serves as the primary resource for the development of the report on the guidelines. For example, the 2005 DGAC Report was used to form the recommendations that are used by the USDA and HHS for programs and public policy development (80).

The Dietary Guidelines summarize and synthesize knowledge regarding nutrient and food components into recommendations for a pattern of eating that can be adapted by the general public. The Dietary Guidelines provide key recommendations based on the scientific evidence for lowering the risk of chronic disease and promoting health. A basic premise of the Dietary Guidelines is that nutrient needs should be met primarily through food consumption. Foods provide various nutrients and other compounds that may have beneficial effects on health and reduce disease risk. Fortified foods and dietary supplements may be useful sources for one or more nutrients that otherwise might be consumed in less than recommended amounts. Though recommended in some instances, dietary supplements cannot replace a healthful diet (80).

The USDA Food Guide (http://www.cnpp.usda.gov/) and the DASH Eating Plan (45) are intended to combine the dietary recommendations from the Dietary Guidelines into a healthy way of eating for most individuals. The USDA Food Guide and DASH Eating Plan are based on age and gender and have a wide range of calorie levels to meet the needs of different groups of people. The USDA Food Guide uses population food intake to create the nutritional content for the different food groups. The DASH Eating Plan is based on selected foods chosen for a sample 7-day menu (45).

Recommended calorie intake for each plan will differ for individuals based on age, gender, and activity levels. Individuals who eat nutrient dense foods may be able to meet their **dietary reference intake** (DRI) of nutrients without consuming their full calorie allowance. The Dietary Guidelines are organized by specific themes and provide key recommendations for specific population groups that are used together to plan an overall healthy diet. The Dietary Guidelines for 2005 are organized according to the following themes (80):

1. Adequate nutrients within calorie needs
2. Weight management
3. Physical activity
4. Food groups to encourage
5. Fats
6. Carbohydrates
7. Sodium and potassium
8. Alcoholic beverages
9. Food safety

The Dietary Guidelines are updated every 5 years and used to develop programs for the general public. The most recent guidelines can be found at www.cnpp.usda. gov/. The creation of MyPyramid and MyPyramid for Kids allows individuals to create diets and alter nutritional intake to promote health. Figure 6.7 illustrates the specific components of MyPyramid for adults. Recent changes to MyPyramid have led to the inclusion of the following categories of food groups: grains, vegetables, fruits, oils, milk, and meat and beans. Children often have different nutritional requirements than adults and require information to be presented in a format that is easy to understand. As a result, the MyPyramid for Kids was created to promote healthy eating and active living among children aged 6 to 11 years. Figure 6.8 illustrates the design of MyPyramid for Kids. Exercise science professionals can play an important role in promoting healthy nutrition because of the close interaction with people, young and old, who are interested in making positive changes in their nutritional intake and eating behaviors.

> ➤ *Thinking Critically*
> *Why should individuals be careful about where nutritional information is obtained from when trying to consume a healthier diet?*

Current Nutritional Issues for Health

There are numerous nutritional issues for promoting good health that remain unresolved and will require additional research and study. One example is the effectiveness of diets with different macronutrient composition (e.g., low carbohydrate

---

Dietary reference intake A system of nutrition recommendations that are used to promote good nutrition by the general public and health professionals.

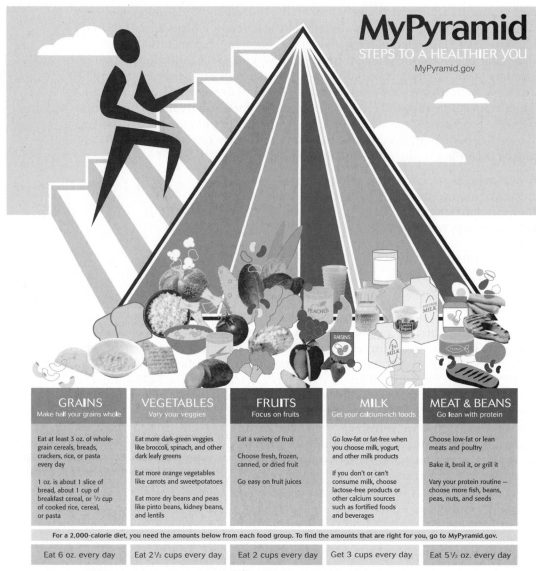

FIGURE 6.7 ▼ MyPyramid: The current recommendations for healthy eating. (From MyPyramid.gov.)

or high protein) in achieving and maintaining a healthy body weight and reducing the risk of disease. It will also be important to identify the most appropriate and effective educational strategies for promoting healthy eating by individuals in general and society as a whole. Considerable discussion among nutrition and health experts and scholars also exits in the following areas: the role of high glycemic index foods on disease risk, whether vitamin and mineral supplements can prevent chronic disease, and whether herbal supplements can enhance health and reduce disease risk (66).

➤ *Thinking Critically*
What nutritional information might you provide to an individual just beginning an exercise program to improve health and fitness?

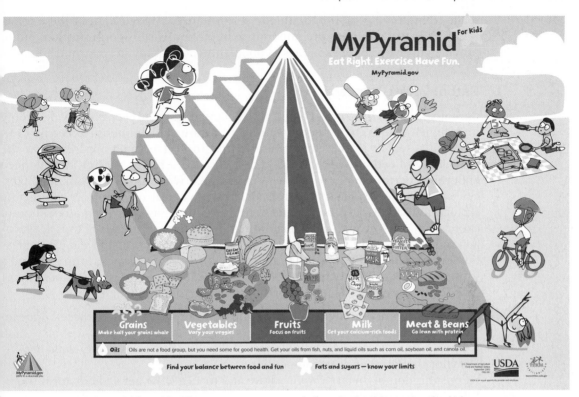

FIGURE 6.8 ▼ MyPyramid for Kids: The current recommendations for healthy eating for kids. (From MyPyramid.gov.)

NUTRITION FOR SPORT AND ATHLETIC PERFORMANCE

In order for athletes to perform at optimal levels, proper nutritional intake during both training and competition is very important. Athletes across the sports spectrum, from ultra-endurance performers to athletes who must rely on high levels of strength and power production to be successful, work closely with sport nutritionists to ensure proper macronutrient and micronutrient intake. For example, during training, athletes must have adequate energy supplies to insure that the proper intensity and duration of individual workouts can be maintained so that improvements in performance can occur. In various sports, it is critical that prior to and during competition fluid and food intake strategies be appropriate for maintaining peak performance. Exercise science professionals, as well as sport nutritionists, play important roles in determining how nutritional intake influences sports and athletic performance. The role of nutrition as it affects sport and athletic performance can be studied from several perspectives including training versus competition; macronutrient intake versus micronutrient intake; endurance athlete versus strength athlete). In this section, we will examine several primary areas of sport nutrition: the influence of dietary carbohydrate, protein, and fat intake; vitamin and mineral intake; fluid replacement; and ergogenic aids as they relate to improving sport and athletic performance. The selection of these topics is not meant to minimize the importance of other areas of sport nutrition, but to provide you with some examples of popular areas of study in sport nutrition.

Carbohydrate Intake

Carbohydrates in the form of blood glucose and **muscle glycogen** provide energy for muscle contraction, especially during moderate to high intensity exercise (33). Through research in the early twentieth century, it became apparent that the availability of carbohydrate to working muscles is a limiting factor in prolonged endurance performance (19,34,55). The research work of many prominent exercise science professionals demonstrated that glycogen depletion in contracting skeletal muscle resulted in a decrease in exercise intensity or even a cessation of exercise (9,10). Through daily dietary manipulation, the storage of muscle glycogen can be returned to normal levels or elevated above normal levels. This elevation in muscle glycogen results in an improvement of exercise performance and a subsequent delay in fatigue (76). Important nutrition and exercise components of muscle glycogen loading for competition include the following (13):

• A tapered reduction in the intensity and duration of training the week prior to the competition
• Consumption of dietary carbohydrate at 5 to 7 g CHO per kg body mass per day for the week prior to competition
• Consumption of dietary carbohydrate at 7 to 12 g CHO per kg body mass the day prior to competition
• Rest the day prior to competition
• High carbohydrate meal before the competition

Adequate daily intake of dietary carbohydrate is also important for athletes participating in sports that rely on strength and power production by the muscles of the body. This is particularly true during periods of high intensity and high volume training. Sufficient daily carbohydrate intake is necessary to replenish muscle glycogen levels following training and help create an anabolic environment that will promote skeletal muscle repair and protein synthesis (18,37,82). It is generally recommended that 60% to 70% of an athlete's total calorie intake should consist of carbohydrates (21,61). Other recommendations suggest that the replenishment of muscle glycogen is enhanced within 24 hours if between 5 and 12 g of carbohydrate per kg body mass are consumed (13). This amount of dietary carbohydrate intake provides sufficient carbohydrate for energy production and saves amino acids for protein synthesis in the body (13).

Complex carbohydrates including grains, pasta, whole grain breads, potatoes, rice, and bagels are the best food sources for replenishing muscle glycogen and providing other nutrients needed by the body. Complex carbohydrates provide a sustained release of glucose into the blood, result in a lower insulin release

Muscle Glycogen The storage form of glucose in skeletal muscle.

Table 6.7	Benefits of Carbohydrate Consumption Prior to and During Prolonged Exercise
CONSUMPTION OF CARBOHYDRATE	**BENEFICIAL EFFECTS**
Prior to exercise	• Increases muscle and liver glycogen concentrations • Delays muscle and liver glycogen depletion • Improves exercise performance
During exercise	• Delays muscle and liver glycogen depletion • Maintains blood glucose concentration • Improves exercise performance
Following exercise	• Enhances muscle and liver glycogen synthesis • Improves recovery from exercise

from the pancreas, and provide more nutrients than do simple carbohydrates. An insufficient supply of carbohydrates will potentially leave an athlete feeling fatigued, lethargic, and unable to train at the desired intensity and duration (21).

During exercise, carbohydrate ingestion is important for maintaining blood glucose concentrations within normal ranges, especially when the exercise duration is long. During prolonged exercise, the body uses its available stores of muscle glycogen and increasingly relies on blood glucose supplied by the liver. As liver glycogen stores are depleted, the athlete may experience low blood glucose levels (59). This condition, called hypoglycemia, can result in feelings of anxiety, nervousness, and tremor, and can affect the functioning of the central nervous system (54). If blood glucose and muscle glycogen levels become depleted, then exercise intensity may need to be decreased resulting in a reduction of exercise performance. Glucose ingestion during long-duration exercise (over 60 minutes) has been shown to reduce the rate of muscle and liver glycogen depletion, maintain normal blood glucose concentrations, delay the onset of fatigue, and improve endurance performance (59). Table 6.7 provides some of the beneficial effects of consuming carbohydrates prior to and during prolonged exercise.

Protein Intake

The regular consumption of adequate amounts and types of protein is important for ensuring the optimal performance of individuals during sport and athletic competition. The DRI for protein is 0.8 g protein per kg body mass per day (35). This level, however, may not be sufficient for athletes who need more protein than sedentary individuals. This greater requirement arises because athletes have increased needs for energy during training and competition, must repair tissue damaged during exercise, and must build new skeletal muscle to meet the demands of exercise training (14). Endurance athletes may require between 1.2 to 1.4 g of protein per kg body mass per day, whereas strength and power athletes may require between 1.6 and to 1.7 g of protein per kg body mass per day (58). Table 6.8 illustrates the differences in protein requirements for a nonathletic

Table 6.8	Daily Protein Requirements for a Nonathletic Person, an Endurance Athlete, and an Offensive Lineman in Football

INDIVIDUAL	BODY WEIGHT	PROTEIN REQUIREMENTS
Nonathlete	150 lb (68 kg)	Approx. 55 g protein/day
Endurance athlete	140 lb (63.5 kg)	76–90 g protein/day
Offensive lineman in football	300 lb (136 kg)	218–231 g protein/day

person, an endurance athlete, and an offensive lineman in football using the protein requirements discussed above. The amount of daily protein intake required varies by individual and is dependent on the factors shown in Figure 6.9 (53).

Foods high in protein content include many animal and dairy products. It is probably best to consume protein in several meals throughout the day so that the individual amino acids are readily available to the body tissues for continued protein synthesis (14,53,71). This practice is common place for athletes who are trying to either maintain or increase skeletal muscle mass. Dietary protein intake should closely match protein needs. Too much protein in the diet may lead to increased urinary calcium excretion (42), but there is no clear consensus on the significance of this issue on health and performance (25).

Processed protein supplements are frequently viewed by athletes and coaches as an economical and convenient source of dietary protein (Figure 6.10). This is particularly true of athletes who would rather "mix a shake" than prepare or purchase a meal. Commercial companies often claim that processed protein supplements provide improved and faster absorption of the amino acids over food protein. These processed protein supplements are available in the form of whey protein powders, free hydrolyzed amino acids, and free form amino acids. Though protein supplements may be a convenient source of protein, good food sources provide the necessary dietary protein, are usually less expensive, and contain other nutrients that can help athletes maximize their sport and athletic performance (4). Athletes must also be careful about consuming too much protein as this practice can lead to excess calorie intake, reduced carbohydrate intake, and possibly abnormal kidney function (52).

➤ **Thinking Critically**

Where can an athlete or coach receive knowledge about proper nutrition for increasing lean body mass and enhancing muscular strength?

Fat Intake

Excess dietary fat intake is generally not considered to be of benefit for enhancing sport and athletic performance. Most athletes consume sufficient amounts of dietary fat and therefore receive sufficient amounts of the fat-soluble vitamins for normal physiologic function (61). Athletes who are involved in sports where excess body weight may be detrimental to performance must closely monitor total

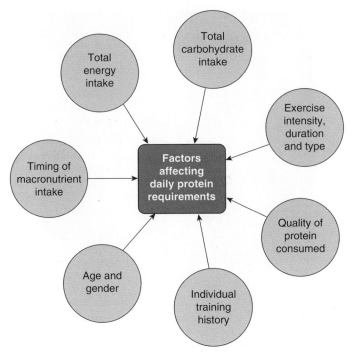

FIGURE 6.9 ▼ Factors affecting daily protein requirements (53).

calorie and dietary fat intake in an effort to maintain a body weight conducive to successful performance.

There has been some interest in the use of high fat diets for improving long-duration aerobic endurance performance (12,72). Fatigue during aerobic endurance events, such as a marathon or triathlon, is often related to muscle glycogen depletion and low blood glucose levels (76). The chronic consumption of high fat diets can result in the increase of fat stores in skeletal muscle and an improvement in the ability to use fat as a fuel source (32). When a 2 to 4 week high fat diet is combined with a high carbohydrate diet for 1 to 3 days immediately prior to competition, there are increases in fat oxidation and a reduction in muscle glycogen utilization in prolonged aerobic endurance events such as a marathon or ultra-endurance events lasting longer than 4 hours (51,72). Continued study and research in this subject by exercise science professionals should provide additional insight into this area of nutritional intake.

Vitamin and Mineral Intake

Vitamins and minerals are not a direct source of energy for the body. They are important, however, in the regulation and control of the metabolic reactions in the body. Vitamins and minerals are contained in the various foods we consume. Most athletes consuming an adequate amount of total calories receive sufficient amounts of vitamins and minerals in their diets (61). Athletes who are consuming a low calorie diet or a specialty diet (e.g., vegetarian) must be careful to eat foods

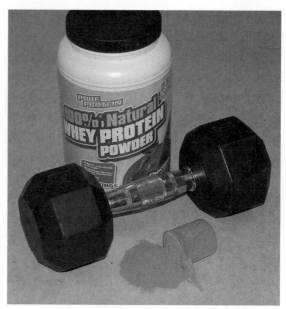

FIGURE 6.10 ▼ Processed protein supplements.

from a variety of different food groups to ensure that they are receiving the vitamins and minerals needed for normal physiologic function (61).

Vitamins play an important role in energy production and tissue metabolism. The B-complex vitamins, niacin, pantothenic acid, folate, biotin, and vitamin C play essential roles in using carbohydrate and fat for energy. Vitamins B_6 and B_{12}, vitamin C, folate, and biotin play an essential role in protein metabolism. In general, vitamin supplementation in excess of the daily recommended intake has not been shown to improve exercise performance in individuals consuming a nutritionally well-balanced diet (61). Athletes on a low-calorie diet or a vegetarian diet, however, may become deficient in certain vitamins if appropriate food choices are not made (61).

Vitamins E, C, and beta-carotene are referred to as **antioxidant vitamins** because of their ability to protect the body from damage caused by **oxygen free radicals**. Free radicals are produced during cellular metabolism when an oxygen molecule is combined with an unpaired electron making them highly reactive to other compounds. Free radicals attack the cellular membrane and have been linked to damage associated with aging, cancer, coronary artery disease, and other chronic diseases (20). Antioxidants, such as vitamin E and vitamin C and enzymes such as glutathione peroxidase, catalase, and superoxide dismutase, protect the

Anti-oxidant vitamins Vitamins that work to limit the formation of oxygen free radicals.

Oxygen free radicals Compounds produced during cellular metabolism when an oxygen molecule is combined with an unpaired electron making them highly reactive and potentially damaging to the cell.

Female athlete triad A combination of disordered eating, amenorrhea, and osteoporosis that is prevalent in female athletes who participated in sports where low body weight is an important factor in success.

Hemoglobin An iron-containing protein present in red blood cells that carries oxygen.

Table 6.9	Vitamins and Potential Benefits to Athletic Performance
VITAMIN	**ROLE IN ATHLETIC PERFORMANCE**
E	Functions as an antioxidant to prevent cell damage
B_1	Involved in carbohydrate metabolism
B_2	Involved in carbohydrate metabolism
B_3	Involved in energy metabolism
B_6	Involved in amino acid and glycogen metabolism
Pantothenic Acid	Involved in energy metabolism
Folate	Important in amino acid metabolism
B_{12}	Important in amino acid metabolism
Biotin	Involved in amino acid and glycogen metabolism
Vitamin C	Functions as an antioxidant to prevent cell damage

tissues of the body (70). These vitamins and enzymes react directly with free radicals to reduce their reactivity and thus help to protect the cells of the body from damage (20). Table 6.9 provides some examples of vitamins that may be important for improving athletic performance.

Minerals are an important component of numerous metabolic reactions in the body including energy production and muscle contraction (61). Minerals serve three broad roles in the body: structural, functional, and regulatory. Structural roles for minerals include the formation of bones and teeth. Functional roles include maintaining normal heart rhythm, initiating muscle contraction, creating nervous system conductivity, and promoting normal acid-base balance. Regulatory roles of minerals include becoming components of the enzymes and hormones that moderate cell activity (61). In general, athletes do not require more minerals than healthy physically active people (61). However, athletes who do not receive sufficient minerals from foods owing to low calorie intake or specialty diets may be at risk for certain disease conditions. Osteoporosis and anemia are two common health conditions experienced by athletes not consuming sufficient calcium and iron.

Osteoporosis can result from insufficient calcium intake and is of particular concern among athletes involved in endurance and weight control sports such as long distance running, dance, and gymnastics (47). The **female athlete triad** is a condition linked with eating disorders and menstrual irregularities and with the development of osteoporosis at a young age (Figure 3.7). A key issue in the prevention of osteoporosis is the regular sufficient intake of calcium. The ACSM has published position stands on this potentially very serious health condition (3,47,65). A more detailed discussion of osteoporosis and the female athlete triad is found in Chapter 3.

The mineral iron is very important for ensuring proper oxygen transport to tissues of the body (35). Iron is an important component of **hemoglobin**, which is a fundamental component of red blood cells. An insufficient intake of iron can lead to reduced hemoglobin concentration, red blood cell number, and anemia (35). Female endurance athletes frequently exhibit low levels of hemoglobin, which results in **sports anemia** (7,27). Iron supplementation to iron deficient athletes has been shown to improve blood measures of iron status, maximal oxygen consumption, and endurance performance times (40). Iron supplementation improves the iron status of athletes and has the potential to improve aerobic endurance performance (68).

Hydration Status and Fluid Replacement

Normal physiologic function depends on a proper water and electrolyte balance. Water is the medium in which all cells exist and functions occur. Even small decreases in total body water can impair sport and athletic performance (75). For example, a loss of just 2% of total body water can significantly impact athletic performance (8). Electrolytes important for normal body function include sodium, potassium, and chloride (8). Electrolytes are lost predominately in sweat and a significant reduction in electrolytes can impair both sport and athletic performance (75). If an individual loses too much body water or electrolytes and cannot regulate body temperature adequately, there is the potential for serious injury arising from heat exhaustion and heat stroke (75).

Athletes sweat considerably during training and competition and therefore must pay close attention to replacing fluids (Figure 6.11). Athletes train and compete during hot and humid weather conditions and athletes who participate in prolonged endurance events such as marathons, ultramarathons, triathlons, and long distance cycling require both water and electrolytes to maintain normal hydration levels (75). Consuming only water during prolonged training and competition

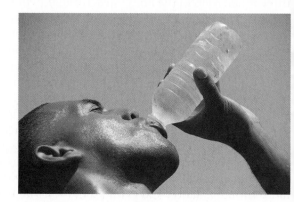

FIGURE 6.11 ▼ Sweating and fluid replacement. (Photo from Comstock/Getty Images.)

Sports anemia A condition of low blood hemoglobin that is the result of increases in blood volume.
Euhydration A state of normal levels of body water.
Hyponatremia An abnormally low concentration of sodium ions in blood.

Table 6.10	Fluid Replacement Recommendations to Maintain Normal Hydration Status (75)
TIME PERIOD	**RECOMMENDATION**
Before Exercise	• Prehydrate at least several hours before exercise to allow fluid absorption and urine output to return to normal • Consuming beverages with sodium and/or small snacks or meals may stimulate thirst and fluid intake
During exercise	• Develop an individualized fluid replacement strategy that will prevent excessive dehydration • Consuming beverages with electrolytes and carbohydrates can help maintain fluid and electrolyte balance
After exercise	• Consume 1.5 L of fluid for each kilogram of body weight lost • Consuming beverages with sodium and/or small snacks or meals may stimulate thirst and fluid retention

may help maintain **euhydration**, but it will not replace the electrolytes lost in sweat (75). A condition called **hyponatremia** (low sodium concentration) can arise if normal levels of sodium in the blood get too low. Hyponatremia can result in seizures, respiratory arrest, very low blood pressure, coma, and even death (75). It is important that athletes consume carbohydrate and electrolyte beverages when competing in long-duration activities, especially in hot and/or humid conditions.

The ACSM position stand on exercise and fluid replacement is an excellent resource for understanding the implications of dehydration and the correct procedures for maintaining euhydration, especially during exercise (75). Athletes should develop individualized fluid and electrolyte replacement strategies to maintain euhydration and reduce the risk for dehydration (75). Table 6.10 provides fluid replacement strategies to maintain normal hydration status.

Athletes engaged in training and competition that result in excessive sweating can monitor hydration status by performing two simple tasks. First, athletes should monitor their weight before and after practice and throughout the day. For each pound of weight lost during practice, approximately 16 oz of water or fluid should be consumed. A second strategy for maintaining hydration status is to monitor the frequency of urination and the color of the urine. Repeated urination that is of a light color typically indicates that the athlete is euhydrated. Athletes who urinate infrequently and who have dark-colored urine are generally dehydrated (75).

Ergogenic Aids

Ergogenic aids are substances or devices that work to improve performance during training or competition. Ergogenic aids may be classified as biomechanical, nutritional, pharmacologic, physiologic, and psychological (85). The use of many ergogenic aids is considered illegal by various sports governing associations. Consequently, many sports governing associations have list of banned substances, equipment, or aids. Many athletes, however, continue to use ergogenic aids as a means to improve performance during training and competition.

Nutritional ergogenic aids work to enhance sport and athletic performance by improving energy production, enhancing anabolic activities in the body, influencing exercise metabolism, and aiding in recovery from exercise (4,15). Carbohydrate, protein, vitamin, and mineral supplementation are often considered nutritional ergogenic aids. Athletes and coaches working to enhance sport and athletic performance work with sport nutrition and other exercise science professionals to examine the influence of various nutritional ergogenic aids on physiologic, biochemical, and performance factors. Conversely, other exercise science and sports medicine professionals continue to work to detect the use of illegal and banned ergogenic aids by athletes. Numerous ergogenic aids are classified as nutritional, and some of the more common ones are presented in Table 6.11 (4,15).

> ### ➤ *Thinking Critically*
>
> *How might coursework in nutrition prepare an individual for a career as a registered dietician, exercise physiologist, strength and conditioning coach, or a fitness instructor?*

Table 6.11	Nutritional Ergogenic Aids (4,15)
ERGOGENIC AID	**POTENTIAL BASIS FOR ENHANCING PERFORMANCE**
Creatine	• Improves energy production during high intensity exercise • Increases body weight and lean body mass
Caffeine	• Increases alertness and wards off drowsiness • Increases fat oxidation and reduces carbohydrate utilization
Sodium bicarbonate and sodium citrate	• Increase the body's ability to buffer lactic acid production
L-carnitine	• Improves fat oxidation • Decreases lactic acid formation
Aspartic acid	• Decreases ammonia formation in muscle
Ginseng	• Increases fat oxidation and reduces muscle glycogen utilization
Omega-3 fatty acids	• Improve oxygen delivery to muscles thereby enhancing aerobic metabolism
Antioxidants (superoxide dismutase and catalase)	• Protect tissues from the damage caused by oxygen free radicals
Coenzyme Q_{10}	• Increases aerobic energy production
Glycerol	• Improves hydration and may decrease dehydration
Chromium picolinate	• Enhances muscle protein development

I N T E R V I E W

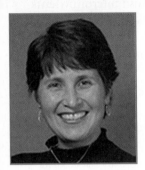

Stella Volpe, PhD, RD, LD/N, FACSM, Associate Professor of Nursing and Nutrition, University of Pennsylvania, Philadelphia

Brief Introduction

I received a bachelor of science degree in exercise science from the University of Pittsburgh, a master of science degree in exercise physiology from Virginia Polytechnic Institute and State University, and a doctor of philosophy from Virginia Tech in Nutrition. I completed a postdoctoral fellowship at the University of California at Berkeley. I am a registered dietician and certified as an ACSM Exercise Specialist.

➤ **Why did you choose to become involved in your work as an exercise and sport nutritionist?**

I have been an athlete my entire life. I am still a competitive rower and field hockey player, and I work out a lot. It was always difficult for me to separate food and performance. I always felt the need to combine them, because they are so influential on each other. I was very much influenced, as well, by Dr Janet Walberg Rankin, my MS thesis advisor and PhD committee member. She has a PhD in nutrition, but was in an Exercise Physiology department and did research related to both areas. She was and still remains a big inspiration to me.

➤ **Which individuals or experiences were most influential in your career development?**

I have been influenced by several exceptional individuals including my sixth grade teacher, Miss Margie Cullen, Dr Fred Goss, University of Pittsburgh (my undergraduate advisor), Dr Janet Walberg Rankin, Virginia Tech University, my MS thesis advisor, Dr Janette Taper, Virginia Tech University, my PhD dissertation advisor, and professional colleagues Dr Priscilla Clarkson, at the University of Massachusetts and Dr Gary Foster, at the University of Pennsylvania.

➤ **What are your most significance professional accomplishments?**

Writing grants and obtaining them are always fun for me. It is a challenge, but I really like to write.

I enjoy the collaboration with others on my grants and I on their grants. Therefore, getting that first NIH grant was very special for me. Seeing all of my students excel is so special to me. I get a joy out of seeing them present and do well in research and in the classroom. Also, being selected for a Distinguished Teaching Award at the University of Massachusetts meant so very much to me, because this is a university-wide award. My service to scientific organizations is important to me. I must admit, ACSM is the one organization to which I give most of my time. I was a member-at-large then president of the New England Chapter. I have been and am still on several committees at the national level (and associate editor of *ACSM's Health and Fitness Journal*).

➤ **What advice would you have for an undergraduate student beginning to explore a career in exercise science?**

My advice is to be as collaborative as possible. The more connections that you make will help you flourish in more ways than just your career. It is my friends and colleagues who I can turn to for advice. Your career is so important, but do not let it envelope you. Family is so important, and they should come first, before your career. I think that when people are trying too hard to succeed, it may not happen. That is not to say that a person should not work hard—not at all! A strong work ethic will get a person far in life! But, in general, have a good balance in your life, keep your priorities, be honest, work hard, enjoy what you do!

SUMMARY

- The consumption of appropriate amounts of the macronutrients and micronutrients is important for promoting health and successful performance in sport and athletic competition.
- Proper nutritional intake can reduce the risk of certain diseases and allow individuals to derive health benefits from participating in physical activity and exercise.
- Dietary guidelines have been established to help individuals make food choices that will enhance health and reduce disease risk.
- Aerobic endurance and strength-power athletes have an increased need for some nutrients including carbohydrate, protein, and certain vitamins and minerals.
- It is important for athletes to monitor nutrition and water intake so that successful performance can be derived during training and competition.

FOR REVIEW

1. What are some nutritional intake habits that could lead to an increased risk for hypertension, heart disease, breast cancer, colon cancer, osteoporosis, and obesity?

2. How has NHANES contributed to the understanding of nutritional patterns of people living in the United States?

3. What is the main function of the ADA and the SCAN?

4. What are the differences between simple and complex carbohydrates?

5. What is the difference between type 1 diabetes mellitus and type 2 diabetes mellitus?

6. What role do vitamins and minerals play in enhancing health?

7. Describe the differences between a dietary recall and a dietary record.

8. Why must endurance and strength and power athletes be concerned about daily carbohydrate intake?

9. Why do endurance and strength and power athletes need more protein than the RDI?

10. Why are vitamins E, C, and beta-carotene considered antioxidants?

11. What benefits are derived from consuming carbohydrate during prolonged exercise?

12. Which ergogenic aids would be beneficial for an endurance athlete?

13. Which ergogenic aids would be beneficial for a strength athlete?

REFERENCES

1. Abbasi F, McLaughlin T, Lamendola C, et al. High carbohydyrate diets, triglyceride rich lipoproteins, and coronary heart disease risk. *Am J Cardiol*. 2000;85:45–8.
2. Ahlborg B, Bergstrom J, Ekelund LG, Hultman E. Muscle glycogen and muscle electrolytes during prolonged physical exercise. *Acta Physiol Scand*. 1967;70:129–42.
3. American College of Sports Medicine. Osteoporosis and exercise. *Med Sci Sports Exerc*. 1995;27:i–vii.
4. Applegate E. Effective nutritional ergogenic aids. *Int J Sport Nutr*. 1999;9:229–39.
5. Applegate EA, Grivetti LE. Search for the competitive edge: A history of dietary fads and supplements. *J Nutr*. 1997;127:869S–73S.
6. Astrup A, Buemann B, Western P, Toubro S, Raben A, Christensen NJ. Obesity as an adaptation to a high-fat diet: Evidence from a cross- sectional study. *Am J Clin Nutr*. 1994;59:350–5.
7. Balaban EP, Cox JV, Snell P, Vaughan RH, Frenkel EP. The frequency of anemia and iron deficiency in the runner. *Med Sci Sports Exerc*. 1989;21:643–8.
8. Barr SI, Costill DL, Fink WJ. Fluid replacement during prolonged exercise: Effects of water, saline, or no fluid. *Med Sci Sports Exerc*. 1991;23:811–7.
9. Bergstrom J, Hermansen L, Hultman E, Saltin B. Diet, muscle glycogen and physical performance. *Acta Physiol Scand*. 1967;71:140–50.
10. Bergstrom J, Hultman E. Nutrition for maximizing sports performance. *JAMA*. 1972;221:999–1006.
11. Binkley JK, Eales J, Jekanowski M. The relation between dietary change and rising US obesity. *Int J Obes*. 2000;24:1032–9.
12. Burke LM, Hawley JA, Angus DJ, et al. Adaptations to short-term high-fat diet persist during exercise despite high carbohydrate availability. *Med Sci Sports Exerc*. 2002; 34:83–91.
13. Burke LM, Kiens B, Ivy JL. Carbohydrates and fat for training and recovery. *J Sports Sci*. 2004;22:15–30.
14. Butterfield G. Amino acids and high protein diets. In: Lamb DL, Williams MH, editors. *Ergogenics:Enhancement of Performance in Exercise and Sport*. Ann Arbor (MI): Wm C. Brown; 1991. p. 87–122.
15. Butterfield G. Ergogenic aids: Evaluating sport nutrition products. *Int J Sport Nutr*. 1996;6:191–7.
16. Calle EE, Rodriguez C, Walker-Thurmond K, Thun MJ. Overweight, obesity, and mortality from cancer in a prospectively studied cohort of U.S. adults. *N Engl J Med*. 2003;348:1625–38.
17. Cassell JA. *Carry the Flame: A History of the American Dietetic Association*. Sudbury (MA): Jones and Bartlett; 1990.
18. Chandler RM, Byrne HK, Patterson JG, Ivy JL. Dietary supplements affect the anabolic hormones after weight-training exercise. *J Appl Physiol*. 1994;76:839–45.
19. Christensen EH, Hansen O. Respiratorischen quotient und O2-aufnahme. *Skandinavisches Archive fur Physiologie*. 1939;81:180–9.
20. Close DC, Hagerman AE. Chemistry of reactive oxygen species and antioxidants. In: Alessio HM, Hagerman AE, editors. *Oxidative Stress, Exercise and Aging*. London: Imperial College Press; 2006. p. 1–8.
21. Costill DL. Carbohydrates for exercise: Dietary demands for optimal performance. *Int J Sports Med*. 1988;9:1–18.
22. Courtice FC, Douglas CG. The effect of prolonged muscular exercise on the metabolism. *Proc Royal Soc Lond*. 1935;119:381–3.
23. Coyle EF, Montain SJ. Benefits of fluid replacement with carbohydrate during exercise. *Med Sci Sports Exerc*. 1992;24:S324–30.
24. Darden E. Olympic athletes view vitamins and victory. *J Home Econ*. 1973;65:8–11.
25. Dawson-Hughes B, Harris SS, Rasmussen H, Song L, Dallal GE. Effect of dietary protein supplements on calcium excretion in healthy older men and women. *J Clin Endocrinol Metab*. 2004;89:1169–73.
26. Després JP, Moorjani S, Lupien PJ, Tremblay A, Nadeau A, Bouchard C. Regional distribution of body fat, plasma lipoproteins, and cardiovascular disease. *Arteriosclerosis*. 1990;10:497–511.
27. Eichner ER. Fatigue of anemia. *Nutr Rev*. 2001;59: S17–9.
28. Flegal KM, Williamson DF, Pamuk ER, Rosenberg HM. Estimating deaths attributable to obesity in the United States. *Am J Public Health*. 2004;94:1486–9.
29. Fowles ER, Sterling BS, Walker LO. Measuring dietary intake in nursing research. *Can J Nurs Res*. 2007;39:146–5.
30. Fuchs CS, Willett WC, Colditz GA, et al. The influence of folate and multivitamin use on the familial risk of colon cancer in women. *Cancer Epidemiol Biomarkers Prev*. 2002;11:227–4.
31. Glueck CJ, Gartside P, Laskarzewski PM, Khoury P, Tyroler HA. High-density lipoprotein cholesterol in blacks and whites: Potential ramifications for coronary heart disease. *Am Heart J*. 1984;108:815–26.
32. Goedecke JH, Christie C, Wilson G, et al. Metabolic adaptations to a high-fat diet in endurance cyclists. *Metabolism*. 1999;48:1509–17.
33. Gollnick PD. Metabolism of substrates: Energy substrate metabolism during exercise and as modified by training. *Federation Proc*. 1983;44:353–7.
34. Gordon B, Kohn LA, Levine SA, Matton M, Scriver WDM, Whiting WB. Sugar content of the blood in runners following a marathon race. *JAMA*. 1925;85: 508–9.
35. Gropper SS, Smith JL, Groff JL. *Advanced Nutrition and Human Metabolism*. 5th ed. Belmont (CA): Thompson Brooks/Cole; 2009.
36. Guyton AC, Hall JE. *Textbook of Medical Physiology*. Oxford (UK): Elsevier; 2006.
37. Haff GG, Koch AJ, Potteiger JA, et al. Carbohydrate supplementation attenuates muscle glycogen loss during acute bouts of resistance exercise. *Int J Sport Nutr Exerc Metab*. 2000;10:326–39.
38. Heaney RP. Calcium, dairy products, and osteoporosis. *J Am Coll Nutr*. 2000;19:88S–99S.
39. Hegsted DM. A look back at lessons learned and not learned. *J Nutr*. 1994;124:1867S–70S.
40. Hinton PA, Giordano C, Brownlie T, Haas JD. Iron supplementation improves endurance after training

in iron-depleted, nonanemic women. *J Appl Physiol.* 2000;88:1103–11.

41. Hu FB, Rimm EB, Stampfer MJ, Ascherio A, Spiegelman D, Willett WC. Prospective study of major dietary patterns and risk of coronary heart disease in men. *Am J Clin Nutr.* 2000;72:912–21.

42. Itoh R, Nishiyama N, Suyama Y. Dietary protein intake and urinary excretion of calcium: A cross-sectional study in a healthy Japanese population. *Am J Clin Nutr.* 1998;67:438–44.

43. Ivy JL, Lee MC, Brozinick JT, Reed MJ. Muscle glycogen storage after different amounts of carbohydrate ingestion. *J Appl Physiol.* 1988;65:2018–23.

44. Kannel WB, Larson M. Long-term epidemiologic prediction of coronary disease. *Cardiology.* 1993;82: 137–52.

45. Karanja NM, Obarzanek E, Lin PH, et al. Descriptive characteristics of the dietary patterns used in the Dietary Approaches to Stop Hypertension trial. *JADA.* 1999;99:S19–27.

46. Keys A, Brozek J, Henschel A, Mickelsen O, Taylor HL. *The Biology of Human Starvation.* Minneapolis (MN): The University of Minnesota Press; 1950.

47. Kohrt WM, Bloomfield SA, Little KD, Nelson ME, Yingling VR, American College of Sports Medicine. Physical activity and bone health. *Med Sci Sports Exerc.* 2004;36:1985–96.

48. Koushik A, Hunter DJ, Spiegelman D, et al. Fruits, vegetables, and colon cancer risk in a pooled analysis of 14 cohort studies. *J Natl Cancer Inst.* 2007;99: 1471–83.

49. Kraut H, Muller EA, Muller-Wecker H. Die abhangigkeit des muskeltrainings und eiweissbestand des korpers. *Biochem Z.* 1954;324:280–94.

50. Krogh A, Lindhard J. The relative value of fats and carbohydrates as sources of muscular energy. *Biochem J.* 1919;14:290–4.

51. Lambert EV, Goedecke JH, van Zyl C, et al. High-fat diet versus habitual diet prior to carbohydrate loading: Effects on exercise metabolism and cycling performance. *Int J Sport Nutr Exerc Metab.* 2001;11:209–25.

52. Lemon PWR. Do athletes need more dietary protein and amino acids? *Int J Sport Nutr.* 1995;5:S39–61.

53. Lemon PWR. Beyond the zone: Protein needs of active individuals. *J Am Coll Nutr.* 2000;19:513S–21S.

54. Levin BE, Dunn-Meynell AA, Routh VH. Brain glucose sensing and body energy homeostasis: Role in obesity and diabetes. *Am J Physiol.* 1999;276:R1223–31.

55. Levine SA, Gordon B, Derick CL. Some changes in the chemical constituents of the blood following a marathon race. *JAMA.* 1924;82:1778–9.

56. Lindquist CH, Gower BA, Goran MI. Role of dietary factors in ethnic differences in early risk of cardiovascular disease and type 2 diabetes. *Am J Clin Nutr.* 2000;71:725–32.

57. Liu S, Manson JE, Lee IM, et al. Fruit and vegetable intake and risk of cardiovascular disease: The Women's Health Study. *Am J Clin Nutr.* 2000;72:922–8.

58. Manore MM, Barr SI, Butterfield GE, American College of Sports Medicine, American Dietetic Association and Dieticians of Canada. Nutrition and athletic performance. *Med Sci Sports Exerc.* 2000;32: 2130–45.

59. Maughan RJ. Physiology and Nutrition for Middle Distance and Long Distance Running. In: Lamb DL, Knuttgen HG, Murray R, editors. *Perspectives in Exercise Science and Sports Medicine: Physiology and Nutrition for Competitive Sport.* Carmel (IN): Cooper Publishing Group; 1994. p. 329–71.

60. Mayer J, Bullen B. Nutrition and athletic performance. *Physiol Rev.* 1906;40:369–97.

61. McArdle WD, Katch FI, Katch VL. *Sports and Exercise Nutrition.* Baltimore (MD): Lippincott Williams & Wilkins; 2005.

62. McCullough ML, Feskanich D, Rimm EB, et al. Adherence to the Dietary Guidelines for Americans and risk of major chronic disease in men. *Am J Clin Nutr.* 2000;72:1223–31.

63. McCullough ML, Feskanich D, Stampfer MJ, et al. Adherence to the Dietary Guidelines for Americans and risk of major chronic disease in women. *Am J Clin Nutr.* 2000;72:1214–22.

64. National Health and Nutrition Examination Survey. National Health and Nutrition Examination Survey. 2007. *http://www cdc gov/nchs/nhanes htm.*

65. Nattiv A, Loucks AB, Manore MM, Sanborn CF, Sundgot-Borgen J, Warren MP. The female athlete triad. *Med Sci Sports Exerc.* 2007;29:i–x.

66. Nestle M, Dixon LB. *Taking Sides: Clashing Views on Controversial Issues in Food and Nutrition.* Guilford (CT): McGraw-Hill/Dushkin; 2004.

67. Nichols BL. Atwater and USDA nutrition research and service: A prologue of the past century. *J Nutr.* 1994; 124:1718S–27S.

68. Nielsen P, Nachtigall D. Iron supplementation in athletes. *Sports Med.* 1998;25:207–16.

69. Paffenbarger RS, Wing AL, Hyde RT. Physical activity as an index of heart attack risk in college alumni. *J Epidemiol.* 1978;108(3):161–75.

70. Quindry J, Powers SK. Aging, exercise, antioxidants, and cardioprotection. In: Alessio HM, Hagerman AE, editors. *Oxidative Stress, Exercise and Aging.* London: Imperial College Press; 2006, p. 125–44.

71. Rennie MJ, Tipton KD. Protein and amino acid metabolism during and after exercise and the effects of nutrition. *Annu Rev Nutr.* 2000;20:457–83.

72. Rowlands DS, Hopkins WG. Effects of high-fat and high-carbohydrate diets on metabolism and performance in cycling. *Metabolism.* 2002;51:678–90.

73. Sanjoaquin MA, Appleby PN, Thorogood M, Mann JI, Key TJ. Nutrition, lifestyle and colorectal cancer incidence: A prospective investigation of 10998 vegetarians and non-vegetarians in the United Kingdom. *Br J Cancer.* 2004;90:118–21.

74. Sawin CT. Eugene F. DuBois (1882–1959), Basal Metabolism, and the Thyroid. *Endocrinologist.* 2003;13: 369–71.

75. Sawka MN, Burke LM, Eichner ER, et al. Exercise and fluid replacement. *Med Sci Sports Exerc.* 2007; 39:377–90.

76. Sherman WM. Carbohydrate feedings before and after exercise. In: Lamb DL, Williams MR, editors. *Perspectives in Exercise Science and Sports Medicine.* New York (NY): McGraw-Hill Companies; 1991.

77. Slattery ML, Schumacher MC, Smith KR, West DW, Abd-Elghany N. Physical activity, diet, and risk of colon cancer in Utah. *Am J Epidemiol.* 1988;128:989–99.

8. Tipton CM. Exercise Physiology, part II: A contemporary historical perspective. In: Massengale JD, Swanson RA, editors. *The History of Exercise and Sport Science*. Champaign (IL): Human Kinetics; 1997. p. 396–438.

9. Todhunter EN. Reflections on nutrition history. *J Nutr*. 1983;113:1681–5.

0. U.S. Department of Health and Human Services and U.S. Department of Agriculture. *Dietary Guidelines for Americans, 2005*. Washington (DC): U.S. Government Printing Office; 2005. p. 1–85.

1. Van Itallie TB, Sinisterra L, Stare FJ. Nutrition and athletic performance. *JAMA*. 1956;162:1120–6.

2. Volek JS, Kraemer WJ, Bush JA, Incledon T, Boetes M. Testosterone and cortisol in relationship to dietary nutrients and resistance exercise. *J Appl Physiol*. 1997; 82:49–54.

3. Volpe SL. Sports nutrition. In: Brown SP, editor. *Introduction to Exercise Science*. Philadelphia (PA): Lippincott, Williams & Wilkins; 2001. p. 162–91.

84. Westerterp KR. The assessment of energy and nutrient intake in humans. In: Bouchard C, editor. *Physical Activity and Obesity*. Champaign (IL): Human Kinetics Publishers, Inc; 2000. p. 133–49.

85. Williams MH. *Beyond Training: How Athletes Enhance Performance Legally and Illegally*. Champaign (IL): Leisure Press; 1989.

86. Wright DA, Sherman WM, Dernbach AR. Carbohydrate feedings before, during or in combination improve cycling endurance performance. *J Appl Physiol*. 1991;71:1082–8.

87. Yu-Poth S, Zhao G, Etherton T, Naglak M, Jonnalagadda S, Kris-Therton PM. Effects of the National Cholesterol Education Program's step I and step II dietary intervention programs on cardiovascular disease risk factors: A meta-analysis. *Am J Clin Nutr*. 1999;69:632–46.

Exercise and Sport Psychology

After completing this chapter you will be able to:

1. Define exercise and sport psychology and provide examples of how each area contributes to the understanding of physical activity, exercise, sport, and athletic performance.

2. Identify the important historic events in the development of both exercise psychology and sport psychology.

3. Discuss the different areas of study that are related to sport psychology.

4. Discuss the different psychological factors that influence participation in regular physical activity and exercise.

Exercise psychology and sport psychology are areas of study concerned with the behavior, thoughts, and feelings of healthy, disabled, and diseased individuals engaging in physical activity, exercise, sport, and athletic competition. Many of the theories and methodologies from the parent discipline of psychology are used in the basic and applied studies of exercise and sport psychology. A conceptual framework for exercise and sport psychology is shown in Figure 7.1 (58, 59). The relationship between exercise psychology, sport psychology, and the parent discipline of psychology can be delineated using the following assumptions:

1. content knowledge in exercise psychology and sport psychology is fundamentally linked to the discipline of psychology

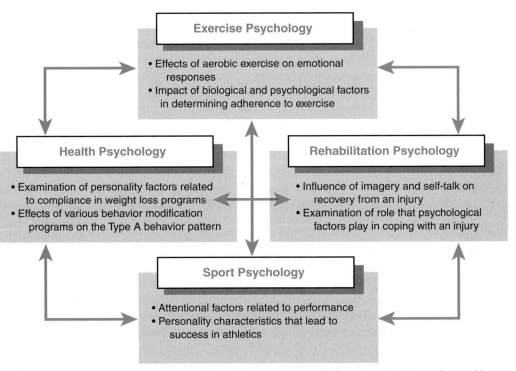

FIGURE 7.1 ▼ Conceptual framework of exercise and sport psychology (58,59). (From Brown SP. *Introduction to Exercise Science.* Baltimore (MD): Lippincott Williams & Wilkins; 2000. 312 p. Originally modified from Rejeski WJ, Brawley LR. Defining the boundaries of sport psychology. *Sport Psychol.* 1988;2:231–42.)

Exercise psychology Concerned with the cognitions, emotions, and behaviors that are related to perceptual and objective changes in cardiovascular fitness, muscular strength and endurance, flexibility, and body composition.
Sport psychology Concerned with the application of psychological principles to performance in the areas of sport and athletic competition.

2. examination and study of relevant issues in exercise psychology and sport psychology involves the use of a wide range of models and techniques from various aspects of psychology

3. exercise psychology and sport psychology have distinct areas of study, but also important relationships with each other (53,58)

Both exercise psychology and sport psychology use the educational, scientific, and professional contributions of psychology to help understand the mental aspects of physical activity, exercise, sport, and athletic competition. Exercise psychology is the study of the **cognitions**, emotions, and behaviors that are related to the **perceptual** and **objective** changes in cardiovascular fitness, muscular strength and endurance, flexibility, and body composition (58). Sport psychology is specifically concerned with the application of psychological principles to performance in the areas of sport and athletic competition (58,59). The principles of exercise and sport psychology can be used on both the individual and group levels. Health psychology is another area of study that has a close association with both exercise and sport psychology. Health psychology seeks to advance the understanding of health and illness in individuals of all age ranges.

The principles of exercise psychology and sport psychology can be used in a variety of professional environments. Exercise science professionals working to generate new knowledge in the areas of exercise and sport psychology may be concerned with developing methods for enhancing exercise adherence, self-esteem, leadership skills, and group or team cohesion. Exercise science and allied-healthcare professionals working with patients in a clinical setting may use various principles from exercise psychology to enhance exercise program adherence or reduce anxiety and depression associated with participation in a cardiac rehabilitation program. Personal trainers and coaches working with healthy individuals or athletes in an applied environment may apply the principles of sport psychology to promote improvement in psychological well-being or performance during training and competition (53,74).

Assessing psychological phenomena in exercise and sports psychology requires a variety of research and analytic methods not often used in other areas of exercise science. The most common method has been to use a **constructionist approach** in which considerable emphasis is given to the individual's subjective experience. The self-report, using standardized questionnaires or psychological inventories, is the predominant research and analytic strategy used in both exercise and sport psychology. Most of the questionnaires measure specific forms of thoughts, feelings, or behaviors (3). Individuals are frequently asked to complete questionnaires prior to and following participation in an exercise session

Cognition Mental faculty of knowing, which includes perceiving, recognizing, conceiving, judging, reasoning, and imagining.

Perceptual Recognition and interpretation of sensory stimuli based chiefly on memory.

Objective Interpretation of facts based on observable phenomena.

Constructionist approach Belief that individuals construct new knowledge from their experiences.

Hypnotic catalepsy A state of physical rigidity induced by hypnosis.

athletic practice, or competition, or as part of an acute or chronic intervention strategy (53).

Observing individuals and recording what they do during exercise or sport activities has also been used to enhance the understanding of behavior and psychological traits. The use of observation techniques requires extensive training for the individuals viewing the participants so that all observers are recording behaviors in the same manner and fashion. Personal interviews are also used in exercise and sport psychology when a greater understanding of beliefs, experiences, or values of the individual is required. Interviews, like other scientific methods of collecting information, must be structured to be systematic and individuals must be trained in the proper use of interview techniques to ensure accuracy and effectiveness (72). Although both exercise psychology and sport psychology have only recently developed into well-defined professional fields of study, the basis for their development has a rich history.

HISTORY OF EXERCISE AND SPORT PSYCHOLOGY

Early writings by the ancient Greeks extolled the virtues of a strong relationship between the mind and the body (32,73). It was not until the nineteenth century, however, that a fundamental knowledge base in exercise and sport psychology was established. Most of the significant developments of exercise and sport psychology have occurred since the mid 1960s leading to exercise and sports psychology emerging as professional areas of study in exercise science (32).

Early Influences

The foundation for the development of exercise and sport psychology as fields of study originated during the late nineteenth and early twentieth centuries. The discipline of psychology arose from philosophy during the mid nineteenth century and ultimately became the parent discipline to exercise and sport psychology (73). Early work establishing relationships between the mind and the body was largely a result of individuals trained in psychology examining factors related to physical activity and exercise. For example, in 1884, Conrad Rieger published what is considered to be the first article related to psychology and exercise in which he reported that the mental state of **hypnotic catalepsy** enhanced muscular endurance (47). Shortly thereafter, Norman Triplett (1861–1931) published the first true experimental study that was directly related to exercise and sport psychology (70). Triplett, a bicycling enthusiast, was interested in how direct competition between two individuals affected performance. Triplett observed that when two individuals competed against each other, a social factor that seemed to motivate cyclists to perform better existed that was not observed when individuals performed alone (32). In the early twentieth century, several scholars studied various relationships between physical activity and sport and the responses of the brain and the nervous system. In 1908, the president of the American Psychological Association (APA), G. Stanley Hall highlighted the advancements in these areas in a report that described the psychological benefits from participating in physical education (35).

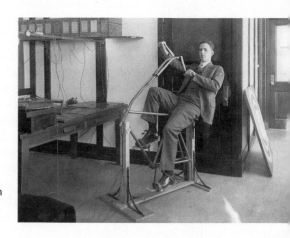

FIGURE 7.2 ▼ Coleman R. Griffith (ca. 1920). (Photo used with permission from University Archives, University of Illinois, Urbana.)

One of the early true pioneers of exercise and sport psychology was Coleman R. Griffith (Figure 7.2), who in 1925 became the director of the Research in Athletics Laboratory at the University of Illinois (73). Griffith, who is often recognized as the "Father of North American Sport Psychology" studied various psychological factors related to participation in American football and basketball. Griffith published two classic textbooks about his work with athletes and coaches; *Psychology of Coaching* in 1926 and *Psychology and Athletics* in 1928. Likely the first practicing sport psychologist, Griffith was hired in 1938 by Philip Wrigley owner of the Chicago Cubs to help improve the performance of the professional baseball team (34).

The expansion of the foundation of exercise and sport psychology occurred throughout the mid-twentieth century. In 1938, Franklin Henry established a graduate program in the psychology of physical activity at the University of California-Berkley. Henry, a scholar in motor behavior, advocated the scientific development of sport and exercise psychology (74). During the early years of World War II, Dorothy Hazeltine Yates engaged in mental training interventions with boxers and aviators, primarily focusing on a "relaxation set-method" and mental preparation for performance (73). Yates published two books and developed a psychology course for athletes and aviators at San Jose State University (73). Throughout the 1940s and 1950s, research in the areas of physical activity, exercise, sport, and athletic competition examined personality traits in athletes, emotions and stress related to youth sport competition, college athletic performance, competition, motor performance, and exercise (73).

Recent Influences

The period of 1965 to 1980 saw tremendous advances in exercise and sport psychology including the development of a research knowledge base that was distinct and separate from the closely related disciplines of motor behavior and motor learning (73). Contributing to this growth were several important historic events. The International Society of Sport Psychologists (founded in 1965) and the meeting of the First World Congress of Sport Psychology in Rome, Italy in the same year were instrumental in bringing together scholars interested in the use of psychological techniques for improving sport and athletic performance. Professional organizations also emerged in America to help promote exercise and sport psychology. The first meeting of the North American Society for the Psychology of Sport and Physical Activity (NASPSPA) occurred during the 1967 American Alliance for Health, Physical Education, and Dance (AAHPER) National Conference in Las Vegas, Nevada. Early on NASPSPA continued to meet during the annual AAHPER conferences until 1975 when it began to hold independent meetings.

Many national and international scholars played key roles in the development of exercise and sport psychology from the 1960s through the 1980s. Noteworthy first generation American scholars included Ranier Martens, Dan Landers, William Morgan, and Dorothy Harris. Prominent international scholars included Paul Kunath, Peter Roudik, Miroslav Vanek, Morgan Olsen, and John Kane. Of particular importance is Ferruccio Antonelli, who was instrumental in the establishment of the International Society of Sport Psychologists and spearheaded the first sport psychology research journal, *International Journal of Sport Psychology*. Additional prominent journals helped to disseminate exercise and sport psychology research, and facilitate its development as a field of study, particularly the *Journal of Sport Psychology* (1979) that was renamed the *Journal of Sport and Exercise Psychology* in 1988; *The Sport Psychologist* (1987); *Journal of Applied Sport Psychology* (1989); and *Health Psychology* (1996) (73).

During the mid-1980s, there was a shift in the research and application interests of many exercise and sport psychologists from laboratory activities to more field-based experimentation and practice (32). This shift resulted in a significant increase in the number of individuals working to enhance psychological skills training with competitive athletes. As a result of this movement, the formation of the Association for Applied Sport Psychology was established in 1985. Another key event in the development of exercise and sport psychology occurred in 1986 when the APA recognized Division 47—Exercise and Sport Psychology as a formal division within the APA. At about the same time, there was an increase in the publication of research in exercise psychology (73). Systematic research investigations provided evidence that exercise decreased stress, anxiety, and depression (15), improved mood and positive emotion (8), and enhanced **self-efficacy**, **self-concept**, and **self-esteem** (65). Additional research work in the area of exercise adherence (18) and interventions to change physical activity behavior (22) was also being performed. A key step in the professionalization of exercise and sport psychology occurred in 1991

> ➤ *Thinking Critically*
> *In what ways has exercise psychology contributed to a broader understanding of physical fitness and health?*

> ➤ *Thinking Critically*
> *In what ways has sport psychology contributed to a broader understanding of sport and athletic performance?*

Self-efficacy An impression that an individual is capable of performing in a certain manner or attaining certain goals.

Self-concept The sum total of an individual's knowledge and understanding of his or her self.

Self-esteem The way individuals think and feel about themselves and how well they do things that are important to them.

when the Association of Applied Sport Psychology began to confer the title "Certified Consultant" on individuals who met specific training criteria (32). This certification designation limits the certified consultant's role to an educational one, emphasizing psychological skills training (32).

At the end of the twentieth century and into the twenty-first century, exercise and sport psychology continued to further define the knowledge base, expand into new areas of study, and clarify professional practice-related issues (73). Additional study and research is being performed in the areas of interpretive approaches to knowledge construction (10), feminist methodology (31), developing a pragmatic research philosophy (30), and developing an **ecologic meta-theoretical approach** (23). The areas of exercise and sport psychology continue to grow and develop as needs evolve for having a better understanding of the mental and psychological factors that affect physical activity and exercise and performance in sport and athletic competition. Table 7.1 provides some of the significant events in the historic development of exercise and sport psychology.

Table 7.1	Significant Events in the Development of Exercise and Sport Psychology
DATE	**SIGNIFICANT EVENT**
1884	Conrad Rieger published the first article related to psychology and exercise
1898	Norman Triplett published the first true experimental study in exercise and sport psychology
1908	APA President G. Stanley Hall issued a report highlighting the psychological benefits from participating in physical education
1925	Coleman R. Griffith established the Research in Athletics Laboratory at the University of Illinois and studied sport psychology
1938	Franklin Henry established a graduate program in the psychology of physical activity at the University of California-Berkley
1965	Formation of the International Society of Sport Psychologists and the First World Congress of Sport Psychology in Rome, Italy
1967	NASPSPA was founded
1970	First publication of the *International Journal of Sport Psychology*
1979	First publication of the *Journal of Sport and Exercise Psychology*
1985	Formation of the Association for the Advancement of Applied Sport Psychology
1986	APA formally recognized Division 47 – Exercise and Sport Psychology
1988	First publication of the *Journal of Sport and Exercise Psychology*
1989	First publication of the *Journal of Applied Sport Psychology*
1991	Association for the Advancement of Applied Sport Psychology began to confer the title Certified Consultant, AAASP

STUDY OF THE MIND AND BODY

articipation in physical activity, exercise, sport, and athletic competition involves coordinated efforts of the body and the mind. The study of mental aspects of physical activity, exercise, sport, and athletic competition is the foundation of exercise and sport psychology. Exercise and sport psychology include the study and application of the affect (i.e., emotion), behavior, and cognition (i.e., thought) of individuals as they prepare to engage in planned movement. Although they are distinct areas of study in exercise science, exercise and sport psychology continue to have close connection to the parent discipline of psychology specifically as it relates to cognitive and **behavioral psychology**. Exercise and sport psychology has three primary objectives linked to physical activity, exercise, sport, and athletic competition:

1. Understanding the social-psychological factors that influence individual behavior
2. Understanding the psychological effects derived from participation
3. Enhancing the experiences of individuals prior to, during, and following participation (72)

To accomplish these objectives, exercise and sport psychology professionals focus primarily on the following areas of study: personality, motivation, arousal and performance, and attention. A solid understanding of these areas will assist many exercise science professionals in their attempts to fulfill their professional job responsibilities.

Personality

Personality is defined as the entire qualities and traits, including character and behavior that are specific to someone. Individual personality plays an important role in the behaviors that individuals' exhibit during participation in physical activity, exercise, sport, and athletic competition. Personality research in exercise and sports psychology has been a popular area of study (73) and underlies much of what exercise and sports psychology professionals study (71). Personality is conceptualized in different ways with one example of a model shown in Figure 7.3 (37).

At the center of an individual's personality is the psychological core, thought to be the most stable and least modifiable aspect of personality. The psychological core is developed from early interactions with the environment (parents and objects) and includes such aspects of personality as perceptions of the external world, perceptions of self and basic attitudes, values, interests, and motives (53).

Ecologic meta-theoretical approach Belief in an understanding that the individual is part of a larger group and this influences the actions and behaviors of the individual.
Behavioral psychology A branch of psychology based on the proposition that all things that organisms do can and should be regarded as behaviors.
Personality The complete qualities and traits, including character and behavior, which are specific to a person.

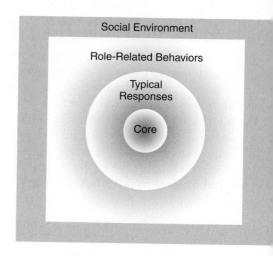

FIGURE 7.3 ▼ Conceptualization of personality. (From Brown SP. *Introduction to Exercise Science*. Baltimore (MD): Lippincott Williams & Wilkins; 2000. 314 p.)

Our core personality is the basis for our thoughts, feelings, and behaviors. Arising from the core are actions and behaviors that are consistent with the core and usually fairly consistent over time. Our behaviors can change as a result of influences from the social environment, such as being a member of a recreational sport team, and these are often referred to as role-related behaviors. These role-related behaviors represent the most dynamic aspect of an individual's personality because behaviors can vary based on the situation or surroundings the individual is involved in at a particular moment in time. These role-related behaviors remain consistent with an individual's psychological core. In general, personality is relatively stable over time, but can be changed and modified according to the environment and situations. The two most common approaches to studying personality are the dispositional approach, which is focused on the person and the learning approach, which is focused on the environment (53).

Dispositional Approach

A popular approach to studying personality is the trait theory approach. **Traits** are enduring and consistent internal attributes that an individual possesses and exhibits. Considerable information has been generated on individual traits and individuals can be described as having traits such as temperamental, nervous, sensitive, restless, confident, dynamic, gregarious, lighthearted, composed, and poised. Two individuals who helped develop our current understanding of personality and traits were Raymond B. Cattell (1905–98) and Hans J. Eysenck (1916–97). Cattell proposed that personality consisted of 16 factors and he developed the 16 Personality Factor (16PF) Questionnaire to assess them (12). Use of this questionnaire was widely popular for studying and describing personality in the sports domain during the 1960s and 1970s (53,71). Some examples of questions used in the 16PF questionnaire are shown in Figure 7.4.

Traits Relatively enduring, highlyn consistent internal attributes that an individual possesses and exhibits.

1. On social occasions I:
   - ☑ Readily come forward
   - ☐ In between
   - ☐ Prefer to stay quietly in the background
2. I sometimes cannot get to sleep because and idea keeps running through my head.
   - ☐ True
   - ☐ Uncertain
   - ☐ False
3. In my personal life I reach the goals I set almost all of the time.
   - ☐ True
   - ☐ Uncertain
   - ☐ False
4. I would prefer to have an office of my own, not sharing it with another person.
   - ☐ Yes
   - ☐ Uncertain
   - ☐ No
5. When I am in a small group, I am content to sit back and let others do most of the talking.
   - ☐ True
   - ☐ Uncertain
   - ☐ False

FIGURE 7.4 ▼ Examples of the 16PF Questionnaire (12).

Eysenck developed another approach to examine relationships among traits (24). He believed that personality could be captured most effectively with only three dimensions: extroversion–introversion, neuroticism–stability, and psychoticism–superego. An important aspect in this approach to examining personality is that each dimension has a biologic basis and that each personality trait is intimately linked with biologic processing (53). Eysensck's model was commonly used in attempts to characterize success in exercise, sport, and athletic performance. For example, individuals who are extroverts tend to seek out sensory stimulation and are well able to tolerate pain. Consequently, it is hypothesized that extroverts would be more likely to participate in sport and athletic competition and would be more successful in sports than individuals who are introverts (25). The current research indicates, however, that no distinguishable personality exists for athletes compared to nonathletes. Furthermore, there appears to be no consistent personality differences between athletic subgroups (e.g., team athletes vs. individual sport athletes, contact sport versus non-contact sport). There have been several differences identified in personality characteristics between successful and unsuccessful athletes (53). Specifically, successful athletes are

- More self-confident
- Better able to retain optimal competition focus in response to obstacles and distractions
- Efficiently self-regulate activation
- Have more positive thoughts, images, and feelings about sport
- More highly determined and committed to excellence in their sport (72)

Sport psychology is also concerned with whether participation in sports and athletic competition can influence personality development and change. For example, are independent, extroverted individuals developed through sport and athletic participation or are independent, extroverted people attracted toward sport and athletics? Research suggests that independent, extroverted people are more interested in participating in sport and athletics. Furthermore, it appears that engaging in structured sports programs can lead to positive changes in personality and behavior (53,74).

With respect to physical activity and exercise, no set of personality characteristics have been identified that predict adherence to a physical activity or exercise program. Personality type cannot be used to predict regular exercisers from sedentary individuals; however, two personality characteristics are strong predictors of exercise behavior. Individuals more confident in their physical abilities are likely to exercise more than those who are less physically confident. Additionally, individuals who express self-motivation are more likely to begin and continue with regular exercise, and less motivated individuals are more likely to never start regular exercise or discontinue a program that has been started (72).

Participation in regular physical activity or exercise programs causes positive changes in several personality traits. Negative factors (e.g., neuroticism) are reduced and positive factors (e.g., extroversion) are enhanced following participation in regular exercise programs (53). Participation in long-term physical activity and exercise programs can result in reductions in both anxiety and neuroticism (54). Children, adolescents, and adults show improvement in self-esteem with improvement in physical fitness parameters (28). Regular physical activity is also associated with decreases in depression and a reduction of depressive symptoms in individuals who are clinically depressed at the beginning of the exercise treatment (53,72).

> ➤ **Thinking Critically**
> *In what ways might exercise enhance the mental state of an individual?*

Motivation

Motivation is an important component for participation in physical activity, exercise, sport, and athletic competition. Motivation is defined as a complex set of internal and external forces that influence individuals to behave in certain ways (72). **Extrinsic motivation** is the predominant influence that occurs when individuals engage in a certain behavior to gain some external reward from that participation. **Intrinsic motivation** is the predominant factor that causes an individual to engage in behavior because the individual enjoys the process and gains pleasure and satisfaction from that participation. The study of motivation in exercise psychology and sports psychology has most often used an achievement framework. The McClelland-Atkinson model is one of the earliest and most influential models used to study motivation, and many of the current motivational models are derived from this model (53). The McClelland-Atkinson model employs a complex approach to predict and explain the need to achieve success and avoid failure. In this model, both individual and environmental factors play an important role in determining success or failure (74).

Numerous social-psychological theories of motivation have been developed. Many of these theories use a cognitive approach to achievement motivation, such that individual desire for achievement is assumed to be caused by cognitive mechanisms. Self-confidence or an individual's perception of their own ability to perform a skill or activity is one of the most important cognitive concepts. Self-confidence and self-efficacy have been shown to be significantly related to successful sport and athletic performance with some experts believing that it is the most important factor determining success in sport and athletic competition. The two most prominent social-psychological theories in exercise and sport psychology are Bandura's social cognitive theory (4) and Weiner's attribution theory (75).

Social Cognitive Theory

Social cognitive theory suggests that components of an individual's knowledge attainment can be directly related to observing others within the context of social interactions, experiences, and outside media influences (26). Self-efficacy is a major component of the social cognitive theory. Self-efficacy is the cognitive mechanism mediating motivation and thus an individual's behavior. The convictions or beliefs an individual has that he or she is capable of performing in a certain manner or attaining certain goals provide consistent support for that individual to be successful. Self-efficacy is not a measure of the skills that individuals actually possess, but is instead a measure of an individual's own judgment of what he or she can do with those skills and the self-confidence specific to a particular situation. Self-efficacy has been shown to be an important factor in an individual's choice of activity, effort exerted in those activities, and persistence in the activity when faced with challenges (53). A model of self-efficacy is presented in Figure 7.5 (53).

Self-efficacy is derived from four factors: past performance, observing others, social persuasion, and physiologic arousal. The most prominent of these factors is past performance in an activity. Past performance is the most dependable and influential factor affecting self-efficacy. Past success leads to an increased feeling of self-efficacy, whereas past failures, especially repeated failures, lead to decreased feelings of self-efficacy. Observing others engaging in the same physical movement or activity can also affect efficacy judgments. This is particularly important if an individual has limited experience with the movement skill or activity. Social persuasion, although a relatively weak source, is the influence of a social situation on self-efficacy. The final influence on efficacy is physiologic arousal, which is the appraisal by individuals of their own physiologic states. An individual may have an increased heart rate, nervousness, muscle fatigue, or pain prior to performance, each of these may lead to a decrease in self-efficacy (53).

Motivation Psychological feature that arouses an organism to action toward a desired goal.
Extrinsic motivation Motivation that comes from factors outside an individual.
Intrinsic motivation Motivation that comes from factors within an individual.
Social cognitive theory Belief that portions of an individual's knowledge acquisition can be directly related to observing others within the context of social interactions, experiences, and outside media influences.

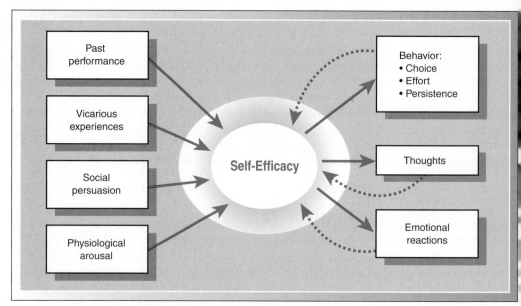

FIGURE 7.5 ▼ Model of self-efficacy. (From Brown SP. *Introduction to Exercise Science.* Baltimore (MD): Lippincott Williams & Wilkins; 2000. 318 p.)

Self-efficacy can determine individual behavior as it relates to choice, effort, persistence, thoughts, and emotional reactions. A key aspect of social cognitive theory is the reciprocal relationship between self-efficacy and behavior. Behaviors, thoughts, and feelings have a reciprocal influence on self-efficacy, which, can in turn, influence the sources of efficacy information. Self-efficacy is dynamic and can be constantly changed as new information is presented to the individual (53). Self-efficacy is an important determinant of behavior in physical activity and sports. It accounts for approximately 25% of all the available possibilities for explaining individual performance (26). Self-efficacy has been shown to predict the adoption and the maintenance of moderate and vigorous physical activity and exercise programs in a variety of populations (26,53).

Exercise and sport psychology professionals, as well other exercise science professionals can use the knowledge about self-efficacy to enhance performance in physical activity, exercise, sport, and athletic competition. By using appropriate interventions to enhance self-efficacy, there is an increased probability that an individual will adopt physical activity and exercise behaviors that are consistent with good health. Additionally, the enhancement of self-efficacy in an athlete will likely improve that individual's performance during a sport or athletic competition.

Attribution Theory

The second prominent theory for explaining motivation is Weiner's **attribution theory**. This theory explains how an individual interprets achievement outcomes and how that interpretation influences future behavior (68). The basic principle of attribution theory claims that after engaging in a behavior that results in some outcome, an individual begins to search for reasons why the outcome happened as it did (53). These reasons for the outcome are referred to as causal attributions.

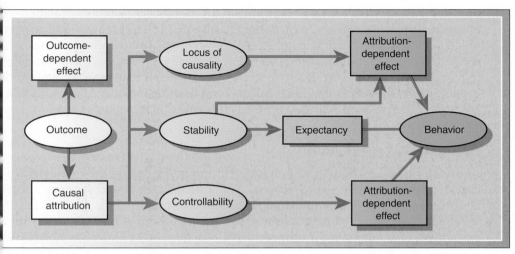

FIGURE 7.6 ▼ The outcome-dependent effect. (From Brown SP. *Introduction to Exercise Science.* Baltimore (MD): Lippincott Williams & Wilkins; 2000. 319 p.)

Individuals predominately use four common attributions: ability, effort, task difficulty, and luck or chance (53). The attribution theory focuses on identifying common dimensions underlying the attributions. Weiner (75) identified three causal dimensions: locus of causality, stability, and controllability:

• Locus of causality refers to whether the cause of attribution is perceived to reside internally or externally to the individual.
• Stability refers to the variability of the attribution over time with some attributions relatively permanent (stable), whereas others are relatively temporary (unstable).
• Controllability refers to whether the attribution is under the individual's control or controlled by someone or something else.

When an outcome occurs, an individual experiences an emotion, referred to as an outcome-dependent effect. Figure 7.6 illustrates the outcome-dependent effect. If the outcome was successful, the individual will have good emotions; if the outcome was a failure, the individual will have bad emotions. The individual then engages in a causal search to determine the factors that were responsible for the outcome. The factors or causes are then processed in terms of placement along the three dimensions (causality, stability, and controllability) (53).

Individuals who are characterized as chronic exercisers have higher perceptions of individual control over their own health, an internal locus of causality, and more control over exercise behavior. Each of these three causal dimensions can predict negative emotional reactions to discontinuing an exercise program (53). The attributional processes may be significant components of complex behaviors like exercise. In addition to the social cognitive and attribution theories, other popular topics of

Attribution theory Belief that explains how an individual interprets achievement outcomes and how that interpretation influences future behavior.

motivational study have included intrinsic motivation, social-psychological theories of intentions, and achievement goal orientations (53,74). The promotion of positive outcomes during physical activity, exercise, sport, and athletic competitions will result in a positive emotional response of the individual providing further support for continued participation. Exercise science professionals engage in all manner of supportive behaviors in attempts to try and enhance the experience of individuals participating in physical activity, exercise, sport, and athletic competition.

Arousal and Performance

Arousal is a state of heightened physiologic and psychological activity. Participation in physical activity, exercise, sport, and athletic competition requires a level of arousal to energize an individual for movement (Figure 7.7). An individual's state of arousal varies along a continuum from deep sleep at one end to extreme excitement or agitation at the other end. Arousal can also be viewed as a construct with multiple dimensions—having at least the dimensions of valence (degree of attraction or aversion that an individual feels toward a specific object or event) and intensity (the strength of the state of arousal) (53,68).

An individual's level of arousal is constantly changing depending on the situation and environment. The central nervous system, predominately the brain, contains the physical structures involved in the control of arousal. Interactions

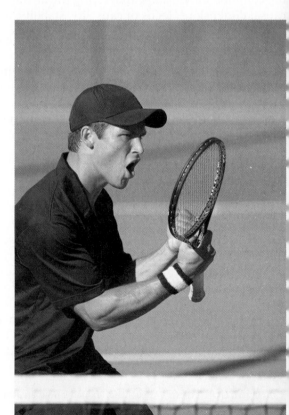

FIGURE 7.7 ▼ Arousal in an athletic competition. (Photo by Digital Vision/Ryan McVay/Getty Images.)

among the reticular-activating system, cerebral cortex, and hypothalamus in the brain interact with the peripheral nervous system, the somatic nervous system, and the autonomic nervous system to regulate arousal. The brain exerts a strong influence on the adrenal glands, which are responsible for releasing epinephrine and norepinephrine into the circulatory system. These hormones are responsible for helping to increase the level of activity (i.e., arousal) in various tissues of the body (53).

A variety of factors can influence the level of arousal. For example, a perceived stressor might initiate the fight or flight response, which increases the level of arousal. Some level of stress is beneficial for enhancing physiologic and psychological functions. Many individuals, however, equate all stressors with negative reactions. This has resulted in arousal being equated with anxiety. Not all stressors should be viewed as creating a negative response in the body. Instead, an individual's interpretation of a stressor determines whether it is viewed as a threat or challenge (17). If an individual believes that a stressor is a threat, arousal leads to anxiety (53,72).

Physiologic and biochemical measures such as brain activity, heart rate, and the stress hormone cortisol have been used to measure arousal. Additionally, questionnaires have been used to specifically measure individual perceptions of arousal. The study of arousal in sport and athletic competition is important because of the role arousal plays in affecting performance. There are two major models proposed to explain the effects of arousal on performance: drive theory and inverted U hypothesis (53).

Drive Theory

Drive theory is used to describe the relationship between an individual's level of arousal and performance. In general, as arousal increases, performance increases in a linear fashion. Figure 7.8 shows the relationship between arousal and performance. Drive theory predicts that individual motor movements or skill performance is a function of the interaction between habit and arousal. Habit is used to describe the dominance of the most well-learned response of an individual to

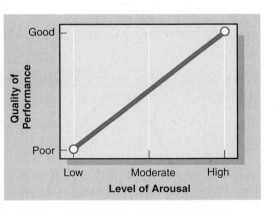

FIGURE 7.8 ▼ Relationship between arousal and performance using the drive theory. (Based on Brown SP. *Introduction to Exercise Science.* Baltimore (MD): Lippincott Williams & Wilkins; 2000. 322 p.)

Arousal A state of responsiveness to stimuli.

a given situation, even if it is an incorrect response (66). Increasing arousal will increase the probability that an individual will select the dominant response for the situation. If it is a correct response, then performance is successful. When a new skill is being learned, there is a higher probability that the dominant response will likely be an incorrect one (53). As an individual becomes better at performing the skill, the dominant response becomes the correct response. In this instance, the increased arousal actually facilitates successful performance (53,74).

For gross motor skills that require muscular strength, speed, and/or endurance a positive linear relationship between arousal and performance exists (53). For example, during the assessment of muscular strength, it is important for the individual being tested to be aroused so that maximal force production is generated during the muscular movement. Professional scholars disagree whether a positive linear relationship exists for those activities requiring the accuracy of fine motor skills. If an individual becomes too aroused, this might result in a decrease in performance. For example, an amateur golfer playing for the local club championship does not want to become too aroused when attempting a short putt that could result in winning the tournament. There appears to be a point of diminishing returns regarding arousal so at the high-intensity end of the arousal continuum, performance is adversely affected by too much arousal (42,53).

Inverted U Hypothesis

The inverted U hypothesis is used to explain changes in performance when there are changes in the level of arousal. As arousal increases from low to moderate levels, there is an increase in skill performance. As arousal continues to increase, there is a point when performance begins to decline. Figure 7.9 shows the relationship between arousal and performance using the inverted U hypothesis (42,53).

To achieve the best possible performance during sport or athletic competitions, optimal arousal must be achieved. At least two factors contribute to obtaining optimal levels of arousal and performance: task characteristics and individual differences. The main features of task characteristics are task complexity and type of task. A simple movement skill requiring few decisions will be less affected by higher levels of arousal than a complex movement skill requiring many decisions. Conversely, a fine movement skill requiring great accuracy or precision would

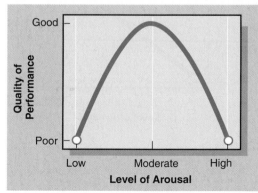

FIGURE 7.9 ▼ Relationship between arousal and performance using the inverted U hypothesis (42, 53). (Based on Brown SP. *Introduction to Exercise Science.* Baltimore (MD): Lippincott Williams & Wilkins; 2000. 322 p.)

require much less arousal for optimal performance than a gross movement skill requiring strength, speed, or endurance (53).

Experience and personality factors can also affect individual performance. A highly experienced athlete can endure higher levels of arousal without an adverse affect on performance. In this instance, the optimal level of arousal is shifted to the right on the arousal continuum. Personality factors associated with arousal have the most influence on the relationship between arousal and performance. Individuals who are more highly aroused in normal situations would not be able to tolerate much additional arousal without an adverse effect on performance. Much of the performance enhancement work in sport psychology deals with helping athletes determine their optimal arousal zones for effective performance and then teaching them skills to assist in achieving and maintaining that optimal arousal level (42,53).

Attention

Attention, as used in exercise and sport psychology, is defined as the ability to focus on a specific skill or activity. Attention may also be more broadly defined as concentration (64) with four components:

* Focusing on the relevant clues in the environment (selective attention)
* Maintaining the attentional focus over time
* Having awareness of the situation
* Shifting attentional focus when necessary (74).

Being able to focus one's attention greatly contributes to success in exercise, sport, and athletic competition. Individuals and especially athletes who can concentrate on certain relevant environmental stimuli, though at the same time ignoring irrelevant stimuli, will have a greater chance at successful performance than individuals who are distracted and unable to concentrate. The amount of effort that is required for such focusing of attention can be important. Typically, as an individual begins to learn a skill, he/she must make a conscious effort to focus attention on the skill and its components. As the individual becomes more proficient at performing the skill, he/she will have to focus less attention on the skill and can focus more on other aspects of the environment (53,74).

Attention is a difficult concept to study in sport and athletic environments because there is no uniform strategy for studying it and because many of the methodologies for studying attention involve the disruption of performance at some level. Additionally, an individual's level of arousal can have an impact on attention, adding another factor that must be considered or controlled. Arousal has its most significant effects on attention by influencing how focused an individual can be. In essence, as individual arousal

> ➤ *Thinking Critically*
>
> *What specific information about an individual would you need to help that individual improve performance during a sport or athletic competition?*

Attention Process whereby a person concentrates on some features of the environment to the (relative) exclusion of others.

Table 7.2	Common Ways to Assess Attention and Limitations Associated with Each (53,74)	
MEASURE OF ATTENTION	**DESCRIPTION**	**LIMITATION**
1. Dual-task paradigm	• Individual is asked to perform two tasks at the same time with the belief that the primary task will require the majority of attention, allowing performance on the second task to be assessed	• The manipulation required fundamentally disrupts performance • It is unclear whether there is a limit to attentional capacity, the assumption of which underlies the technique
2. Self-report	• Individual is asked to provide information about what he/she was focusing on during performance of a skill or task	• It is unclear whether athletes can actually access the cognitive processes that occur during attentionally demanding activities and then put those operations into words • Athletes may not complete assessment questionnaires right before a competition
3. Psychophysiologic measurements	• The psychological construct of attention can be assessed based on physiologic responses of the body immediately prior to performance.	• Measurement of a physiologic variable does necessarily provide the assessment of a psychological variable

increases, the attentional focus narrows and the individual's attention becomes more concentrated. This is required for effective performance. As arousal increases from low to moderate intensity, the individual's attentional field becomes more focused. Performance is generally improved because the narrowing of attention allows the individual to eliminate needless stimuli from the field of attention. However, if arousal is too high it can have an adverse affect on performance. In this instance, attention can become so narrow that the individual misses important information that is central to the performance of the skill or task at hand (53,74). Sport psychology professionals use a variety of techniques and strategies to enhance athletic competition in athletes. Attention can be indirectly assessed using several measurement procedures including behavioral measures of attention, self-report measures of attention, and psychophysiologic measures of attention (53). Table 7.2 provides three of the most common ways to assess attention and limitations associated with each (53,74).

EXERCISE AND MENTAL HEALTH

Mental health problems account for significant hospitalization and medical costs in the United States (38,69,74). For example, treatment for mental health problems had the second highest percentage increase (>7.0%) in medical costs from 1987 to 2000, outgaining treatments for all other disease conditions except heart disease (69). About 15% of all Americans use mental health services, with an estimated 18.1% suffering from **anxiety** and 9.5% suffering from a mood disorder (38). Anxiety and **depression** are significant mental health problems that can also lead to other adverse health conditions (38). Acute and chronic exercises have the potential to influence psychological moods and emotions. Exercise also has the ability to enhance mental health by reducing anxiety and depression (43,49,54) and enhancing psychological well-being (52).

Anxiety

Anxiety is a state of uneasiness and apprehension related to future uncertainties. Acute bouts of physical activity and exercise and participation in regular exercise programs reduce state and trait levels of anxiety. Positive benefits occur in those individuals suffering from normal to moderately high levels of anxiety. Both aerobic exercise and resistance exercise training can reduce anxiety levels with aerobic exercise producing anxiety reductions similar to other commonly used anxiety treatments (53,54,74). Exercise reduces anxiety regardless of an individual's age, gender, fitness level, and health status or anxiety level. Though anxiety levels can be reduced through exercise, there are some general exercise guidelines that should be followed to maximize the influence:

- Exercise intensity should be at least 30% of maximal heart rate
- Exercise durations of up to 30 minutes provide the greatest effects
- Participation in longer training programs has more effect than shorter programs (54,74)

The total volume of exercise required for decreasing anxiety is not entirely clear. Individuals can vary the intensity, duration, and frequency of exercise in an effort to affect psychological status. Depending on the level of anxiety, as little as 5 minutes of exercise may have a positive impact (54).

Depression

Mental depression is a state of general emotional dejection and withdrawal. Though the standard treatment for mental depression is prescription medications or psychotherapy, many individuals use exercise as an effective alternative treatment choice (74). Physical inactivity is also related to higher levels of depression (21). Both aerobic exercise and resistance exercise training can reduce depression, and the reduction occurs for all types of individuals across age, gender, and health status. Exercise produces larger antidepressant effects when the training program is at least 9 weeks in duration and does not depend on changes in fitness level (21,39,53,54). Exercise may work to alleviate depression through psychological or neurobiologic mechanisms. The psychological mechanisms might include enhanced self-efficacy, self-esteem, and improved social support. The neurobiologic mechanisms might include changes in neurotransmitter substances such as norepinephrine, serotonin, and tryptophan, as well as changes in the secretion of hormones from the hypothalamus–pituitary–adrenal axis (39). Future work

---

Anxiety State of uneasiness and apprehension related to future uncertainties.
Depression A reduction in physiologic and psychological activity.

in this area should lead to additional insight into the role of physical activity and exercise as part of the treatment regimen for individuals with depression.

Psychological Well-being

Though much of the past study of psychological changes associated with physical activity and exercise has focused on reductions in negative emotions, there is a significant amount of support for exercise being effective in enhancing and improving many positive psychological states (Figure 7.10) (53). Exercise can have positive effects on mood states such as vigor, clear thinking, energy, alertness, and well-being (74). In some instances, exercise performed for as little as 10 minutes can produce positive psychological benefits (36). One of the most consistently reported effects from acute and chronic exercise is increased feelings of energy (50,68). Physical activity and exercise has also been shown to increase self-confidence, self-esteem, and cognitive function (74). Although it is clear that exercise is related to positive changes in mood (29), it is unclear whether exercise actually causes the enhanced mood (74). The following characteristics and guidelines for physical activity and exercise appear to have the greatest impact on changing an individual's mood:

- Performing rhythmic abdominal breathing
- Relative absence of interpersonal communication
- Performing closed and predictable activities that allow for preplanned movement
- Performing rhythmic and repetitive movements that allow the mind to focus on important issues

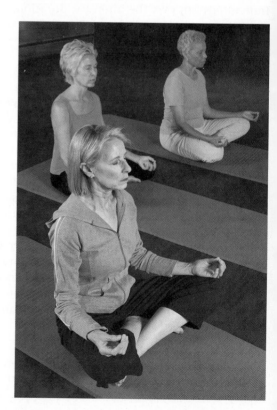

FIGURE 7.10 ▼ Exercise and relaxation. (Photo by Digital Vision/Barry Austin/Getty Images.)

- Performing 20 minutes of a moderate intensity physical activity and exercise
- Performing moderate intensity physical activity or exercise at least two to three times per week
- Performing activities that are enjoyable (7,21,74)

Theories of Exercise and Psychological Well-being

Physical activity and exercise are advocated as a way to maintain and enhance good mental health. In general, exercise can promote improvements in mental health including mood state and self-esteem. Research on acute exercise indicates that 20 to 40 minutes of aerobic activity results in improvements in state anxiety and mood that persist for several hours. Numerous explanations and theories, both physiologic and psychological, have been proposed on how physical activity and exercise enhance mental health. Table 7.3 provides a list of the physiologic and psychological factors that could play a role facilitating improvements in mental health from exercise (74). Although no one theory has support as the sole or primary mechanism producing these positive changes, four explanations are frequently mentioned (50). These include the distraction hypothesis, endorphin hypothesis, thermogenic hypothesis, and monoamine hypothesis (53).

The *distraction hypothesis* is the only true psychological explanation among those hypotheses most commonly proposed. This hypothesis suggests that the reason for an improved emotional profile after exercise is because exercise provides a distraction from the normal everyday occurrences that often lead to stress and negative emotions. This allows the individual to focus on things other than those factors leading to stress and negative emotions (48). The *endorphin hypothesis* is named after a class of stress hormones called endorphins. During exercise, endorphin concentrations are increased and remain elevated for some time after the exercise is finished. Elevated endorphin levels have been positively correlated to individuals feeling better and it has become popular to claim that the endorphins are responsible for this improved mood (67). It has been difficult to prove, however, that the elevation of endorphin levels is responsible for making individuals feel better following exercise. The *thermogenic hypothesis* suggests that exercise of sufficient intensity and/or duration will result in an elevation of body temperature. It is thought that an elevated body temperature will result in a variety of positive changes such as a reduction in

Table 7.3	Physiologic and Psychological Factors That Could Play a Role in the Mental Health Effects of Exercise (53,74)	
PHYSIOLOGIC FACTORS	**PSYCHOLOGICAL FACTORS**
Increases in cerebral blood flow	Enhanced feeling of control
Changes in brain neurotransmitters	Feeling of competency and self-efficacy
Increases in maximal oxygen consumption and delivery of oxygen to brain	Positive social interactions
Reduction in muscle tension	Improved self-concept and self-esteem
Structural changes in the brain	Opportunities for fun and enjoyment

muscle tension after exercise and other psychological changes (11). The *monoamine hypothesis* suggests that changes in brain neurotransmitters can result in exercise-induced emotional changes. The neurotransmitters norepinephrine, dopamine, and serotonin are often localized to brain structures known to have an important role in emotion and are altered with exercise (57). Although each of these hypotheses provides indirect support for a role of physical activity and exercise reducing stress and negative emotions, much more work needs to be done to better understand the mechanisms for how physical activity and exercise enhances mental health.

Exercise and Brain Function

Exercise impacts every system in the body including the brain where it enhances and protects brain function. Aging causes dysfunction and degeneration in neurons and personality changes in some instances. Changes in brain **neurotransmitters** determine how factors like brain blood flow, brain electric activity, and by-products of brain neurotransmitters are linked with emotions and thoughts (14). Blood flow to the brain changes with exercise. As exercise intensity increases from low to moderate levels, the temporal, parietal, and frontal regions of the brain have an increase in blood flow. Recorded electric activity of the brain has been shown to predict how an individual will feel after that exercise (55). Higher-level functions of the brain, especially those associated with frontal lobe and hippocampal regions of the brain, may be selectively maintained or enhanced in humans with higher levels of fitness (13,53).

Regular exercise training can also influence brain function, particularly in older adults. Lifetime exercise enhances several aspects of cognition. Much of this research has employed aerobic exercise such as walking, running, bicycling, and swimming. Cross-sectional studies have shown that aerobic exercise improves both the peripheral and central nervous system components of reaction resulting in a reduced time to recognize and respond to a stimulus. Individuals who have engaged in exercise for a lengthy period of their lives respond more quickly to the presentation of auditory or visual stimuli, discriminate between multiple stimuli, and make faster movements. Additionally, exercisers can outperform non-exercisers on tasks such as reasoning, working memory, and fluid intelligence tests. Differences in performance on seemingly similar tasks between lifetime exercisers and non-exercisers, however, have not always been found (13,53).

> ➤ *Thinking Critically*
>
> *How do the various content areas of exercise psychology provide for improvements in healthcare for healthy and diseased individuals?*

EXERCISE BEHAVIOR

Physical inactivity and poor fitness are strong predictors of disease risk. For example, individuals who are physically inactive have a higher risk for certain types of cardiovascular disease and cancer (46). Being physically active promotes good health and decreases the risk of morbidity and mortality (9,40,45,52). Despite national efforts at promoting physical activity, morbidity and mortality rates from lifestyle-related diseases are at an all-time high (27,46). There are numerous physiologic and psychological benefits to be derived from being physically active.

Regular physical activity has been shown to

- Reduce the risk of cardiovascular disease including stroke, high blood pressure, and coronary artery disease
- Reduce the risk of certain cancers including colorectal and breast
- Be an important component for promoting weight loss and maintaining a healthy body weight
- Improve psychological factors such as a reduction in stress and depression and an increase in self-esteem (74)

Despite the many benefits derived from participating in regular programs of physical activity and exercise, approximately 50% of American men and women do not perform sufficient regular physical activities to meet the *Healthy People 2010* objective of at least 30 minutes a day of moderate-intensity activity on 5 or more days a week, or at least 20 minutes a day of vigorous-intensity activity on 3 or more days a week, or both (41). Many barriers to exercise participation are within the control of the individual and hence amenable to change (74). The major barriers to participating in regular physical activity and exercise programs are lack of time, lack of energy, and lack of motivation (51,61,74). If an individual does overcome the barriers and begins an exercise program, the next obstacle he/she will encounter is to continue regular participation with the program. **Exercise adherence** is challenging for most individuals and approximately 50% of those individuals who start a program discontinue or "drop out" within the first 6 months (18). Individuals cite a variety of reasons for discontinuing a regular physical activity and exercise (18,63). In an effort to better understand why people either do not begin a regular program or discontinue a program, exercise psychology professionals have promoted several theories and models of exercise behavior. It is important for exercise science professionals to have a solid understanding of how these theories influence exercise behaviors.

Theories and Models of Exercise Behavior

It is believed that improvements in exercise adoption and adherence can occur if a better understanding of how and why individuals participate in physical activity and exercise is achieved. There are four prominent models used to help explain the process of exercise adoption and adherence (16,74). Table 7.4 illustrates the four models of exercise behavior and the theory associated with each model. Each of the proposed models (**Health Behavior, Theory of Planned Behavior/Reason Action**, Social Cognitive Theory, and **Transtheoretical**) has been used

---

Neurotransmitter A chemical substance that is produced and secreted by a nerve ending and then diffuses across a synapse to cause the excitation or inhibition of another nerve.

Exercise adherence The ability to continue participation in a regular program of exercise.

Health Behavior A theoretical model used to explain and predict individual health behaviors using six constructs of behavior.

Theory of Planned Behavior/Reason Action A theory used to describe and predict deliberate and planned individual behavior.

Transtheoretical Model of Behavior A model used to understand the stages that individuals progress through, and the cognitive and behavioral processes they use while changing health behaviors.

Table 7.4	Models of Exercise Behavior and the Theory Associated with Each Model (74)
MODEL	**THEORY**
Health Belief Model	• Probability of an individual engaging in exercise depends on the person's perception of the severity of the potential illness as well as the appraisal of the costs and benefits of exercise (6)
Theory of Planned Behavior/ Reasoned Action	• Probability of an individual engaging in exercise depends on the individual's attitudes toward a particular behavior and the individual's perceptions of his/her ability to perform the behavior (2)
Social Cognitive Theory	• Probability of an individual engaging in exercise depends on the personal, behavioral, and environmental factors that interact in a reciprocal manner (4)
Transtheoretical model	• Probability of an individual engaging in exercise depends on the stage of change the individual is currently in for establishing and maintaining a lifestyle change (56)

in different settings to help understand why individuals may or may not initiate and continue participation in a regular exercise program.

The *Health Behavior Model* is a psychological model that attempts to explain and predict individual health behaviors. The original model provides four constructs representing the perceived threat and net benefits of an action or behavior: perceived susceptibility, perceived severity, perceived benefits, and perceived barriers. These concepts were proposed as an explanation for an individual's readiness to take action. Two additional concepts were subsequently added to the model: cues to action and self-efficacy. Cues to action would activate the readiness of an individual and stimulate overt behavior. The most recent addition to the model is self-efficacy, or an individual's confidence in the ability to successfully perform an action. This concept was added to help the Health Behavior Model better fit the challenges of changing habitual unhealthy behaviors, such as being sedentary, smoking, or overeating (60).

The *Theory of Planned Behavior/Reasoned Action* is used to describe and predict deliberate behavior because behavior can be deliberative and planned. The Theory of Planned Behavior/Reasoned Action is based on the belief that an individual's behavior is determined by his/her intention to carry out the behavior and that this intention is, in turn, a function of his/her attitude about the behavior and his/her subjective norm. The best predictor of an individual's behavior is the intention to perform the behavior. Intention is the cognitive representation of an individual's readiness to perform a given behavior, and it is considered to be the immediate antecedent of behavior. This intention is determined by three factors: attitude toward the specific behavior, subjective norms, and perceived behavioral control. The Theory of Planned Behavior/Reasoned Action maintains that only specific attitudes toward the behavior in question can be expected to predict that behavior (1).

Social Cognitive Theory explains how individuals acquire and maintain certain behavioral patterns and can also be used to provide the basis for intervention strategies (5). Evaluating behavioral change depends on the environment, the individual, and the behavior. This theory provides a framework for designing, implementing, and evaluating programs. The environment refers to the factors (social and physical) that can affect an individual's behavior. The social environment refers to individual and group interactions that could influence behavior and includes family members, friends, and colleagues. The physical environment refers to the factors in the built environment the individual encounters and includes, for example, the size and shape of a room, the weather conditions, or the availability of specific foods. The environment combined with the individual situation provides the framework for understanding an individual's behavior. The situation refers to the mental representations of the environment that may affect an individual's behavior. The situation includes an individual's perception of the place, time, physical features, and activity (33). The social and physical environments constantly influence each other. Individual behavior is not simply the result of the environment and the individual (33). The environment provides models for behavior, and individuals do certain things in response to the environmental and social factors (5).

The *Transtheoretical Model* has been used to understand the stages that individuals progress through, and the cognitive and behavioral processes they use while changing health behaviors. The Transtheoretical model is effective at predicting and explaining the exercise behaviors of individuals (44). In this model, there are five stages of change in which individuals progress through as a behavior is adopted (44). The five stages are shown in Figure 7.11. The model postulates that individuals engaging in a new behavior move through the stages of precontemplation, contemplation, preparation, action, and maintenance. Movement through these stages does not always occur in a linear manner, but may also be cyclic as many individuals must make several attempts at behavioral change before their goals are realized. The amount of progress people make as a result of intervention tends to be a function of the stage they are in at the start of treatment. Instruments have been developed to measure the stages and processes of exercise adoption and maintenance

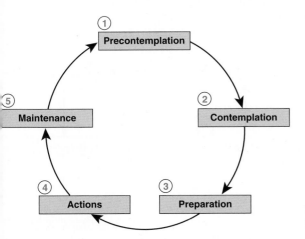

FIGURE 7.11 ▼ Cyclic pattern of stages of change (56,74).

and the related constructs of exercise specific self-efficacy and decision making (33). Movement through the stages is cyclic and can be affected by many factors outside a person's control. Individuals use numerous strategies and techniques to change behaviors, and the strategies are their processes of change (74).

Determinants of Exercise Adherence

Exercise psychology is used to help better understand the thought process of individuals adopting and maintaining a regular exercise program. This is critical for developing strategies that will enhance individual exercise adherence. The natural progression for an individual wishing to participate in an exercise program is illustrated in Figure 7.12. Movement into and out of each major phase can be affected by numerous factors (62). These determinants can be categorized into personal and environmental factors that can have positive, negative, or no influence on exercise adherence (19,20,74). The personal determinants can be further divided into demographic, cognitive and personality variables, and behaviors whereas the environmental determinants can be divided into social environment, physical environment, and physical activity characteristics (74). Examples of personal determinants include age, education level, exercise knowledge, attitude, and level of self-confidence. Examples of environmental determinants include access to facilities, cost, family influences, and perceived available time (62).

> ➤ **Thinking Critically**
>
> *How might coursework in exercise and sport psychology prepare an individual for a career as a healthcare specialist, personal trainer, or athletic coach?*

Using the information about an individual's personal and environmental determinants in conjunction with the theories of behavior change, exercise and sport psychology professionals as well as other exercise science professionals can develop effective strategies for enhancing exercise adherence. Table 7.5 illustrates some of the major approaches and strategies for enhancing exercise adherence (74). It is important to effectively match the theories and models of exercise behavior with the appropriate strategy for enhancing adherence to increase the probability of an individual adopting regular exercise as a healthy behavior. By not effectively promoting adherence, there is a greater likelihood that an individual will discontinue a regular program of physical activity and exercise and thereby not derive the associated health benefits (53,74).

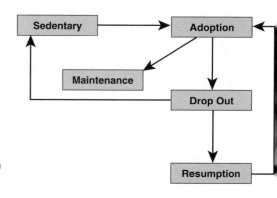

FIGURE 7.12 ▼ Natural progression phases of exercise (62).

Table 7.5	Major Approaches and Strategies for Enhancing Exercise Adherence (74)	
STRATEGY	**EXAMPLES**	
Behavior modification approaches	• Prompts • Contracting	
Reinforcement approaches	• Charting attendance and participation • Rewarding attendance and participation • Feedback	
Cognitive and behavioral approaches	• Goal setting • Association and dissociation	
Decision-making approaches	• Decision balance sheet	
Social support approaches	• Social and family actions	
Intrinsic approaches	• Focus on the experience • Process orientation • Engagement in purposeful and meaningful activity	

INTERVIEW

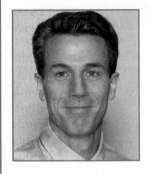

Jack Raglin, PhD, FACSM, Professor, Department of Kinesiology, Indiana University-Bloomington.

Brief Introduction

My career as an undergraduate college student began in 1975 at the University of Nebraska. I was looking forward to college and was interested in many academic topics, but devoted to none. My initial plan was to major in biology with a general goal of working in the medical field, but I found myself unmotivated by the idea of a focus on a career path that would inevitably be preoccupied with some aspect of illness. I ended up switching my major to psychology as a junior, with an academic minor in life sciences and art. But again, if I was going to go on in graduate school I saw the career options dealing once again with illness, and whether it be psychological or physical, it did not appeal to me.

➤ **Why did you choose your professional career?**

My work in the field of sport psychology has focused on the intersection of physiology and psychology as it applies to both sport and physical exercise. By unplanned but fortuitous circumstances, my undergraduate education in psychology with a minor in life science left me well prepared for graduate study in sport psychology.

Although this coursework was enjoyable and intellectually stimulating, I had no interest in pursuing a career in counseling or social work, and was unsure of what direction to take if I went on for graduate school. By chance, I learned about Dr Jim Crabbe, a faculty member in physical education who was doing psychological research on athletes. This piqued my curiosity because I had a personal interest in sport and physical fitness but

(Continued)

even more so because I had no inkling that an academic field in sport psychology actually existed. I contacted Dr Crabbe who graciously allowed me to work with him on several research projects. He also provided me information about graduate programs in sport psychology and advised me to take courses in exercise physiology and anatomy, which would likely be prerequisites. After graduating, I began graduate school at the University of Wisconsin-Madison under the preeminent sport psychologist Dr William P. Morgan. In retrospect, I could not have chosen a better department or mentor, but the main reason for applying was that Dr Fran Nagle, an exercise physiologist in the department, strongly recommended the program to my father, who had long known Dr Nagle from his days as the All-American quarterback at the University of Nebraska.

➤ Which individuals or experiences were most influential in your career development?

The experiences I had at Wisconsin set the stage for my professional career. The faculty and students were uniformly outstanding and a strong commitment to research permeated the department. The range of Dr Morgan's research was unprecedented in the field; it not only addressed traditional issues in sport but also the psychology of exercise. Another important influence on me at Wisconsin was Dr Henry Montoye. Monty, as he was referred to by his fellow faculty (but never students), ran a team-taught course on exercise and health that I was assigned to serve as a teaching assistant. He also sat on my thesis and dissertation committee and helped me immensely, never failing to identify the critical issues or limitations in my research despite his own work in physiology and epidemiology. For me it was a formative lesson that the well-trained researcher was not relegated to a single field, but could work across a variety of disciplines. Today I greatly enjoy the challenges and rewards of working with students and faculty whose research falls outside my own specialization.

➤ What are your most significance professional accomplishments?

To one extent or another, my most productive lines of research have their roots at the University of Wisconsin. It was there I first became involved with Dr Morgan's studies with swimmers and other endurance athletes, which were done in an effort to understand and prevent the occurrence of overtraining syndrome. The findings of this work revealed that changes in mood state are among the most reliable means of determining if athletes are adapting to intense training. My own research on overtraining has involved, among other things, examining the association between mood changes during overtraining with relevant biologic variables. Another line of research which began under Dr Morgan examined the psychological benefits of single bouts of exercise, and my recent work on this topic has centered on quantifying how different exercise modes and dosages influence state anxiety. For example, we have found that aerobic exercise consistently results in significantly greater anxiety reduction than anaerobic activity, even after controlling for intensity and duration, but combining both modes in a single session yields positive benefits.

➤ What advice would you have for an undergraduate student beginning to explore a career in exercise science?

My advice to the undergraduate student who is exploring career options or considering graduate school is simple. Explore! The more students and faculty you meet, the greater the number of academic settings you experience and the more eclectic your courses, the wider your vista will become. My own career path in sport psychology began after a serendipitous meeting with a professor from a school and department completely removed from my major. Learning about different fields and research topics will not only help you make more informed decisions about your career path but will make you more adaptable in whatever field of research or work setting you choose. The pace of science insures that during your career you will witness the creation of entirely new fields of research. The more transdisciplinary your training and more adaptable your own perspective, the more easily you will be able to negotiate the ever-changing tides of research.

SUMMARY

- Exercise psychology and sport psychology are areas of study concerned with the behavior, thoughts, and feelings of healthy, disabled, and diseased individuals engaging in physical activity, exercise, sport, and athletic competition.
- Individual factors of personality, motivation, arousal, and attention each have a strong influence on the successful performance of exercise and sport.
- Regular physical activity and exercise can influence mental health by reducing anxiety and depression, enhancing psychological well-being, and improving various aspects of brain function
- Exercise adherence is important for achieving significant physical and mental health benefits but it can be affected by several personal and environmental factors.

FOR REVIEW

1. What are the specific areas of study in exercise psychology and sport psychology?
2. Describe the first experimental research study that directly impacted exercise and sport psychology.
3. What are the primary professional organizations in exercise psychology and sport psychology?
4. Name the primary research journals in exercise psychology and sport psychology.
5. Describe how personality plays a role in exercise, sport, and athletic competition.
6. What two personality characteristics are strong predictors of exercise behavior?
7. Describe the difference between extrinsic and intrinsic motivation as they relate to participation in physical activity and exercise?
8. How does self-efficacy influence performance in sport and athletic competition?
9. What individual characteristics do chronic exercisers display?
10. Describe why a level of arousal that is too high can adversely affect performance?
11. Why is attention difficult to study during a sport or athletic competition?
12. Describe how acute and chronic exercises might influence an individual's level of anxiety and depression.
13. List five factors or characteristics that physical activity and exercise should possess to impact an individual's mood.
14. Describe how each of the following theories enhances psychological well-being:
    a. Distraction
    b. Endorphin
    c. Thermogenic
    d. Monoamine
15. How does the transtheoretical model predict and explain the exercise behavior of individuals?

REFERENCES

1. Ajzen I. The theory of planned behavior. *Organ Behav Hum Decis Process*. 1991;50:179–211.
2. Ajzen I, Madden TJ. Prediction of goal-directed behavior: attitudes, intentions, and perceived behavioral control. *J Exp Social Psychol*. 1986;22:453–74.
3. Anastasi A. *Psychological Testing*. New York (NY): Macmillan; 1988.
4. Bandura A. *Social Foundations of Thought and Actions: A Social Cognitive Theory*. Englewood Cliffs (NJ): Prentice-Hall; 1986.
5. Bandura A. *Self-efficacy: The Exercise of Control*. New York (NY): Freeman; 1997.
6. Becker MH, Maiman LA. Sociobehavioral determinants of compliance with health care and medical care recommendations. *Med Care*. 1975;13:10–24.
7. Berger BG, Motl RW. Physical activity and quality of life. In: Singer R, Hausenblas HA, Janelle CM, editors. *Handbook of Sport Psychology*. New York (NY): Wiley; 2001. p. 636–70.
8. Berger BG, Owen DR. Stress reduction and mood enhancement in four exercise modes: Swimming, body conditioning, hatha yoga, and fencing. *Res Q Exerc Sport*. 1988;59:148–59.
9. Bish CL, Blanck HM, Serdula MK, Marcus M, Kohl HW, Khan LK. Diet and physical activity behaviors among americans trying to lose weight: 2000 behavioral risk factor surveillance system. *Obes Res*. 2005;13:596–607.
10. Brustad R. A critical analysis of knowledge construction in sport psychology. In: Horn TS, editor. *Advances in Sport Psychology*. Champaign (IL): Human Kinetics; 2002. p. 21–37.
11. Bulbulian R, Darabos BL. Motor neuron excitability: The Hoffman reflex following exercise of high and low intensity. *Med Sci Sports Exerc*. 1986;18:697–702.
12. Cattell RB. *The Scientific Analysis of Personality*. Baltimore (MD): Penguin; 1965.
13. Churchill JD, Galvez R, Colcombe S, Swain RA, Kramer AF, Greenough WT. Exercise, experience and the aging brain. *Neurobiol Aging*. 2002;23:941–55.
14. Cotman CW, Engesser-Cesar C. Exercise enhances and protects brain function. *Exerc Sport Sci Rev*. 2002;30:75–9.
15. Crews DJ, Landers DM. A meta-analytic review of aerobic fitness and reactivity to pscyhological stressors. *Med Sci Sports Exerc*. 1987;19:114–20.
16. Culos-Reed SN, Gyurcsik NC, Brawley LR. Using theories of motivated behavior to understand physical activity. In: Singer RN, Hausenblaus HA, Janelle CM, editors. *Handbook of Sport Psychology*. New York (NY): Wiley; 2001. p. 695–717.
17. Dienstbier RA. Arousal and physiological toughness: Implications for mental and physical health. *Psychol Rev*. 1989;96:84–100.
18. Dishman RK. *Exercise Adherence: Its Impact on Public Health*. Champaign (IL): Human Kinetics; 1994.
19. Dishman RK, Buckworth J. Adherence to physical activity. In: Morgan WP, editor. *Physical Activity and Mental Health*. Philadelphia (PA): Taylor & Francis; 1997. p. 63–80.
20. Dishman RK, Sallis JF. Determinants and interventions for physical activity and exercise. In: Bouchard C, Shepard RJ, Stephens T, editors. *Physical Activity,*

Fitness, and Health. Champaign (IL): Human Kinetics; 1994. p. 214–38.
21. Dunn AL, Trivedi MH, O'Neal HA. Physical activity dose-response effects on outcomes of depression and anxiety. *Med Sci Sports Exerc*. 2001;33:S587–97.
22. Dzewaltowski DA. Toward a model of exercise motivation. *J Sport Exerc Psychol*. 1989;11:251–69.
23. Dzewaltowski DA. The ecology of physical activity and sport: Merging science and practice. *J Appl Sport Psychol*. 1997;9:254–76.
24. Eysenck HJ, Eysenck SBG. *Eysenck Personality Inventory Manual*. London: University of London Press; 1968.
25. Eysenck HJ, Nias DK, Cox DN. Sport and personality. *Adv Behav Res Ther*. 1982;4:1–56.
26. Feltz DL. Self-confidence and sports performance. In: Pandolf KB, editor. *Exercise and Sport Science Reviews*. New York (NY): MacMillan; 1988. p. 423–57.
27. Flegal KM, Williamson DF, Pamuk ER, Rosenberg HM. Estimating deaths attributable to obesity in the United States. *Am J Public Health*. 2004;94:1486–9.
28. Fox KR. Self-esteem, self-perceptions and exercise. *Int J Sport Psychol*. 2000;31:228–40.
29. Gauvin L, Rejeski WJ, Reboussin BA. Contributions of acute bouts of vigorous physical activity to explaining diurnal variations in feeling states in active middle-aged women. *Health Psychol*. 2000;19:265–75.
30. Giacobbi PR, Poczwardowski A, Hager P. A pragmatic research philosophy for applied sport psychology. *The Sport Psychol*. 2005;19:18–31.
31. Gill DL. Feminist sport psychology; a guide for our journey. *The Sport Psychol*. 2001;15:363–72.
32. Gill DL. Sport and exercise psychology. In: Massengale JD, Swanson RA, editors. *The History of Exercise and Sport*. Champaign (IL): Human Kinetics, Inc; 2003. p. 293–320.
33. Glanz K, Rimer BK, Lewis FM. *Health Behavior and Health Education. Theory, Research and Practice*. San Francisco (CA): Wiley & Sons; 2002.
34. Green CD. Psychology strikes out: Coleman R. Griffith and the Chicago Cubs. *Hist Psychol*. 2003;6:267–83.
35. Hall GS. *Physical Education in Colleges: Report of the National Education Association*. Chicago (IL): University of Chicago Press; 1908.
36. Hansen CJ, Stevens LC, Coast JR. Exercise duration and mood state: How much is enough to feel better? *Health Psychol*. 2001;20:267–75.
37. Hollander EP. *Principles and Methods of Social Psychology*. New York (NY): Oxford University Press; 1967.
38. Kessler RC, Chiu WT, Demler O, Walters EE. Prevalence, severity, and comorbidity of twelve-month DSM-IV disorders in the National Comorbidity Survey Replication. *Arch Gen Psychiatry*. 2005;62:617–27.
39. Knubben K, Reischies FM, Adli M, et al. A randomised, controlled study on the effects of a short-term endurance training programme in patients with major depression * Commentary. *Br J Sports Med*. 2007;41:29–33.
40. Kohrt WM, Bloomfield SA, Little KD, Nelson ME, Yingling VR, American College of Sports Medicine. Physical activity and bone health. *Med Sci Sports Exerc*. 1996;36:1985–96.

41. Kruger J, Miles IJ. Prevalence of regular physical activity among adults—United States, 2001 and 2005. *Morb Mortal.* 2007;56:1209–12.

42. Landers DM, Boutcher SH. Arousal performance relationships. In: Williams JM, editor. *Applied Sport Psychology: Personal Growth to Peak Performance.* Mountain View (CA): Mayfield; 1993. p.197–218.

43. Landers DM, Petruzzello SJ. Physical activity, fitness, and anxiety. In: Bouchard C, Shepard RJ, Stephens T, editors. *Physical Activity, Fitness, and Health.* Champaign (IL): Human Kinetics; 1994. p. 868–82.

44. Marcus BH, Dubbert PM, Forsyth LH, et al. Physical activity behavior change: Issues in adoption and maintenance. *Health Psychol.* 2000;19:32–41.

45. Mazzeo RS, Cavanagh PR, Evans WJ, et al. Position Stand: Exercise and physical activity for older adults. *Med Sci Sports Exerc.* 1998;30:992–1008.

46. Minino AM, Heron MP, Murphy SL, Kochanek KD. *Deaths: Final Data for 2004.* Washington (DC): U.S. Department of Health and Human Services; 2007. p. 55–19, 1–120.

47. Morgan WP. Hypnosis and muscular performance. In: Morgan WP, editor. *Ergogenic Aids and Muscular Performance.* New York (NY): Academic Press; 1972. p. 193–233.

48. Morgan WP. Affective beneficence of vigorous physical activity. *Med Sci Sports Exerc.* 1985;6:422–5.

49. Morgan WP. Physical activity, fitness, and depression. In: Bouchard C, Shepard RJ, Stephens T, editors. *Physical Activity, Fitness, and Health.* Champaign (IL): Human Kinetics; 1994. p. 851–67.

50. Morgan WP, O'Connor PJ. Exercise and mental health. In: Dishman RK, editor. *Exercise Adherence: Its Impact on Public Health.* Champaign (IL): Human Kinetics; 1988. p. 91–121.

51. Myers RS, Ross DL. Perceived benefits of and barriers to exercise and stage of exercise adoption in young adults. *Health Psychol.* 1997;16:277–83.

52. Pate RR, Pratt M, Blair SN, et al. A recommendation from the Centers for Disease Control and Prevention and the American College of Sports Medicine. *JAMA.* 1995;273:402–7.

53. Petruzzello SJ. Exercise and sports psychology. In: Brown SP, editor. *Introduction to Exercise Science.* Philadelphia (PA): Lippincott, Williams & Wilkins; 2001. p. 310–33.

54. Petruzzello SJ, Landers DM, Hatfield BD, et al. A meta-analysis on the anxiety reducing effects of acute and chronic exercise: Outcomes and mechanisms. *Sports Med.* 1991;11:143–82.

55. Petruzzello SJ, Tate AK. Brain activation, affect, and aerobic exercise: An examination of both state-independent and state-dependent relationships. *Psychophysiology.* 1997;34:527–33.

56. Prochaska JO, Johnson SS, Lee P. The v change. In: Schron E, Ockene J, Schumaker S, Exum WM, editors. *The Handbook of Behavioral Change.* New York (NY): Springer; 1998. p. 159–84.

57. Ransford CP. A role for amines in the antidepressive effect of exercise: A review. *Med Sci Sports Exerc.* 1982;14:1–10.

58. Rejeski WJ, Brawley LR. Defining the boundaries of sport psychology. *Sport Psychol.* 1988;2:231–42.

59. Rejeski WJ, Thompson A. Historical and conceptual roots of exercise psychology. In: Seraganian P, editor. *Exercise Psychology: The Influence of Physical Exercise on Psychological Processes.* New York (NY): John Wiley & Sons; 1993. p. 3–35.

60. Rosenstock IM, Strecher VJ, Becker MH. Social learning theory and the health belief model. *Health Educ Behav.* 1988;15:175–83.

61. Russell SJ, Craig CL. *Physical Activity and Lifestyles in Canada.* Ottawa (ON): Canadian Fitness and Lifestyle Research Institute; 1996. p. 1–7.

62. Sallis JF, Hovell MF. Determinants of exercise behavior. In: Pandolf KB, Holloszy JO, editors. *Exercise and Sport Science Reviews.* Baltimore (MD): Williams & Wilkins; 1990. p. 307–30.

63. Sallis JF, Hovell MF, Hofstetter CR, et al. Distance between homes and exercise facilities related to Frequency of exercise among San Diego residents. *Public Health Rep.* 1990;105:179–85.

64. Solso RL. *Cognitive Psychology.* Boston (MA): Allyn & Bacon; 1995.

65. Sonstroem RJ, Morgan WP. Exercise and self-esteem: Rationale and model. *Med Sci Sports Exerc.* 1989;21:329–37.

66. Spence JT, Spence KW. The motivational components of manifest anxiety: Drive and drive stimuli. In: Spielberger CD, editor. *Anxiety and Behavior.* New York (NY): Academic; 1966.

67. Steinberg H, Sykes EA. Introduction to symposium on endorphins and behavioral processes: Review of literature on endorphins and exercise. *Pharmacol Biochem Behav.* 1985;23:857–62.

68. Thayer RE. *The Biopsychology of Mood and Arousal.* New York (NY): Oxford University Press; 1989.

69. Thorpe KE, Florence CS, Joski P. Which medical conditions account for the rise in health care spending? *Health Aff.* 2004;26:678–686.

70. Triplett N. The dynamogenic factors in pacemaking and competition. *Am J Psychol.* 1898;9:507–53.

71. Vealey RS. Personality and sport: A comprehensive view. In: Horn TS, editor. *Advances in Sport Psychology.* Champaign (IL): Human Kinetics; 2002.

72. Vealey RS. Introduction to Kinesiology. In: *Sport and Exercise Psychology.* 3rd Ed. Champaign (IL): Human Kinetics; 2005. pp. 269–300.

73. Vealey RS. Smocks and jocks outside the box: The paradigmatic evolution of sport and exercise psychology. *Quest.* 2006;58:128–59.

74. Weinberg RS, Gould D. *Foundations of Sport and Exercise Psychology.* Champaign (IL): Human Kinetics; 2007.

75. Weiner B. *An Attributional Theory of Motivation and Emotion.* New York (NY): Springer; 1986.

CHAPTER

Motor Behavior

After completing this chapter, you will be able to:

1. Define motor behavior and provide examples of how motor development, motor learning, and motor control contribute to the understanding of physical activity, exercise, sport, and athletic performance.

2. Identify the important historic events in the development of motor behavior as a scientific discipline.

3. Discuss the important areas of study in motor development, motor learning, and motor control.

4. Describe some of the important topics in the fields of motor development, motor learning, and motor control.

The basic and applied knowledge found in the discipline of **motor behavior** impacts exercise science professionals in many important ways. Motor behavior is an umbrella term that describes the study of the interactions between many of the physiologic and psychological processes of the body. Motor behavior helps provide exercise science and allied health professionals with an understanding of how the body develops, controls, and learns movement skills that individuals use not only in physical activity, exercise, sport, and athletic competition but in everyday activities as well. Exercise science professionals use the knowledge gain from the study of motor behavior to improve physical activity and exercise performance and enhance success in sport and athletic competition. Motor behavior is comprised of three related areas of study: motor development, motor learning, and motor control (22).

Motor development is the study of change in motor behavior over a life span and the various processes, which underlie these changes (8). Motor development is an area of study that examines the alterations in motor behavior that result from the maturation of the individual, rather than those alterations that occur owing to practice or experience. Motor development is concerned with how individuals learn and control movement as physical and mental changes occur over the lifespan. Originally, motor development involved the study of developmental changes from infancy to adulthood, but it now also includes changes that occur to the aged individual (22).

Motor learning is the study of how individuals learn skilled movements from practice or experience (46). When individuals learn how to move in efficient motor patterns, there is often a permanent change in the neural control of muscle actions. Motor learning has evolved primarily from the disciplines of psychology and education. The application of its principles, however, is found in all areas of exercise science and sports medicine (22).

Motor control is the study of the neurologic, physiologic, and behavioral aspects of movement (46). The neuromuscular system commands complex and coordinated movements by individuals, and motor control is concerned with how our brain and spinal cord plan and perform those movements. Motor control includes the study of how the central nervous system controls the body prior to as well as during movement (22).

Each of the areas comprising motor behavior is interrelated and all have application to the performance of physical activity, exercise, sport and athletic competition. The development of knowledge and the study of motor development, learning and control is, however, generally performed separately. This is partially because the individuals studying these areas come from different fields of science. It is also important to understand that the broad application of motor behavior

Motor behavior An umbrella term that includes the disciplines of motor control, motor learning, and motor development.

Motor development The study of motor performance throughout the life span from birth through old age.

Motor learning The study of the acquisition of basic and advanced movement skills that are used in everyday activities.

Motor control The study of the understanding of the mechanisms by which the nervous and muscular systems coordinate body movements.

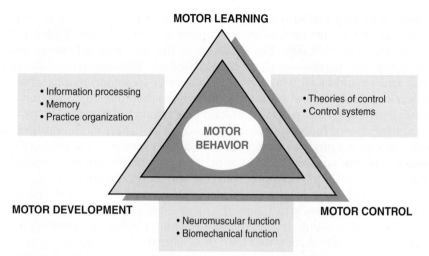

MOTOR LEARNING

- Information processing
- Memory
- Practice organization

MOTOR BEHAVIOR

- Theories of control
- Control systems

MOTOR DEVELOPMENT

- Neuromuscular function
- Biomechanical function

MOTOR CONTROL

FIGURE 8.1 ▼ A schematic of the general organizational structure of motor behavior (22). (From Brown SP. *Introduction to Exercise Science.* Baltimore (MD): Lippincott, Williams & Wilkins; 2000. 335 p.)

goes beyond the study of movement associated with exercise, sport, and athletic competition. The principles of motor behavior are applied to a variety of other skills such as factory work, operating equipment and machinery, and performing complex movements associated with leisure activities. Figure 8.1 provides a schematic of the general organizational structure of motor behavior (22). Exercise science and allied health professionals working in a variety of employment settings use the principles of motor behavior to enhance performance in a variety of activities, as well as promote recovery from injury or medical interventions. The historic development of motor behavior is derived from an interaction of the parent disciplines of biology, psychology, and education.

BRIEF HISTORY OF MOTOR BEHAVIOR

Similar to many of the other areas of study in exercise science, the history of motor behavior begins with the writings of ancient scholars who provided the framework for many of the principles associated with nervous system control over muscle contraction. Trying to provide an overview of the history of motor behavior is challenging, however, because much of the historic development of the three areas is interrelated. Only recently have distinct separations of the areas of motor development, motor control, and motor learning occurred.

Early Influences on Motor Development

The area of motor development had its early foundational period from 1787 to 1928. During this time, contemporary developmental psychology and motor development had established a basis for study. Most of the prominent information in motor development came from observing the activities of babies and their changes in reflexes, movements, and feeding behaviors on a day-to-day basis (8). The publication of the book *Infancy and Human Growth* (21) in 1929 marked a period of increased

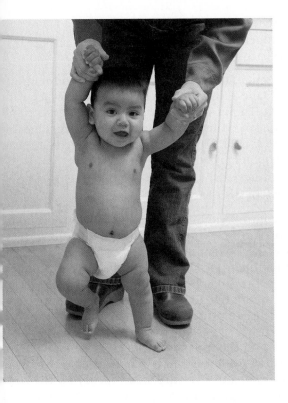

FIGURE 8.2 ▼ Motor development of a young infant. (Photo by Digital Vision/Steven Puetzer/Getty Images.)

research and study in motor development. Throughout the early twentieth century, important work in motor development was being conducted on infants and children (Figure 8.2). For example, a classic study by Myrtle B. McGraw (1899–1988) provided a thorough description of the behavior sequences that occur in infants and young children (36). Significant work was also performed on the role of maturation on motor development and the ability of children to reach, sit, and stand (10,51). During the mid-twentieth century, much of the research and scholarly activity performed in motor development was conducted by physical educators who had an interest in the growth, strength, and motor performance in children (51).

Recent Influences on Motor Development

Beginning in the mid-1960s, a shift in the focus of motor development occurred from an emphasis on developmental psychology and the understanding of the influence of maturation to a physical education emphasis on how to improve children's motor behavior (8). This allowed motor development to become part of the study of physical activity (51). During the late 1960s and early 1970s, there were four influential books published by scholars that served to define motor development (9,12,41,53). During the 1980s and 1990s, there was a shift in major areas of research and study in motor development that resulted in an expansion of knowledge in the following subjects:

- Variations in performance associated with age and gender
- Variation in performance associated with maturation

- Physical activity as a factor in growth and maturation
- Racial/ethnic and social factors influencing motor performance
- Cognitive factors in children's skill acquisition (51)

Individuals who have been instrumental in the advancement of motor development include G. Lawrence Rarick, Jane E. Clark, Robert M. Malina, Mary Ann Roberton, Vern Seefeldt, and Jerry R. Thomas (51). The Motor Development and Learning Special Interest Area within the American Alliance for Health, Physical Education, Recreation, and Dance (AAHPERD) is considered a primary professional organization for motor development scholars and professionals (51).

Early Influences on Motor Control and Motor Learning

Much of the early work in motor control and motor learning focused on understanding and explaining the control of muscle contraction by the nervous system. Claudius Galen (ca. 129–ca. 216 AD), a Roman physician, proposed that muscle contraction was controlled by a fluid that passed down the nerves to the muscles, causing them to inflate. Galen termed the fluid, the key component to this hydraulic system, as "animal spirits." This theory remained until Rene Descartes (1596–1650) expanded on Galen's proposed hydraulic system in the mid-seventeenth century. According to Descartes, a sensory signal caused the movement of "animal spirits" from the heart and arteries into the muscles responsible for movement. Even though many scientists provided evidence that contradicted the hydraulic system of muscle control, this model remained the dominant theory for the control of muscle contraction until the late eighteenth century when it was replaced with a model that centered on the concept of bioelectricity (29,42,49).

In the late eighteenth century, Luigi Galvani (1737–1789) conducted a series of experiments that resulted in the formation of the concept of bioelectricity. When Galvani applied an electric stimulus to a nerve or muscle of a frog, it caused a contraction. Galvani also demonstrated that muscle contraction in a frog could be caused by lightning or by contacting the nerve of one frog with the nerve of another frog. Galvani was convinced that certain tissues could generate electricity, which in turn resulted in muscle contraction. Figure 8.3 illustrates Galvani's experiment with a frog that helped establish the neurophysiologic concept of bioelectricity, which provided the foundation for the development of motor learning and motor control.

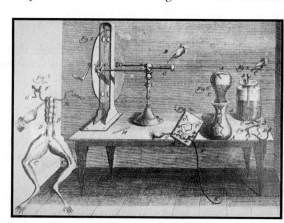

FIGURE 8.3 ▼ Galvani's experiment with a frog leads to the concept of bioelectricity.

The mid nineteenth century saw the birth of motor control and motor learning as they are presently understood. By the end of the nineteenth century, several significant research experiments started to shape the fields of motor control and motor learning. In the late 1890s, William L. Bryan (1860–1955) and Noble Harter (5,6) reported on the existence of human learning curves and plateaus and different characteristics of novice and expert telegraph conductors (51). The study of motor control was further enhanced in 1903 with the publication of the book *Le Mouvement* by R.S. Woodworth (1869–1962). This book was critical in establishing and expanding the field of motor skills research (51,54). The law of effect, which holds that stimuli that produce a pleasant or satisfying effect during a particular situation are likely to occur repeatedly during that situation (52), was developed during the late 1920s and significantly impacted motor learning research (51). In 1925, Coleman Griffith became the director of the Research in Athletics Laboratory at the University of Illinois and conducted motor skills research on athletes. As with many other areas of study in exercise science, World War II had a positive influence on the development of motor control and motor learning as disciplines of study. In particular, the training of air force pilots (Figure 8.4) was instrumental in creating some of the early theories on memory, muscle control, movement, transfer of learning, and practice (51).

Recent Influences on Motor Control and Motor Learning

Franklin M. Henry (1904–1993) played an instrumental role in the emergence of motor behavior as an area of study in exercise science (51). In particular, his approach to memory (commonly referred to as the "memory drum" theory) spurred on our understanding of cognitive activity in motor control and learning (27,51). Henry is often known as the "Father of motor skills research (47)." Other individuals who played a significant role in the development of motor control and learning included Alfred Hubbard (University of Illinois) and Arthur Slater-Hammil (Indiana University), who are well-known for starting graduate programs in motor behavior at their respective universities during the late 1960s. The *Journal of Motor Behavior*, the first journal devoted entirely to the publishing of scholarly research in motor learning and control, was first published in 1969. Other journals that have been instrumental in disseminating research and knowledge in motor behavior include the *Journal of Human Movement Studies*, (founded

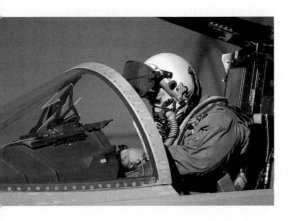

FIGURE 8.4 ▼ The training of air force pilots leads to the development of motor learning and motor control as disciplines of study. (Photo by Stocktrek Images/Getty Images.)

➤ **Thinking Critically**
In what ways has each of the areas of motor behavior (motor development, motor control, and motor learning) contributed to a broader understanding of health, physical fitness, and exercise?

➤ **Thinking Critically**
In what ways has each of the areas of motor behavior (motor development, motor control, and motor learning) contributed to a broader understanding of how individuals can become successful in sport and athletic competition?

in 1970), *Research Quarterly for Exercise and Sport* (first published in 1930) and *Motor Control* (founded in 1997) (51).

Several professional organizations have been instrumental in the professional development of motor control and motor learning. The primary organization that has served all areas of motor behavior has been the North American Society for Psychology of Sport and Physical Activity (NASPSPA). Though many individuals associate NASPSPA primarily with exercise and sport psychology, there are actually three major components of NASPSPA: motor control and learning, motor development, and sport psychology. Additional information on the founding of NASPSPA is contained in the chapter on "Exercise and Sport Psychology." The Society for Neuroscience (founded in 1969), Society for Neural Control of Movement (founded 1989), and the International Society of Motor Control (founded 2002) all support motor control and learning by supporting development activities in the form of professional conferences and workshops (51).

The development of knowledge that forms the basis of motor behavior has occurred through the interactions and efforts from individuals comprising several academic disciplines. Each of the areas that collectively constitute motor behavior has significant application to the activities of exercise science professionals. Table 8.1 provides some of the significant historic events in the development of motor behavior.

Table 8.1	Significant Events in the Historic Development of Motor Behavior
DATE	**SIGNIFICANT EVENT**
1903	Publication of the book *Le Mouvement*, which established the field of motor skills research
1925	Coleman Griffith established the Athletics Research Laboratory at the University of Illinois
1929	Publication of the book *Infancy and Human Growth*
1960	Franklin Henry proposed his "memory drum" theory
1967	Establishment of the NASPSPA
1969	Publication of the *Journal of Motor Behavior*
1970	Publication of the *Journal of Human Movement Studies*
1978	Formation of the Motor Development Academy in the AAHPERD
1997	Publication of the Journal *Motor Control*

MOTOR DEVELOPMENT

Motor development is concerned with the study of motor performance throughout the life span and has several different aspects that distinguish it from motor learning and motor control. First, the origins of motor development arise primarily from the discipline of education, with contributions from the disciplines of educational psychology and physiology. Second, motor development has a much closer association with the discipline of physiology than either motor learning and motor control. Because physical maturation and growth play an important role in an individual's motor development, these factors require considerable attention. Finally, the research methods employed in motor development are different from motor learning and control. In motor development, **longitudinal** and **cross-sectional** studies of individuals or groups of individuals are more prevalent than in the areas of motor learning and motor control (22). Motor development is the continual change in motor behavior throughout the lifespan. These changes occur as a result of the requirements of the movement task, the biology of the individual, and the specific environmental conditions (20). Many exercise science professionals will encounter individuals from across the lifespan during their work making the understanding of motor performance important for ensuring the success of individuals involved in physical activity, exercise, sport, and athletic competition.

Life Span Stages

Human development encompasses all aspects of behavior and can only artificially be separated into stages (20). The separation into stages, however, allows for a partitioning of motor development activities into the following: infancy, childhood, adolescence, adulthood, and older adult. Each of these stages is characterized by either developmental markers or a chronologic age; however, there is not always agreement between motor development experts as to when these stages begin and end. Some experts suggest adding an additional prenatal stage and splitting childhood into early childhood and later childhood stages (14,22). The following sections provide a brief overview of each developmental stage.

Prenatal

Several prenatal factors affect motor development during infancy and throughout later years. Many of these factors can lead to birth defects or developmental abnormalities that can affect normal motor development in the later stages of development. Some of the more common influences include malnutrition and the use of drugs, alcohol, and tobacco by the birth mother; hereditary factors that include chromosome-based and gene-based disorders; environmental factors

---

Longitudinal Following a sample of individuals over a period of time.

Cross-sectional Selection of a sample of subjects to represent the population as a whole.

including radiation and chemical pollutants; and medical problems including sexually transmitted diseases, maternal infection, and stress experienced by the birth mother during pregnancy (18).

Infancy

Much of the information about child infancy comes from describing what movements and activities infants engage in during the early period of development. Much of this information describes the primitive reflexes of infants, which are associated with the basic human needs of nourishment and security. Not all movements performed by infants, however, are reflexive in nature. For example, **maturational theorists** have identified and described several landmark activities that occur during an infant's early development of locomotion and manual control. Locomotion for infants involves movement and includes crawling, creeping, and walking. Each of these forms of locomotion is important for the normal development of an infant. Manual control is the movement of the hands and arms to manipulate an object. The stages of manual control include reaching, grasping, and releasing behaviors. The development of locomotion and manual control progresses in an organized and orderly fashion during the normal growth and development of a child (2,14,18).

Early Childhood and Later Childhood

Early childhood is considered the period of 2 to 6 years of age, whereas later childhood is the period of 6 to 10 years of age. Motor development in childhood involves the improvements in fundamental movement skills and the practice of these movements in everyday activities as well as for participation in physical activity, exercise, sport, and athletic competition. Common fundamental movement

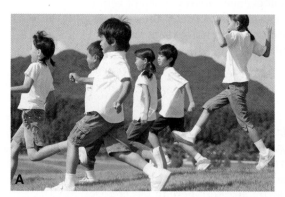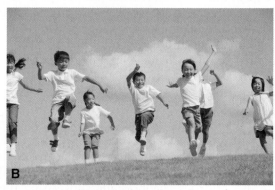

FIGURE 8.5 ▼ The development of fundamental movement patterns such as running (**A**) and jumping (**B**) occurs in early childhood. (Photos by BLOOMimage/Getty Images.)

Maturational theorists Individuals who believe that the chief principle of developmental change in an individual is maturation.

patterns during childhood involve specific movements such as walking, running, jumping, and throwing (Figure 8.5). By 3 years of age, children should display some acceptable level of fundamental movement patterns; however, confusion often exists in body direction, temporal, and spatial adjustments. Gross motor control is developing rapidly during this period. By 6 years of age, the child should refine many of these movement patterns to the degree that they would be classified as mature. Children should become aware of body shape, body size, and physical capacity at this point, and basic mechanical principles of movement are being developed during this time. This period marks a transition from refining fundamental movement abilities to the establishment of transitional movement skills to simple games and athletic skills (18,22).

Adolescence

As a child progresses into and through adolescence, significant improvements in motor performance occur as a result of substantial physical and physiologic changes. Many of these changes are the result of body growth and changes in body structure. Many of the differences between males and females are the result of structural changes that give males several physical advantages over females. For example, as a result of sexual maturation and the increased production of anabolic hormones, males start to produce more muscle mass and there are physical changes in the arms, hips, and shoulders that give a mechanical advantage in certain activities to males over females. These changes result in widening of the gap in motor performance between boys and girls during adolescence. Adolescents advance through different maturation levels and stages of learning new movement skills at different rates of development (2,14). The changes that occur during adolescence lead to physical differences later in life (Figure 8.6).

Adulthood

Early adulthood is the period when most individuals reach their peak physical performances. Peak motor performance occurs around 22 to 25 years of age for women and around 29 years of age for men (14). Though very few changes in motor performance occur throughout early and middle adulthood, there is large individual variation in

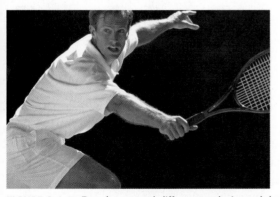 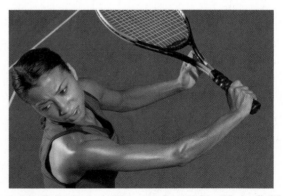

FIGURE 8.6 ▼ Developmental differences during adolescence lead to physical differences later in life. (Photo **[left]** by Comstock Images/Getty Images and photo **[right]** by Stockbyte/Wendy Hope/Getty Images.)

achieving peak performance. Time to peak physical performance and changes in movement patterns are a result of the type of motor skill or movement performed and the frequency of opportunities to perform the motor skill. The maintenance of motor skills through adulthood is a function of the motivation and opportunity to participate in physical activity, exercise, sport, and athletic competition (14).

Older Adulthood

As adults continue to age, there is an increase in the number of health-related problems that occur. This is due in part to a decrease from peak performance of various physical and physiologic functions (22). Decreases in performance commonly begin to occur in cardiorespiratory function, muscular function, and psychomotor function at around 50 to 60 years of age. Older adults tend to decrease more rapidly in physiologic function as they age, with some of the changes occurring differently between genders. There are many factors that can affect the rate of decline such as genetic predisposition, level of physical activity, participation in regular exercise, and nutritional intake (14,22). It has been demonstrated that the older adult responds favorably to the intervention and practice of motor skills (Figure 8.7). Table 8.2 shows the primary changes in the cardiovascular, musculoskeletal, and psychomotor functions that occur with aging.

Of particular interest to the motor development changes that occur with aging is the alteration that transpires in **psychomotor function** or the ability to integrate cognition with motor abilities (22). Two types of intelligence play an important role in psychomotor function: crystal intelligence and fluid intelligence. **Crystal intelligence** is derived largely from education experiences and knowledge. Crystal intelligence is primary about storing information and it can increase until an individual reaches about 60 years of age. **Fluid intelligence** is primary about reasoning and abstract thought. Learning is considered a mechanism of fluid

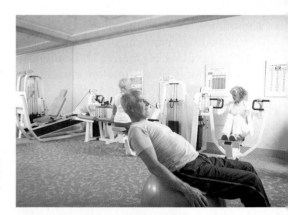

FIGURE 8.7 ▼ Older adults respond favorably to exercise and motor skill development. (Photo by Photodisc/Rob Melnychuk/Getty Images.)

Psychomotor function The ability to integrate cognition with motor abilities.
Crystal intelligence The ability to store information in the brain.
Fluid intelligence The ability to perform reasoning and abstract thought.

Table 8.2	Primary Changes in Cardiovascular, Musculoskeletal, and Psychomotor Function with Aging (14,22)
SYSTEM	**PRIMARY CHANGES**
Cardiovascular	• Decreased cardiac output, heart rate, myocardial muscle mass, peripheral blood flow, and maximal oxygen consumption • Increased cardiac mass and time to return to resting heart rate
Musculoskeletal	• Decreased lean body weight, bone mass, muscle mass, strength, muscle fibers, and motor neurons • Increased body fat and muscle collagen
Psychomotor	• Decreased attention to motor tasks • Decreased motor unit recruitment • Increased reaction time

ntelligence. Essentially, fluid intelligence is a measure of the state of the brain because it is a measure of an individual's ability to make new and unique connections. Crystal intelligence is a state of the mind based on education, because it s a measure of well-established pathways in the brain not the formation of new ones. Fluid intelligence starts to decrease when an individual enters the fourth decade of life and continues to decline as the individual ages. Older individuals do not learn as quickly as younger adults, but they can and do learn new motor skills and movements. The rate at which an individual loses fluid intelligence is related to the amount that an individual uses their fluid intelligence. The more an individual uses his or her mind, the slower the decline in psychomotor function 7,22).

Use of Motor Development Knowledge

The knowledge gained through the study of motor development can assist exercise science professionals working across a broad age range of individuals. For example, exercise science professionals working with young children must be aware of the various developmental progressions so that age-appropriate activities and games can be used to enhance fundamental movement skill development and acquisition (Figure 8.8). Issues such as the rate of physical growth and readiness to learn are key components in movement skill development (15). For those professionals working with older children, knowledge of how physical and motor development characteristics are developed is critical for ensuring that children refine the fundamental movement abilities in the areas of locomotion, manipulation, and stability (16). As children move to the adolescent period of growth and development, numerous physiologic and psychological changes occur that influence the acquisition of mature fundamental movement skills. It is during this period of development that gender differences begin to significantly appear. Individuals working with adolescents must ensure the mastery of the mature fundamental movement skills before the introduction of specialized movement skills occurs (19). As individuals move through adulthood, individual characteristics, the demands of the movement skill, and the environmental circumstances are major factors that

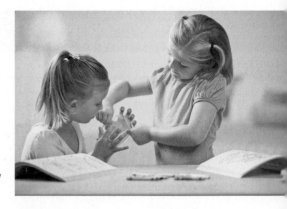

FIGURE 8.8 ▼ Motor development knowledge can be used to establish age-appropriate games for children. (Photo by Stockbyte/Andersen Ross/Getty Images.)

determine the level of success experienced by the adult in the performance of a motor task (17). As an individual moves into old age, the changes to the various systems of the body can have a significant impact on the ability to perform motor skills. In much the same manner that children cannot do many adult activities, many older adults cannot do many of the motor skill activities of a younger person (17). It is important for the exercise science professional to be aware of those motor development changes that occur across the lifespan so that appropriate measures can be taken to ensure safe and successful participation in physical activity, exercise, sport, and athletic competition.

> ### Thinking Critically
> *What specific information about motor development is necessary for an individual attempting to improve a motor skill associated with exercise?*

MOTOR LEARNING

Motor learning is the study of how we become skilled at basic and advanced movements that are used in everyday activities including those involved with physical activity, exercise, sport, and athletic competition. Knowledge and content study in motor learning require an understanding of the process of learning, processing information, organizing practice to make learning efficient, and the process of memory. Exercise science professionals must understand the principles of motor learning to enhance the success of individuals beginning an exercise program, as well as for putting athletes in the best position to be successful during sport and athletic competition. There are several important components to understanding motor learning including information processing, memory, and practice organization and learning.

Information Processing

The study of information processing comes from the parent academic discipline of **cognitive psychology**. Information is constantly presented to individuals during everyday activities and that information must be processed in a manner that often requires a response or action. The focus of material in this section is on how information is processed efficiently and effectively during participation in physical activity, exercise, sport, and athletic competition. Individuals must determine what information is critical for movement and then organize the information so that the muscles can respond in a coordinated and efficient movement pattern. For example, an individual who is running outside must process information about the environment and then make a decision about what action the body should take. If during the run, the individual encounters a hill, information about the slope of the hill and the length of the hill must be processed so that appropriate body lean and stride length can be achieved and the individual can run to the top of the hill. Information processing is customarily organized into three stages (22,46,47):

1. **Stimulus recognition**—collecting information from the environment, which is then identified or recognized as a pattern.
2. **Response selection**—deciding what response to make with the information including determining the stimulus–response compatibility.
3. **Response programming**—organizing and initiating an action after a stimulus has been identified and a response has been selected.

Information processing occurs in the brain and cannot be directly observed or easily studied. An assortment of indirect observation methods are therefore used to create hypotheses about brain activity during information processing. A commonly used method is to record how quickly an individual responds to a stimulus. This method requires an individual to receive an external cue from the environment and then make a response to that cue. The time required to make the response is referred to as **reaction time** and is an indirect measurement of how long it takes for an individual to process the information involved in making a decision and to respond. Using reaction time to analyze a person's mental processing is called the **chronometric method** (2,22,46).

Traditionally, information processing has been viewed as occurring in series or one stage at a time, a position that has continued to define experimentation and study within the field. To accurately study, this method of information processing involves changing and controlling each of the stages individually to see how a particular stage affects overall reaction time. The manipulation of processes in one stage allows researchers and scholars to hypothesize on the role of that individual stage in processing information for a particular movement skill (2,22,47).

The stimulus recognition stage requires an individual to recognize that something has changed in the environment, and that some stimulus has appeared. This is followed by the individual deciding on an appropriate response to that stimulus. The brain organizes a specific set of instructions for muscle actions to send out to the body to cause a particular movement to occur. These instructions give specific

Cognitive psychology Branch of psychology studying the mental processes involved in perception, learning, memory, and reasoning.

Stimulus recognition When an individual collects information from the environment.

Response selection When an individual decides what to do after collecting and processing information.

Response programming When an individual intitiates an action after a response has been selected.

Reaction time The time it takes to receive and respond to a stimulus.

Chronometric method Using reaction time to measure an individual's response to a stimulus.

commands about **body stabilization** and positioning. The recognition and identification of a stimulus is strongly affected by the intensity and clarity of the stimulus. For a stimulus to be identified, the brain must be aroused to the point at
which it contacts memory; which makes an association between the stimulus and
something meaningful (2,22,47). For example, Figure 8.9 shows how a runner
approaching a hill must recognize the hill, including identifying the grade or slope
of the hill, and then process the information so that appropriate muscle actions
may occur and the runner can successfully run up the hill.

The response selection stage of information processing requires an individual to decide on a suitable response to the stimulus. Factors such as the number
of choices (called stimulus–response alternatives) and the similarity of choices
(called stimulus–response compatibility) available to the individual affect the
response selection. Practice may affect both of these factors. Generally, the
more closely related the stimulus is to the response, the quicker the individual
decides on a response (2,22,39). Using the example from above, a runner can
select the appropriate body position, stride length, and running speed based on
the information derived from the stimulus recognition stage. If the runner has
encountered the same type of hill during a previous run, then the practice of
running up that hill will help guide the appropriate response selection of body
position, stride length, and speed for successfully running up the hill.

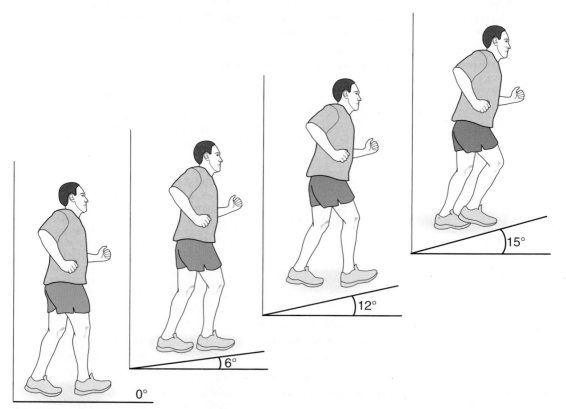

FIGURE 8.9 ▼ To be successful a runner must process information about running up a hill.

In the response programming stage, the commands to the muscles are organized and the response is initiated by the brain and spinal cord. The complexity of the response and the duration of the response affect response programming. As the complexity of the response increases, the reaction time of the individual also increases (31). The amount of time an individual has to organize muscular commands also affects response programming (2,25,31). If a runner encounters a hill after a long stretch of flat running during which the hill can be seen, there is time for the runner to make the appropriate programming response. If, however, the runner encounters the hill after coming around a curve that blocked the view of the hill, then the response programming can be affected and it may be that the runner has to start up the hill before the appropriate body position, stride length, and running speed are selected.

Information processing can be influenced by various factors, and these factors cause reaction time to increase or decrease. For example, during sport and athletic competitions, anticipating a movement by an opponent can decrease the time required by an athlete to respond to a movement by an opponent. In sport and athletic competitions, an individual or team can gain an advantage by using strategies to influence each of the three components of information processing (2,22):

1. **Stimulus identification**—conducting different plays from the same formation
2. **Response selection**—increasing the options opponents must respond to
3. **Response programming**—making the opponent perform a more complicated task

Each of these strategies can significantly influence the stages of information processing. When individuals are challenged at each stage of information processing, there are increases to the overall reaction time. Some disagreement exists as to whether the stages of information processing are separate and different, or if information is processed in a sequential order, so that individuals are able to perform the processing of more than one stage concurrently (2,43,50).

Memory

Memory is important for retaining and recalling facts, events, impressions, and remembering or recognizing previous experiences. A commonly used model to explain memory is called the **multistore memory model** (3). This model has three stores: short-term sensory store, short-term memory, and long-term memory. Information going from short-term store (also known as working memory) to long-term memory signifies information going into the long-term memory. This process is known as **encoding**. Going from long-term memory to short-term memory signifies information moving from the permanent memory to the working memory. This process is called **decoding** (2).

Body stabilization The process of holding the body in a desired position.
Multistore memory model The most widely used model to explain memory storage in humans.
Encoding The process of moving information from short-term store to long-term memory store.
Decoding The process of moving information from long-term memory store to short-term memory store.

Each memory store has a specific function and capacity for keeping information. The capacity of a memory store is the amount of information it can effectively hold. The duration is the length of time that the information remains in the memory store. The short-term sensory store collects information from the environment through the senses. The short-term sensory store has an unlimited capacity for storing information but has a storage duration that is very short. This means individuals can hold a lot of information from the senses but for less than a second. The short-term sensory store holds information while a decision is made on the importance of the information. This decision is made by a process called **selective attention,** a process that requires an individual to actively choose one unit of information to pay attention to at a time. The information that is attended to is sent to the short-term memory store (2,46,47).

There has been considerable interest in the role of regular physical activity and exercise in psychological function. The principal interest area has been in the role cardiovascular fitness and aerobic fitness have on various markers of cognitive function including memory, attention, reaction time, and crystallized and fluid intelligence (Figure 8.10). The working theory has been that age-associated reductions in cardiovascular function lead to lower oxygen levels in the brain and that high levels of cardiovascular fitness and regular aerobic exercise can slow or retard cognitive declines because of an increased oxygen delivery to the brain (35). Though many observational studies suggest that physical activity reduces the rate of cognitive decline, more experimental evidence is still required before a definitive conclusion can be made (33). For example, recent evidence suggests that modest improvements in cognitive function can be observed in those individuals with Alzheimer disease who participated in a 6-month physical activity intervention (33).

Short-term memory store is an individual's conscious or working memory (4). Units of information are collected from either the short-term sensory store or from the long-term memory and stored for short periods of time. The presentation of information and the organization of practice can affect how an individual organizes information in the short-term memory store. Units of information can be

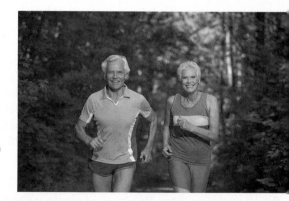

FIGURE 8.10 ▼ Regular exercise can lead to improvements in cognitive function in older adults. (Photo by Westend61/Getty Images.)

Selective attention A process that requires an individual to actively choose one unit of information to pay attention to at a time.

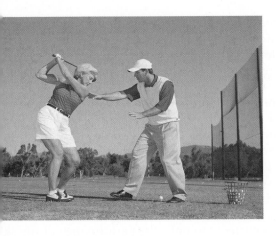

FIGURE 8.11 ▼ Repeatedly practicing a movement skill will commit the movement pattern to memory. (Photo by Lifesize/Mike Powell/Getty Images.)

remembered more easily if grouped together in some systematic way. The duration of short-term memory is considered 1 to 60 seconds, if the thought process of the individual is uninterrupted (2,4,11). Repeatedly practicing a movement skill with feedback on performance can help an individual remember how to do the skill. If a novice engages in the act of practicing a golf shot, the movement skills and patterns will be more easily remembered the individual continues to repeatedly practice the skill (Figure 8.11). To keep the movement skill in memory, however, an individual must move it to the long-term memory for storage.

> **Thinking Critically**
> What specific information about motor learning is necessary for an individual attempting to improve performance against an opponent during an athletic competition?

Information deemed important enough to store permanently is sent from short-term memory to long-term memory, which is believed to have an unlimited storage capacity and storage duration. Even though capacity and duration are seemingly limitless, individuals can forget information that they used to remember. The information is not lost in the memory but the individual has simply failed to retrieve the information from long-term memory. Memory can also be thought of as retaining information, which by definition is learning. To maximize successful performance when teaching an individual a new movement skill, exercise science professionals, including coaches and healthcare professionals, must have an understanding of how memory works. Motor learning scholars are very interested in understanding how memory functions and identifying ways that practice can be organized to optimize the efficiency with which individuals learn (2,23).

Practice Organization and Learning

To fully understand how individuals learn, it is important to clarify the distinction between practice and learning. Performance is typically defined as observable behavior. Learning is defined as a relatively permanent change in behavior that results from practice or experience. As learning results from a change in an individual's memory and cannot be directly observed, the assessment of how much learning has occurred must be inferred from performance, typically via a physical retention test (22,46,47).

Understanding the distinction between practice and learning is critic because an individual's performance during practice is not necessarily an indic tor of learning (23). A practicing-learning paradox exists because certain variabl affect practice performance and retention performance in an opposite manne For example, practicing variations of a movement, instead of practicing the sar movement repeatedly, hinders practice performance but enhances learning. F example, asking an individual to repeatedly shoot a basketball from the sar spot on the floor will enhance the individual's ability to successfully make th particular shot in practice. However, by asking the individual to repeatedly tak shots from different spots on the floor will enhance the learning of the shootir skill but will likely result in fewer successful shots being made during the practic A practice session that does not sufficiently challenge the individual enhanc practice performance, but restricts learning of the skill. Individuals must strike balance between practicing skills repeatedly to enhance performance of the sk and practicing different skills to enhance learning (22,24).

Contextual Interference

Contextual interference describes the interference that results from practicin several different tasks within the context of a single practice session. A high degre of contextual interference can be established by having the individual practice sev eral different skills during the same practice session. A low degree of contextu interference can be established by having the individual practice only one sk during a practice session. Low contextual interference practice (relative to hig contextual interference) leads to superior practice performance, but much inferic learning (48). For example, a softball infielder who is practicing catching groun balls hit directly at her by a coach will become skilled at catching ground balls i practice, but she does not improve the motor skills required to catch ground bal that are hit to her left or right. A coach could increase the contextual interference b hitting ground balls to the left or right of her and requiring the athlete to move an field the ball (Figure 8.12). A further increase in contextual interference could b accomplished by not informing the athlete as to where the ball will be hit mak ing the athlete learn at a higher level. This practice-retention paradox may b dependent on the experience of the individual. In those individuals with limite experience of a particular motor skill or activity, high levels of contextual interfer ence during practice of the skill does not enhance learning more than low leve of contextual interference. In fact, until the individual is experienced at a move ment task, high levels of contextual interference may be detrimental to efficien learning. After some degree of proficiency is reached, however, high contextua interference is beneficial for learning. From a practical standpoint, decreasin extraneous interference is desired during the beginning stages of learning a moto skill, but as the individual becomes more proficient, greater extraneous interfer ence enhances learning of the skill (22,46,47).

Contextual interference The interference that results from practicing a number of different tasks within the context of a single practice session.

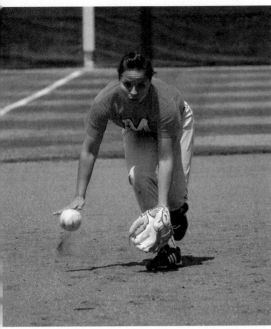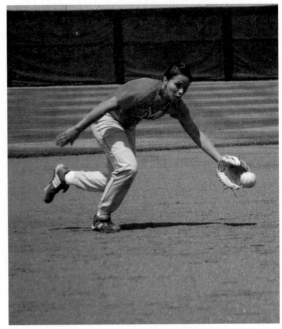

FIGURE 8.12 ▼ Increasing the contextual interference when performing a motor skill enhancing learning.

Variability of Practice

Repeatedly practicing the same movement or motor skill has been shown to impede practice performance but enhance the learning of the skill (46). Similar to that observed with contextual interference, there is substantial variability that appears to be dependent on the individual engaged in the movement or motor skill. Furthermore, practice variability affects children differently than adults and men differently than women, suggesting that an individual's ability and previous knowledge, relative to the practice organization, influences learning (22,46,55).

Knowledge of Results

Providing feedback after a successful motor performance is an extremely important factor affecting both performance and learning. The relationship between performance feedback and learning of motor skills is studied using knowledge of results techniques. Knowledge of results is defined as information about the performance given to the individual by another person observing the motor skill or movement. For example, a physical therapist might provide knowledge of results to a patient with a back injury who is performing a rehabilitation exercise designed to improve lower back and hip flexibility. In this instance, the physical therapist will inform the patient about correct and incorrect movements. The two most commonly used feedback strategies are the summary knowledge of results and fading knowledge of results (22,46,55).

Summary Knowledge of Results

The summary knowledge of results requires individuals to complete several trials of a single skill or movement without receiving any information about his or her performance. After completion of the trials, knowledge of results about those trials is provided to the individual. For example, a basketball player may shoot a total of 10 shots. After completing all shots, a coach will provide feedback to the athlete about various aspects of the technique and movement. Summary knowledge of results can be strongly detrimental to practice performance compared to when knowledge of results is given immediately after each trail (23), but it may facilitate better learning of a motor skill (34).

Some level of knowledge of results is important for motor learning. The appropriate amount of time between when a skill is performed and when the knowledge of results is provided depends on **task complexity** (45,46). Motor skills and movements of greater complexity require more help to solve the motor problem than a simple motor task. If an individual is to learn a complex task, more immediate knowledge of results should be given than if the same individual was learning a simple motor skill or movement. As an individual completes a practice session and improves performance of the movement or motor skill, the optimal time between completion of the movement or skill and the delivery of knowledge of results increases. Inexperienced individuals perform better during both practice and competition if the summary knowledge of results is short; as the individual becomes more skilled, a short summary may lead to better performance during practice but produces less learning (22).

Fading Knowledge of Results

The fading knowledge of results process involves a systematic reduction in the amount of knowledge of results given to an individual during a practice session. This technique benefits learning by helping an individual solve the motor skill problem early in practice. For example, an individual shooting a basketball might receive knowledge of results from the coach after shooting five shots at the beginning of practice. However, as practice progresses, the coach may use fading knowledge of results strategy and only provide feedback after shooting 25 shots. Reducing the knowledge of results as skill proficiency increases results in a highly effective practice schedule (22).

Part-whole Practice

The part-whole practice method is a commonly used to teach complex motor skills and movements. Motor skills high in complexity (i.e., having a high number of components to the skill) and low in organization (i.e., the dependent relationship between components) usually benefit from part-whole practice. Conversely,

Task complexity The level of difficulty required to complete a motor task.

motor skills low in complexity and high in organization benefit from practicing the skill as a whole. As a result, a progressive-part method of practice has emerged for teaching skills and movements. The progressive-part method requires parts of skill to be practiced independently but ordered according to the sequence in which each part occurs in the skill. As components of the skill are learned, they are progressively linked together until the skill is practiced as a whole component. For example, a strength and conditioning coach might teach an athlete the power clean weightlifting skill by breaking the complete skill into two or three components. These components commonly called the beginning phase, clean phase, and jerk phase are practiced in parts until the athlete is sufficiently skilled to begin to link the phases together to perform the complete power clean. The progressive-part practice organization requires limits or boundaries to be established during the initial practice of a skill, when the individual components are practiced independently, but as the skill becomes better learned the boundaries are removed (22).

Learning Difficult Skills

Learning difficult motor skills is obviously important for successful participation in exercise, sport, and athletic competition. Task difficulty is defined as the complexity of the motor problem an individual must resolve to successfully complete a task. Task difficulty is often used to describe the process of learning difficult motor skills. There is a relationship between practice performance and task difficulty that is shown in Figure 8.13 (22). As illustrated in the figure, as the motor task difficulty increases, practice performance of the skill decreases. As the movement skill becomes more challenging, an individual's performance deteriorates. Figure 8.14 shows the hypothetical relationship between learning and task difficulty.

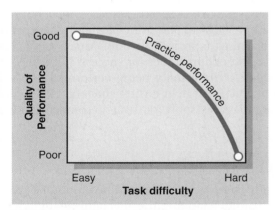

FIGURE 8.13 ▼ The relationship between task difficulty and practice performance (paradox principle). (From Brown SP. *Introduction to Exercise Science*. Baltimore (MD): Lippincott, Williams & Wilkins; 2000. 343 p.)

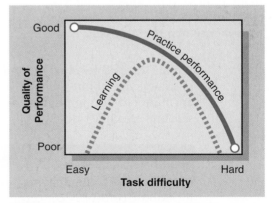

FIGURE 8.14 ▼ A hypothetical relationship between learning and task difficulty (paradox principle). (From Brown SP. *Introduction to Exercise Science*. Baltimore (MD): Lippincott, Williams & Wilkins; 2000. 344 p.)

Motor learning increases with increasing task difficulty to what some experts call the **challenge point**. At this point, the individual is being optimally challenged to enhance learning of the skill or movement. Interestingly, at the challenge point practice performance is not optimal, but learning is optimal. Increasing, the task difficulty beyond this point continues to inhibit practice performance and also begins to inhibit learning (22).

As practice organization becomes more challenging, it leads to poorer practice performance, but superior retention performance (23,48). The performance of motor skills and movements in practice does not necessarily indicate effective learning. Furthermore, too much or too little relative difficulty of the motor skill may hinder learning. As expected, optimal task difficulty depends on the level of the performer and the complexity of the skill or movement. For example, when learning to hit a baseball or softball the initial practice session might involve hitting the ball off of a standing tee. After acquiring a certain level of performance, the individual might move to hitting a tossed or thrown ball. This level of practice is much more difficult as it requires an individual to track the ball and time the swing to hit the ball successfully. This higher level of practice organization will initially lead to poorer practice performance, but provide a higher level of retention performance that ultimately leads to successful acquisition of the skill. If the ball is thrown too fast for the skill level of the individual, then the higher level of difficulty associated with hitting a ball thrown fast may hinder the ability of the individual to hit the thrown ball (22).

Relative task difficulty is defined as the difficulty of the motor problem an individual must resolve to successfully complete a motor task relative to the performance abilities of the individual performing the task. If motor skills or movements are constant, the relative task difficulty depends on the level of ability of the individual performing the task. From a practical aspect, practice organization should be adjusted as the performer's level of performance changes, meaning the difficulty of the required task should increase as the performer becomes more proficient at the movement skill (22,46).

> ➤ *Thinking Critically*
> *What motor behavior information about a sport technique would you need to help an athlete improve performance of a complex skill?*

Exercise science professionals must have a sound knowledge of the principles and concepts of motor learning to provide the individuals they work with the best opportunities for success. Regardless of the age or skill level of the individual or the activity being performed, the use of knowledge about memory and practice will help ensure that the experience encountered during physical activity, exercise, sport, or athletic competition is a safe and effective one.

MOTOR CONTROL

Motor control is the final area of study comprising the discipline of motor behavior. Motor control is concerned with understanding the mechanisms by which the nervous system and muscular system coordinate body movements. Different physical movements and motor skills require different programs of selected muscle actions. The successful performance of physical activity, exercise, sport, and athletic competition depends on the ability to execute the movements required to complete the movement or motor skill. For example, older adults tend to exhibit slower hesitant movements compared with younger adults. This type of muscle action is believed to be owing to a decline in motor movement rather than any developed strategy for caution in the movement (37). The study of neuroanatomy and motor control theories is fundamental to the understanding of motor control and its relationship to performance or movements and motor skills are the study of neuroanatomy and motor control theories.

Neuroanatomy

Neuroanatomy is the study of the structure and function of the central (brain and spinal cord) and peripheral (outside the brain and spinal cord) nervous systems. Figure 8.15 illustrates the components of the nervous system and an explanation of the functions of the nervous system is contained in Chapter 2. The primary functional components of the nervous system are the neurons (i.e., nerve cells). In the brain, neurons transport information among the specialized areas of the brain that allows an individual to do all of the things that make humans unique (e.g., think, react, move, etc.). The anatomy of the brain can be divided into five areas: cerebellum, basal ganglia, supplementary motor cortex, premotor cortex, and motor cortex.

Cerebellum

The **cerebellum** is the area of the brain in humans that serves to coordinate complex voluntary movements, posture, and balance. It is located in the back of and below the cerebrum and consists of two lateral lobes and a central lobe (26). The cerebellum is important for the performance of physical activity, exercise, sport, and athletic completion because it plays a central role in the integration of sensory perception, coordination, and motor control. The cerebellum fine-tunes body movements and motor skills using information derived from the sensory neurons.

Basal Ganglia

The **basal ganglia** are large masses of gray brain matter located at the base of the cerebral hemisphere. The basal ganglia constitute a set of interconnected structures in the forebrain. The basal ganglia serve three main functions: movement

---

Challenge point That point in the learning process where optimal learning is occuring.

Relative task difficulty The level of difficulty required to complete a motor task relative to an individual's level of ability.

Neuroanatomy The study of the structure and function of the central and peripheral nervous systems.

Cerebellum Area of the brain that serves to coordinate complex voluntary movements, posture, and balance in humans.

Basal ganglia Structure in the brain that are responsible for movement organization, scale and amplitude of movement, and perceptual-motor integration.

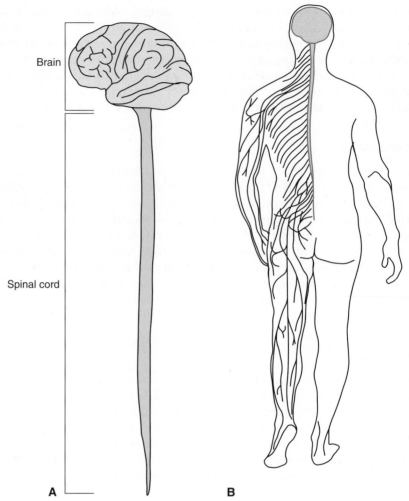

Brain

Spinal cord

A   **B**

FIGURE 8.15 ▼ Components of the nervous system. **A:** The central nervous system consists of the brain and the spinal cord. **B:** The peripheral nervous system consists of cranial nerves and spinal nerves, through which the central nervous system transmits commands to and receives information from the end organs. (From Bhatnagar S. *Neuroscience for the Study of Communicative Disorders.* 3rd ed. Baltimore (MD): Lippincott, Williams & Wilkins; 2008.)

organization, scale and amplitude of movement, and perceptual-motor integration. The basal ganglia are believed to help in choosing and organizing how individuals perform movement. They work in close association with the cerebral cortex and corticospinal system (26). Common diseases associated with improper functioning of the basal ganglia include Huntington disease and Parkinson disease (26).

Supplementary Motor Cortex

The **supplementary motor cortex** is a part of the sensorimotor cerebral cortex, and it is important for planning movements of the body. It collects and processes information from other areas of the brain, such as the basal ganglia and cerebellum, and initiates an organized movement. Information from the supplementary motor cortex is sent to the premotor cortex and primary motor cortex for further processing before and during movement (26).

Premotor Cortex

The **premotor cortex** is an area of motor cortex in the frontal lobe of the brain. The premotor cortex sends nervous signals to the musculature close to the head, like the shoulders and arms, so that the hands become properly oriented to perform specific movements and tasks. The premotor cortex also receives sensory information from neurons that helps with the orientation of the body in space. The premotor cortex evaluates initial conditions of the body and then initiates a plan of action, making sure to stabilize the body or body part before movement begins. The premotor cortex works with the basal ganglia, the thalamus, and the primary motor cortex to control many of the body's more complex patterns of coordinated muscle activity such as those associated with exercise, sport, and athletic competition (22,26).

Motor Cortex

The **motor cortex** is a region within the cerebral cortex involved in the planning, control, and execution of voluntary motor functions. The motor cortex is typically divided into three separate areas: primary motor cortex, premotor area, and supplemental motor area. The motor cortex generates a plan for movement and then executes that plan. It is one of the last areas of the brain to be active before movement of the body begins. The motor cortex also receives feedback from all areas of the body, fine-tunes the motor response to the desired movement, and then sends signals to the skeletal muscles to contract or relax and create the desired movement (22,26).

Peripheral Motor System

The **peripheral motor system** consists of the nerves of the peripheral nervous system and muscles, which those nerves innervate. The primary functional unit of the peripheral motor system is the motor unit. The motor unit is comprised of a motor neuron and all the muscle fibers that the motor neuron innervates. The recruitment of motor units during movement is responsible for the motor patterns that are executed and the force generated by a muscle during contraction (26).

Supplementary motor cortex Area of the brain that collects and processes information from other areas of the brain and initiates an organized movement.

Premotor cortex Works to control many of the body's more complex patterns of coordinated muscle activity.

Motor cortex A region of the cerebral cortex involved in the planning, control, and execution of voluntary motor functions.

Peripheral motor system Component of the nervous system that is responsible for controlling the motor patterns that are executed and the force generated by a muscle during contraction.

Different levels of force can be generated by recruiting different numbers and types of motor units within a whole muscle or group of muscles (13).

General Motor Control Theories

Motor control involves both the sending of information to the muscles to contract and receiving information through afferent neurons from the body's joints, **proprioceptors**, and muscles. The study of motor control during movement must consider both nervous system control of muscle contraction and the influence of the sensory information coming back from the peripheral tissues of the body (46). An individual must be able to coordinate muscle contraction and relaxation to successfully execute a movement or skill. The closed-loop and open-loop theories of motor control are used as explanations of how the brain, nervous system, and muscles coordinate body movement.

Closed-loop Theory

The closed-loop theory of motor control asserts that sensory information necessary to control motor performance is received by the nervous system during the movement. By using this information, muscle activity can be altered during the performance of the movement to correct for changes that need to be made to successfully perform the movement or to respond to something in the external environment (1,30). Figure 8.16 shows an expanded conceptual model of motor performance (47). Corrections and alterations in motor performance can occur because as the movements are being performed feedback is sent to those areas in the brain responsible for correcting and fine-tuning the motor pattern. The closed-loop theory of motor control enhances the accuracy of muscle actions, because movements of the body can be controlled and adjusted as they are occurring. A disadvantage of the closed-loop system is lack of speed by which corrections to muscle actions can be made by the nervous system during the motor performance (22).

Open-loop Theory

An alternative theory describing the control of motor performance is the open-loop theory. This theory suggests that individuals do not receive feedback from the joints, proprioceptors, and muscles of the body during movement (44). The open-loop theory suggests that body movements are completely preplanned prior to the initiation of the movement. Figure 8.17 illustrates an expanded open-loop control system for motor performance (47). In this instance, body movements are controlled by a predefined set of motor commands that once sent to

> ➤ *Thinking Critically*
> *How might information in the area of motor control provide for improvements in preventive and rehabilitative healthcare for those individuals affected by a neuromuscular disease?*

Proprioceptors Nervous structures in the body that are responsible for sensing body position.

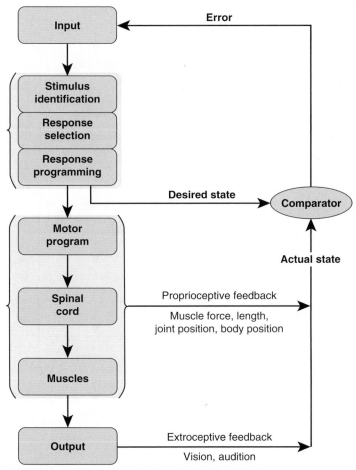

FIGURE 8.16 ▼ An expanded conceptual model of motor performance (47).

he muscles, complete a movement without the involvement of feedback from he muscles. This type of system results in faster movements than the closed-oop system, because the time it takes to provide feedback is eliminated from the rocess. A disadvantage of the open-loop theory is that modifications to mus-le movements cannot be made to correct for errors in the movements being erformed (22).

AREAS OF MOTOR BEHAVIOR APPLICATION

he application of knowledge derived from the study of motor behavior is evident n a wide range of activities and situations for both healthy and diseased individuals. Exercise science professionals should be fundamentally familiar with each area of notor behavior. Understanding the motor development of individuals throughout he lifespan is critical for applying the proper physical activity or exercise interven-ion to enhance health and reduce disease risk and for modifying sport and athletic ompetitions to ensure safety and success. Activities that are not developmentally

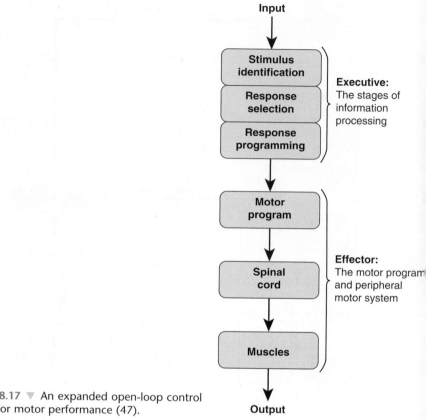

FIGURE 8.17 ▼ An expanded open-loop control system for motor performance (47).

appropriate for a child or an adult may lead to ineffective results and discouragement on the part of the participant. Correct use of motor learning strategies is critical for an athletic coach to make effective use of practice time to enhance sport and athletic competition. The progression of basic and advanced motor skills in a developmentally appropriate sequence is critical for enhancing motor skill acquisition and promoting successful performance of a movement or activity. Understanding how individuals control motor movements is important for ensuring positive patient-based outcomes during the rehabilitation process of those individuals with neurologic disease. Effective rehabilitation strategies must incorporate an understanding of how muscles and movements are controlled by the nervous system. Several examples of how motor behavior can be used by exercise science professionals follow below. The examples provided are not meant to be an exhaustive list, but merely examples of how motor behavior is used in a variety of different situations.

Modification of Equipment, Games, and Playing Environment

To ensure safe and successful participation in exercise and sport activities for individuals of all ages and body size, consideration should be given to modification of the equipment and the exercise or sport environment. Knowledge of how individuals develop skills across the lifespan can assist exercise science and coaching professionals in making appropriate changes to the equipment, the exercise, and sport environment. This process is called scaling (46). For example, many years ago females were expected to participate in basketball using a ball that was of the same size as the men's "regulation" ball even though the average size of the hand of a female is much smaller than a male. Adoption of a ball that was 1 inch small in circumference and 2½ oz lighter than the "regulation" ball occurred in 1984 allowed for improved motor skills and performance. Other examples of equipment modification include the development and use of age and size appropriate tennis rackets and baseball/softball bats for children and adolescents. The use of scaled rackets and bats ensures an enhanced development of motor skills for successfully striking an object. Recreational baseball and softball leagues have employed tee-ball games for young children to enhance skill development (Figure 8.18), and then subsequently allowed older children to bat using pitching machines (Figure 8.19). These types of modifications to the game environment are designed to increase the safety and success of young children playing baseball and softball. The body size scaling of soccer goals and basketball goals allows for improvements in developmentally appropriate skill and motor movement of young children. With an increased emphasis on improving fitness and health in children has come exercise equipment scaled to body size for younger children. Numerous YMCAs, physical therapy facilities, public and private school districts,

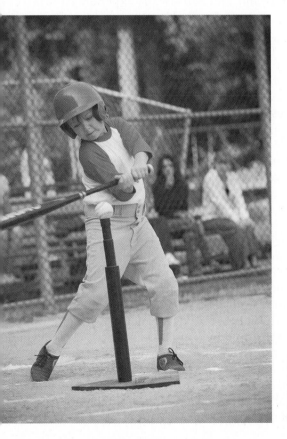

FIGURE 8.18 ▼ The use of a batting tee enhances success in baseball and softball games for young children. (Photo by Digital Vision/Andersen Ross/Getty Images.)

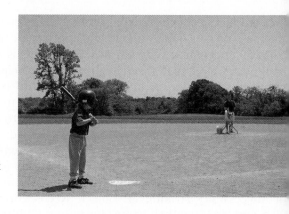

FIGURE 8.19 ▼ Progression to a pitching machine improves the chances for further skill development in baseball and softball games for young children.

youth fitness training facilities, special needs facilities, hospitals, health clubs, and wellness centers have all begun to provide developmentally age-appropriate exercise equipment for use. For older adults, the modification of playing equipment and surfaces can increase participation and enjoyment, improve fitness levels, and increase safety. The use of tennis rackets and golf clubs with larger hitting surfaces provides an increased probability that the tennis ball or golf ball will be struck with accuracy. Increasing the success of the older individual when playing the game will likely lead to a more enjoyable and worthwhile experience (46).

Understanding Parkinson Disease

Parkinson disease is a progressive neurologic disorder characterized by a large number of alterations to motor and nonmotor characteristics that can impact normal physical function. The disease is caused by a decrease in the synthesis of the neurotransmitter dopamine resulting from the death of dopaminergic cells in the brain. The decreased concentration of dopamine results in the following clinical features: muscle tremor at rest, muscle rigidity, an inability to initiate movement (called akinesia), and postural instability. In addition, flexed posture and freezing (called motor blocks) have been included among the classic features of Parkinson disease (28,40).

Parkinson disease affects many aspects of motor control and movement (Figure 8.20). Muscle tremors are evident both at rest and with movement. Muscle rigidity often begins in the neck and shoulders and spreads to the trunk and extremities, making body movement difficult. The ability to move the fingers, hands, arms, or legs rapidly is significantly reduced and motor control to rise from a chair is diminished. Standing posture is characterized by increased hunched shoulders (kyphosis) and fixed knees and elbows, as well as rounded (adducted) shoulders. Individuals with Parkinson disease have a slow and shuffling walking pattern, with shortened steps characterized by legs flexed stiffly at the knees and hips (called festinated), decreased arm swing, and difficulty initiating a step. Postural control and righting reflexes are compromised and lost and as a result, falls can become a recurring problem. Episodes of decreased movement or freezing become more frequent during walking. Individuals with Parkinson disease have problems with the volume and clarity of their speech (40).

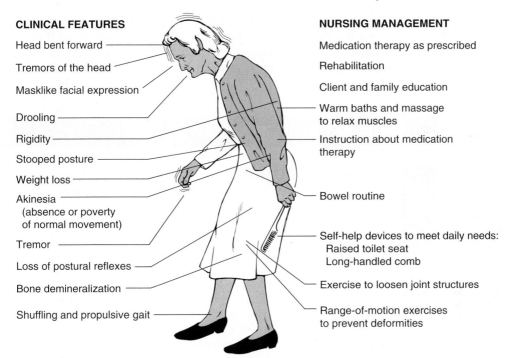

CLINICAL FEATURES

Head bent forward
Tremors of the head
Masklike facial expression
Drooling
Rigidity
Stooped posture
Weight loss
Akinesia
(absence or poverty
of normal movement)
Tremor
Loss of postural reflexes
Bone demineralization
Shuffling and propulsive gait

NURSING MANAGEMENT

Medication therapy as prescribed
Rehabilitation
Client and family education
Warm baths and massage
to relax muscles
Instruction about medication
therapy

Bowel routine

Self-help devices to meet daily needs:
Raised toilet seat
Long-handled comb
Exercise to loosen joint structures
Range-of-motion exercises
to prevent deformities

FIGURE 8.20 ▼ Changes in motor control and movement in Parkinson disease. (LifeArt image © 2010 Lippincott, Williams & Wilkins. All rights reserved.)

The treatment of Parkinson disease involves making adjustments to an individual's lifestyle, participating in regular exercise and physical therapy, eating a healthy diet, and using medications. In some cases, deep brain stimulation may be helpful. Exercise is important for general health, but especially for maintaining good physical function in Parkinson disease. Physical therapy may be advisable and can help improve mobility, joint range of motion, and muscular tone. Although specific exercises cannot stop the progression of the disease condition, improving muscle strength can help an individual feel more confident and capable in his/her movements. Physical therapy can help an individual improve his/her gait and balance. Working with a speech therapist or speech pathologist can improve problems associated with speaking and swallowing. Medications can help manage problems with walking, movement, and tremor by increasing the brain's supply of dopamine (32).

Recent research in the area of Parkinson disease has focused on halting the progression of the disease, restoring lost function, and even preventing the disease. Studying the genes responsible for the disease and identifying gene defects can help researchers understand how Parkinson disease occurs, help develop animal models that accurately mimic the neuronal death in the human disease condition, identify new drug targets, and improve the clinical diagnosis of the disease. Researchers also are conducting many studies of new or improved therapies for Parkinson disease. Although deep brain

> **Thinking Critically**
> *How might coursework in motor development, motor control, and motor learning help prepare an individual for a career as an allied health professional, strength and conditioning coach, or fitness specialist?*

stimulation is now an approved treatment by the Food and Drug Administration there still exists the possibility of other surgical procedures being helpful. Drug therapy, nutritional interventions, gene therapy, and the use of embryonic stem cells to produce dopamine are all areas of research that are currently being investigated (38).

I N T E R V I E W

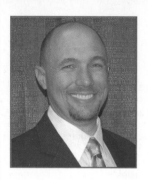

Mark Hoffman, PhD, ATC, FACSM, Associate Professor, Department of Nutrition and Exercise Science, Oregon State University

Brief Introduction

My primary area of scholarship is motor control. Additionally, I am a certified athletic trainer and combine my clinical background and PhD training in the study of motor control. Currently, my research focus is on trying to understand neurologic sex differences and their potential contribution to injuries of the lower extremity. I completed my BS degree in Kinesiology and Athletic Training at Indiana University, my MS degree in human performance at San Jose State University in Human Performance and Athletic Training, and my PhD in Motor Control at Indiana University.

➤ Why did you choose your current profession?

The research work I am pursuing in the area of anterior cruciate ligament injury is the result of being trained both as a motor control specialist and a certified athletic trainer. With a clinical background in sport injury, it has been rewarding to be able to take my research skills and apply them to study a significant clinical problem.

➤ Which individuals or experiences were most influential in your career development?

The two individuals who have influenced me most in the area of motor control have been Dr David Koceja, from Indiana University who served as my PhD advisor and Dr V. Gregory Payne from San Jose State University who served as my Master's thesis advisor.

➤ What are your most significance professional accomplishments?

Although not academic in nature, I lead a group of community volunteers to build a 12,000 sq. ft playground in our neighborhood. It has provided a place for kids to be active and explore, develop physically and socially, and to have fun. The park is a true exhibition of motor control for all ages. Also, having the opportunity to lead the National Athletic Trainers Association's Research and Education Foundation as President has been a significant accomplishment in my professional life.

➤ What advice would you have for an undergraduate student beginning to explore a career in exercise science?

My advice to the undergraduate exercise science student is to get the most you can out of the undergraduate experience. Do not be in a rush to get out of school. As a high school student, I was shocked and almost devastated when I learned I needed a college degree to become a certified athletic trainer. I had never planned on going to a 4-year college, but it ended up being one of the best academic decisions I ever made. It sometimes takes a while for students to understand that having the knowledge of how the body works and the ability to use that knowledge to help people be physically active and healthy is a great asset.

SUMMARY

- Motor behavior is the study of the interactions between the physiologic and psychological processes of the body and includes the disciplines of motor development, motor control, and motor learning.
- The principles of motor behavior are applied to a variety of everyday skills including those involved with work and leisure time activities, physical activity, exercise, sport, and athletic competition, and rehabilitation.
- Motor development includes the study of changes throughout the lifespan and how motor performance is affected by those changes.
- Motor learning is the study of the acquisition of basic and advanced movement skills that are used in everyday activities including those involved with physical activity, exercise, sport, and athletic competition.
- Motor control is the study of the mechanisms by which the nervous and muscular systems coordinate body movements.

FOR REVIEW

1. Define the following terms:
   a. Motor development
   b. Motor control
   c. Motor learning

2. Name the primary professional organizations in the areas of motor control, motor learning, and motor development.

3. What are the three stages of information processing?

4. Describe the following components of the multistore memory model:
   a. Short-term sensory store
   b. Short-term memory
   c. Long-term memory

5. What is the difference between practice and learning?

6. How are summary knowledge of results and fading knowledge of results used to improve motor skill performance?

7. Describe the relationship between practice performance and task difficulty.

8. What are the primary functions of the following neural structures:
   a. Cerebellum
   b. Basal ganglia
   c. Supplementary motor cortex
   d. Premotor cortex
   e. Cortex

(Continued)

9. What is the difference between the closed-loop and open-loop theories of motor control?

10. List the primary stages of motor development.

11. Describe how crystal intelligence and fluid intelligence interact with aging to influence psychomotor function.

REFERENCES

1. Adams JA. A closed loop theory of motor learning. *J Motor Behav.* 1971;3:111–49.

2. Anastasi A. *Psychological Testing.* New York (NY): Macmillan; 1988.

3. Atkinson RC, Shiffrin RM. Human memory: A proposed system and its control processes. In: Spence KW, Spence JT, editors. *The Psychology of Learning and Motivation.* Vol 8. London: Academic Press; 1968.

4. Baddley AD, Hitch G. Working memory. In: Bower GH, editor. *Psychology of Learning and Motivation.* New York (NY): Academic Press; 1974.

5. Bryan WL, Harter N. Studies in the physiology and psychology of the telegraphic language. *Psychol Rev.* 1897;4:27–53.

6. Bryan WL, Harter N. Studies on the telegraphic language: The acquisition of a hierarchy of habits. *Psychol Rev.* 1899;6:345–75.

7. Cattell RB. *Abilities: Their Structure, Growth and Action.* New York (NY): Houghton Mifflin; 1971.

8. Clark JE, Whitall J. What is motor development?: The lesson of history. *Quest.* 1989;41:183–202.

9. Connolly KJ. *Mechanisms of Motor Skill Development.* New York (NY): Academic Press; 1970.

10. Dennis W. The effect of restricted practice upon the reaching, sitting, and standing of two infants. *J Genet Psychol.* 1935;47:17–32.

11. Ericcson KA, Chase WG, Faloon S. Acquisition of a memory skill. *Science.* 1980;208:1181–2.

12. Espenshade A, Eckert HM. *Motor Development.* Columbus (OH): Merrill; 1967.

13. Ferguson RA, Aagaard P, Ball D, Sargeant AJ, Bangsbo J. Total power output generated during dynamic knee extensor exercise at different contraction frequencies. *J Appl Physiol.* 2000;89:1912–8.

14. Gabbard C. *Lifelong Motor Development.* Dubuque (IA): Pearson Education; 2007.

15. Gallahue DL, Ozmun JC. Childhood growth and development. In: *Understanding Motor Development: Infants, Children, Adolescents, Adults.* New York (NY): McGraw-Hill; 2002. p. 164–79.

16. Gallahue DL, Ozmun JC. Fundamental movement abilities. In: *Understanding Motor Development: Infants, Children, Adolescents, Adults.* New York (NY): McGraw-Hill;2002. p. 180–236.

17. Gallahue DL, Ozmun JC. Physiological changes in adults. In: *Understanding Motor Development: Infants, Children, Adolescents, Adults.* New York (NY): McGraw-Hill; 2002. p. 358–80.

18. Gallahue DL, Ozmun JC. Prenatal factors affecting development. In: *Understanding Motor Development: Infants, Children, Adolescents, Adults.* New York (NY): McGraw-Hill; 2002. p. 82–105.

19. Gallahue DL, Ozmun JC. Specialized movement abilities. In: *Understanding Motor Development: Infants, Children, Adolescents, Adults.* New York (NY): McGraw-Hill 2002. p. 304–22.

20. Gallahue DL, Ozmun JC. Understanding motor development: An overview. In: *Understanding Motor Development: Infants, Children, Adolescents, Adults* New York (NY): McGraw-Hill; 2002. p. 2–22.

21. Gesell A. *Infancy and Human Growth.* New York (NY): Macmillan; 1928.

22. Guadagnoli MA. Motor behavior. In: Brown SJ editor. *Introduction to Exercise Science.* Philadelphia (PA) Lippincott, Williams & Wilkins; 2001. p. 334–58.

23. Guadagnoli MA, Dornier LA, Tandy R. Optimal length of summary knowledge of results: The influence of task related experience and complexity *J Exerc Sport Psychol.* 1996;67:239–48.

24. Guadagnoli MA, Holcomb WR, Weber T. The relationship between contextual interference effects and performer experience on the learning of a putting task. *J Hum Mov Stud.* 1999;37:19–36.

25. Guadagnoli MA, Reeve TG. Movement complexity and foreperiod effects on response latencies for aimed movements. *J Hum Mov Stud.* 1992;23:29–9.

26. Guyton AC, Hall JE. *Textbook of Medical Physiology.* Oxford (UK): Elsevier; 2006.

27. Henry FM, Rodgers DE. Increased response latency for complicated movements and a "memory drum" theory of neuromotor reaction. *Res Quar.* 1960;31:448–58.

28. Jankovic J. Parkinson's disease: Clinical features and diagnosis. *J Neurol Neurosurg Psychiatry.* 2008;79 368–76.

29. Jeannerod M. *The Brain Machine.* Cambridge (MA). Harvard University Press; 1985.

30. Keele SW, Posner MI. Processing visual feedback in rapid movement. *J Exper Psychol.* 1968;77:155–8.

31. Klapp ST. Reaction time analysis of central motor control. In: Zelaznick HN, editor. *Advances in Motor Learning and Control.* Champaign (IL): Human Kinetics; 1996. p. 13–35.

32. Kues SHJ, Bloem BR, Hendriks EJM, Bredero-Cohen AB, Munneke M. Evidence-based analysis of physical therapy in Parkinson's disease with recommendations for practice and research. *Mov Disord.* 2007;22:451–60.

33. Lautenschlager NT, Cox KL, Flicker L, et al. Effect of physical activity on cognitive function in older adults at risk for alzheimer disease: A randomized trial. *JAMA*. 2008;300:1027–37.

34. Lavery JJ. Retention of simple motor skills as a function of type of knowledge of results. *Can J Psychol*. 1962; 16:300–11.

35. Mazzeo RS, Cavanagh PR, Evans WJ, et al. Position stand: Exercise and physical activity for older adults. *Med Sci Sports Exerc*. 1998;30:992–1008.

36. McGraw MB. *Growth, A Study of Johnny and Jimmy*. New York (NY): Appleton-Century-Crofts; 1935.

37. Morgan M, Phillips JG, Bradshaw JL, Mattingly JB, Iansek R, Bradshaw JA. Age-related motor slowness: Simply strategic? *J Gerontol*. 1994;49:M133–9.

38. National Institute for Neurological Disorders and Stroke 2008. 2008. Available at http://www.ninds. nih.gov/disorders/parkinsons_disease/detail_ parkinsons_disease.htm#127563159

39. Proctor RW, Reeve TG. *Stimulus-response Compatibility: An Integrated Perspective*. Amsterdam: Elsevier; 1990.

40. Protas EJ, Stanley RK. Parkinson's disease. In: Durstine JL, Moore GE, editors. *ACSM's Exercise Management of Person's with Chronic Diseases and Disabilities*. Champaign (IL): Human Kinetics; 2003. p. 295–302.

41. Rarick GL. *Physical Activity: Human Growth and Development*. New York (NY): Academic Press; 1973.

42. Sabbatini REM. The discovery of bioelectricity. *Brain Mind*. 1998;2:1–4.

43. Sanders AF. Issues and trends in the debate on discrete vs. continuous processing of information. *Acta Psychologica*. 1990;74:123–67.

44. Schmidt RA. A schema theory of discrete motor skill learning. *Psychol Rev*. 1975;82:225–60.

45. Schmidt RA, Lange C, Young DE. Optimizing summary knowledge of results. *Hum Mov Sci*. 1990;9:325–48.

46. Schmidt RA, Lee T. *Motor Control and Learning: A Behavioral Emphasis*. Champaign (IL): Human Kinetics; 2005.

47. Schmidt RA, Wrisberg CA. *Motor Learning and Performance: A Situation-based Learning Approach*. Champaign (IL): Human Kinetics; 2008.

48. Shea CH, Kohl RM, Indermil C. Contextual interference: Contributions of practice. *Acta Psychologica*. 1990;73:145–57.

49. Sherwood DE. Motor control and motor learning. In: Housh TJ, Housh DJ, Johnson GO, editors. *Introduction To Exercise Science*. Scottsdale (AZ): Holcomb Hataway; 2008. p. 234–52.

50. Sternberg S. The discovery of processing stages: Extensions of Donder's method. *Acta Psychologica*. 1969;30:270–315.

51. Thomas JR. Motor behavior. In: Massengale JD, Swanson RA, editors. *The History of Exercise and Sport*. Champaign (IL): Human Kinetics; 2003. p. 203–92.

52. Thorndike EL. The law of effect. *Am J Psychol*. 1927; 39:212–22.

53. Wickstrom R. *Fundamental Movement Patterns*. Philadelphia (PA): Lea & Febiger; 1970.

54. Woodworth RS. *Le mouvement*. Paris: Doin; 1903.

55. Wrisberg CA, Ragsdale MR. Further tests of Schmidt's schema theory: Development of a schema rule for a coincident timing task. *J Motor Behav*. 1979; 11:159–66.

Clinical and Sport Biomechanics

After completing this chapter you will be able to:

1. Define biomechanics and provide examples of the professional relationship between biomechanics and exercise science.
2. Identify the important historic events in the development of biomechanics.
3. Describe the important concepts of kinematics and kinetics.
4. Describe the importance of loading on body tissues.
5. Discuss the differences between clinical biomechanics and sport biomechanics
6. Describe some of the important topics of study in biomechanics

Biomechanics is the study of the human body at rest and in motion using principles and concepts derived from physics, mechanics, and engineering (1). The study of biomechanics involves examining forces acting on and within a biologic structure and the effects produced by such forces (11,12). Biomechanics can be subdivided into static and dynamic movements. **Static biomechanics** examines bodies, masses, and forces at rest or moving at a constant velocity. **Dynamic biomechanics** investigates bodies, masses, and forces when they are speeding up or slowing down (11). The study of **kinematics** and **kinetics** is important for exercise science students trying to understand how the body moves (11). Kinematics is the study of motion, including the patterns and speed of movement of the body segments, without consideration given to the mass of the body or the forces acting upon it. Kinetics is used to describe basic movements and the degree of motor coordination displayed by an individual. Kinetics is concerned with the effects of forces on the motion of a body, especially forces that do not originate within the body itself. Anthropometric factors, such as the size, shape, and weight of the body segments, are principal considerations in a kinetic analysis (11,15).

The examination and understanding of the structural and functional mechanisms underlying human movement are critical to biomechanics. The analyses of biomechanical movement ranges from fundamental motor skills to complex sport activities (11). The relationship between humans and mechanical movement is studied in two primary environments: the clinical setting (called clinical biomechanics) and the sport setting (called sport biomechanics). **Clinical biomechanics** focuses on improving the ability of an injured or disabled individual to perform activities of daily living including work and leisure activities, physical activity, or exercise. For example, exercise science professionals such as athletic trainers and physical therapists use biomechanical principles and techniques to facilitate the recovery of an injured individual. **Sport biomechanics** applies the laws and principles of mechanics and physics to enhance sport performance through the improvement in movement techniques or the development of equipment. For example, athletic coaches and other exercise science professionals may use the knowledge of biomechanical techniques to improve the skilled movements of athletes, whereas manufacturers of sports equipment make alterations to a piece of equipment to improve safety or enhance athletic performance (11). The use of biomechanics and the associated principles of biomechanics has been around for a considerable time.

Static biomechanics   The study of bodies, masses, and forces at rest or in a constant unchanged motion.

Dynamic biomechanics   The study of bodies, masses, and forces when they are in motion.

Kinematics   The study of motion, including the patterns and speed of movement of the body segments, without consideration given to the mass of the body or the forces acting upon it.

Kinetics   The study of the effects of forces on the motion of a body or system of bodies, especially of forces that do not originate within the system itself.

Sport biomechanics   A branch of biomechanics centered on improving sport performance by athletes through the improvement in movement techniques or the development of equipment.

Clinical biomechanics   A branch of biomechanics centered on improving the ability of an injured or disabled individual to perform activities of daily living including work and leisure activities, physical activity, or exercise.

HISTORY OF BIOMECHANICS

Though biomechanics is a relatively young area of scientific study, many of the basic principles that form the foundation of biomechanics can be traced back thousands of years. Similar to many of the other areas of study in exercise science, the developmental history of biomechanics starts with the ancient Greeks and Romans. The writings of many of the Greek scholars provided the framework for the guiding principles of modern biomechanics and the development of both clinical and sport biomechanics. Today, exercise science and other professionals from the disciplines of physics, mechanics, and engineering continue to expand the knowledge base of biomechanics.

Early Influences

The development of mechanical, mathematical, and anatomic models and the first attempt to examine the human body biomechanically were key contributions from scholars and scientists between 700 BC and 200 AD (23). Scholars such as Aristotle (384–322 BC) and Archimedes (287–212 BC) were instrumental in writing about walking, running, and movement in water. One of the early influential books was written by Aristotle and called "De Motu Animalium" or *On the Motion of Animals*. Aristotle viewed the bodies of animals as mechanical systems, and pursued answers to questions such as "What is the physiologic difference between imagining performing an action and actually doing it" (20). Archimedes' essay titled *Floating Bodies* described the principle of water displacement by physical structures and this became the basis for determining the density of an object (23). This principle is used to form the basis for determining the density of a body and ultimately body composition. Galen, a physician to the Roman emperor Marcus Aurelius, wrote *On the Function of the Parts* (meaning the parts of the human body), which was used as the world's standard medical text for over 1,400 years. This text included anatomic descriptions and terminology still used in certain areas of biologic science (23).

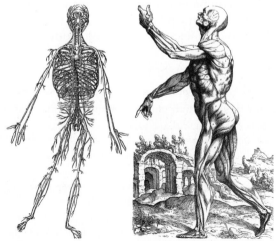

FIGURE 9.1 ▼ Anatomic structure of the body by Andreas Vesalius.

Throughout the Renaissance period of the fourteenth to seventeenth centuries, the science of biomechanics had its foundation further developed by some of the greatest scientists of all time. For example, Leonardo da Vinci examined the structure and function of the human body, analyzed muscle forces as acting along lines connecting origins and insertions, and studied joint function. Andreas Vesalius (1514–64), a Flemish physician furthered the foundational development of biomechanics by publishing his brilliantly illustrated text, *On the Structure of the Human Body* (Figure 9.1) (20,23). Galileo Galilei (1564–1642), an Italian physicist and mathematician, studied the action of falling bodies, the mechanical aspects of bone, and the mechanical analysis of movement. Adding to the work of previous scholars, Giovanni Alphonso Borelli (1608–79) examined various relationships between muscular movement and mechanical principles. Borelli's work *De Moti Animalium* demonstrated how geometry could be used to describe complex human and animal movements such as jumping, running, flying, and swimming (Figure 9.2). For this work, Borelli is often referred to as "the father of biomechanics" (23). Borelli was the first to propose that levers of the musculoskeletal system magnify motion rather than force so that muscles must produce much greater forces than those forces resisting the motion (23). Sir Isaac Newton (1642–1727) published his basic laws in *Philosophia Naturalis Principia Mathematica*

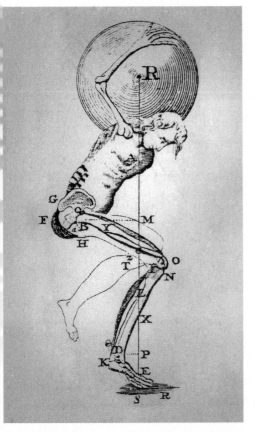

FIGURE 9.2 ▼ Giovanni Borelli's use of geometry to describe movement. (Image as seen in Provencher MT, Abdu WA. Historical perspective: Giovanni Alfonso Borelli: "Father of Spinal Biomechanics." *Spine.* 2000;25:131.)

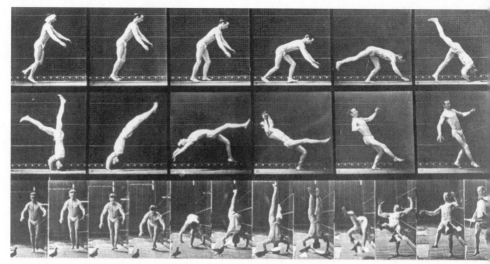

FIGURE 9.3 ▼ Eadweard Muybride's use of pictures to capture human movement. (Photos by Time & Life Pictures/Bernard Hoffman/Getty Images.)

in 1686. Newton's contribution to biomechanics during this time period provides us with a theory for mechanical analysis and an improvement in science through the development of the process of theory and experimentation (23).

During the nineteenth century, the field of biomechanics expanded greatly through several key discoveries including the development of **electromyography**, the development of measuring techniques to examine the kinematics and kinetics of movement, and the beginning of the use of engineering principles in biomechanical analysis (23). During the 1800s, scholars and scientists studied the path of the center of gravity during movement and the influence of gravity on limb movements in walking and running. Several individuals used photographic and cinemagraphic techniques to study the movements of animals and humans. For example, Eadweard Muybridge (1830–1904) used different cameras to capture the movements of animals and humans (Figure 9.3) (10). Further study of movement resulted in a better understanding of gait and led to the development of prosthetic devices for assisting with movement. These developments have led some scholars to refer to the nineteenth century as the "gait century" of biomechanics (23).

Recent Influences

Throughout the twentieth century, biomechanics further evolved into a science-based discipline for the study of animal and human movements. With the expansion of industrial technology came the need to examine the physical and physiologic aspects of industrial work. Jules Amar's book *The Human Motor*, in 1920, focused on the efficiency of human movement and helped establish standards for human engineering in the United States and Europe. Nicholas

Electromyography A technique for evaluating and recording the electrical activity of a muscle or muscle group.

Bernstein (1896–1966) studied the coordination and regulation of movement in both children and adults. This work provided the basis for his theories on motor control and coordination (23). Foundations for the use of biomechanics to examine the efficiency and energy cost of human movement were established by Archibald V. Hill (1886–1977) in the Harvard Fatigue Laboratory and by Wallace O. Fenn (1893–1971) who published the first cinematographic analysis of sprint running in humans (8,23). As the interest in using mechanical and engineering principles to study movement during exercise and sport increased, there was a development of biomechanical laboratories around the United States including those founded by Richard Nelson at the Pennsylvania State University, Charles Dillman at the University of Illinois, and Barry Bates at the University of Oregon. These individuals were instrumental in promoting and developing biomechanics into a scientific discipline for the study of human movement in both clinical and sport environments (26).

> ➤ *Thinking Critically*
> In what ways has the study of biomechanics contributed to a broader understanding of physical fitness and health?

From the mid-1960s until the present day, the study of biomechanics was fueled by several new professional societies and journals, along with national and international conferences in the field. Three main professional societies have been instrumental in promoting biomechanics: the International Society of Biomechanics (1973), the American Society of Biomechanics (1975), and the International Society for Biomechanics in Sport (1982). The *Journal of Biomechanics* began publication in 1968 and the *International Journal of Sports Biomechanics* (now titled *Journal of Applied Biomechanics*) began publication in 1985. The International Society of Biomechanics first published *Clinical Biomechanics* in 1986. These professional organizations and peer-reviewed journals have helped further the development of biomechanics for use in the clinical and sport settings. For additional information on the history of biomechanics, please see the reviews provided by Wilkerson (28) and Nigg (23). Table 9.1 provides a list of some of the significant historic events in the development of biomechanics.

> ➤ *Thinking Critically*
> In what ways has the study of biomechanics contributed to a broader understanding of factors important for improving performance in sport and athletic competition?

STUDY OF BIOMECHANICS

The study and application of biomechanics involves the use of various mechanical and computational principles from the academic disciplines of physics, mathematics, and engineering. The effective analysis of human movement also requires an understanding of the concepts of kinematics and kinetics. Most human movement involves a complex combination of linear and angular motion components where body segments and limbs are moving in different directions at different speeds. Motion of the body or body parts can be classified as linear, angular, or general (21). Exercise science professionals need a solid understanding of these principles to appropriately use biomechanics to assist individuals in improving performance of physical activity, exercise, sport, and athletic performance.

Table 9.1	Historic Events in the Development of Biomechanics
DATE	**HISTORIC EVENT**
ca. 384–322 BC	Aristotle publishes "On the Motion of Animals."
ca. 130–200	Galen publishes "On the Function of the Parts."
1543	Andreas Vesalius publishes "On the Structure of the Human Body."
1679	Giovanni Alphonso Borelli publishes "De Moti Arinalium."
1920	Jules Amar publishes "The Human Motor."
1929	W.O. Fenn publishes the first cinematographic analysis of sprint running in humans.
1968	*Journal of Biomechanics* is first published
1973	International Society of Biomechanics is founded
1975	American Society of Biomechanics is founded
1982	International Society for Biomechanics in Sport is founded
1985	*Journal of Applied Biomechanics* is first published.
1986	*Clinical Biomechanics* is first published

Types of Body Motion

True **linear motion** occurs when all points of the body are moving in the same direction at the same speed and are traveling the same distance. Linear motion may also be thought of as movement along a line of travel. There are two forms of linear motion: rectilinear translation and curvilinear translation. **Rectilinear translation** (sometimes thought of as linear motion) occurs when all points on a body move in a straight line the same distance, with no change in direction. Examples of rectilinear translation might include a downhill skier in a tuck position (Figure 9.4) or a cyclist coasting during a ride. These two examples show how all points of the body can be moving forward in a straight line at the same time. **Curvilinear translation** occurs when all points on a body move in a parallel line the same distance, but the paths followed by the points on the object are curved. An example of curvilinear translation might be the upper body movement, which occurs during jogging or running. In curvilinear translation, the direction of the motion of the object is constantly changing, even though the orientation of the object does not (21). Figure 9.5 illustrates rectilinear and curvilinear translations.

Angular motion, also referred to as rotary motion or rotation, is movement around a central imaginary line known as the axis of rotation, which is oriented perpendicular to the plane in which the rotation occurs. Most voluntary human movement involves the rotation of a body part around an imaginary axis of rotation that passes through the center of the joint to which the body part attaches. Examples of angular motion include the shoulder press and the seated

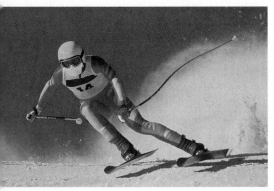

FIGURE 9.4 ▼ A downhill skier in a tuck position provides an example of rectilinear translation. (Photo by Stockbyte/Getty Images.).

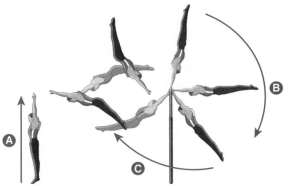

FIGURE 9.5 ▼ Examples of rectilinear (A) and curvilinear translation (B) and whole body rotation (C). (From Dorling Kindersley RF/Getty Images.)

knee extension exercise, which involve movements of a ball and socket joint and a hinge joint, respectively. These movements involve a rotating action, whereby moving portions of the body are constantly in motion relative to other areas of the body (11,21). Figure 9.5C provides an illustration of whole body rotation.

General motion occurs when translation and angular movements are combined. Human movement usually consists of general motion rather than linear or angular motion. Classifying human movement as linear, angular, or general motion simplifies the biomechanical analysis of movement. If a movement can be broken down into the linear and angular components, those components can use the mechanical laws that govern linear and angular motions. The linear and angular analyses are then combined to provide a better understanding of the general motion of the individual or object (11,21). For example, during walking, the body has both angular and translation motions occurring. As steps are taken, the hip joint is performing angular motion, whereas the upper torso is performing translational motion. When analyzing the walking movement for correct form, both types of motion must be considered in the analysis. Exercise science professionals should have a solid understanding of the principles of motion so that effective exercise and rehabilitation programs can be developed. This is especially true for athletic trainers, physical therapists, and occupational therapists.

Linear motion When all points of the body are moving in the same direction at the same speed, and travel the same distance.

Rectilinear translation When all points on a body move in a straight line, the same distance, and with no change in direction.

Curvilinear translation Occurs when all points on a body move the same distance but the paths followed by the points on the object are curved.

Angular motion The motion of a body about a fixed point or fixed axis.

General motion Occurs when the translation and rotation movements are combined.

Mechanical Systems

The complete biomechanical analysis of a movement requires that the system of interest be operationally defined. This helps improve the quality and usefulness of the analysis. In some analyses, the complete body is the system of interest, whereas in other instances only a body segment or limb will be analyzed during the movement. For example, during the analysis of walking patterns in an individual with osteoarthritis of the knee there may be interest in how the person shifts weight from one leg to the other during the movement. This might require the entire body being designated as the system of interest. If only movements of the knee are of interest, then only the affected leg might be designated as the mechanical system of interest (11).

Standard Reference Terminology

The analysis of human movement requires the use of common and specific terminology that precisely identifies body positions and directions of movement. By using consistent terminology, exercise science and allied healthcare professionals can precisely understand the movements describing the actions of the human body (11). This is particularly important for healthcare professionals, such as physical and occupational therapists, who must evaluate body movement and function to help individuals during rehabilitation from injury. Table 9.2 provides a list of terms and definitions commonly used in the biomechanical analysis of human movement.

Joint Movement Terminology

The most effective use of a biomechanical analysis occurs when professionals use consistent joint terminology to describe the movements of bones and joints of the body. When the human body is in the anatomic reference position, all body segments are considered to be positioned at zero degrees. The movement of a body segment occurs in one of the three planes: sagittal, frontal, or transverse. Figure 9.6 illustrates the planes of the body in an anatomic position.

The movement of a body segment away from the anatomic position is described according to the direction of motion and is measured as the angle between the body segment's position and the anatomic position (11). The variou

Table 9.2	Terms and Definitions Used in Biomechanical Analysis
TERM	DEFINITION
Anatomic reference position	An erect standing position with the feet slightly separated, the arms hanging relaxed at the sides, and the palms of the hands facing forward.
Directional terms	Used to describe the relationship of body parts or the location of an external object with respect to the body.
Anatomic reference planes	The division of the body by three imaginary cardinal planes into three dimensions: sagittal, frontal, and transverse.
Anatomic reference axes	The use of three reference axes for describing the rotation of the human body: medio-lateral, antero-posterior, and longitudinal.

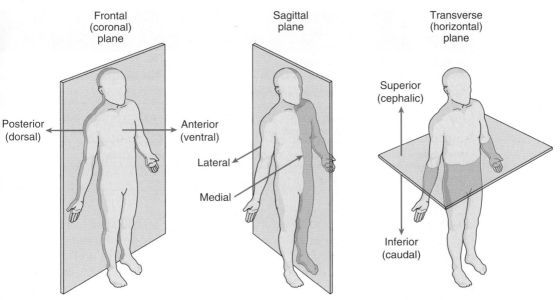

FIGURE 9.6 ▼ Illustration of the planes of the body in an anatomic position. (Adapted from Cohen BJ. *Memmler's The Human Body in Health and Disease.* 10th ed. Baltimore (MD): Lippincott Williams & Wilkins; 2005.)

skeletal muscles and bones of the body are responsible for creating the movement of the body segments and limbs (11,21). Table 9.3 provides the terminologies of the various planes and movements of the body.

Spatial Reference Systems

An understanding of biomechanics and the associated principles requires knowledge of spatial reference systems. During the movement of the body, the three coordinal planes and their associated axes of rotation also move. During a biomechanical analysis of a body movement or sport skill, it is often useful to employ a fixed system of reference. Clinical and sport biomechanics professionals quantitatively describe the movement of humans using a spatial reference system to standardize the measurements collected. The reference system most commonly used is a **Cartesian coordinate system**. In this system, units are measured in the direction of either two or three primary axes. Single direction or planar movements, such as running, cycling, or jumping, can be analyzed using a two-dimensional Cartesian coordinate system (11). Figure 9.7 provides an example of a two-dimensional Cartesian coordinate system. The points of interest are measured in units in the x or horizontal direction and the y or vertical direction. When a biomechanist analyzes human movement, the points of interest are usually the joints of the body, which constitute the end points of the body segments. The position of each joint

Cartesian coordinate system A system in which the location of a point is given by coordinates that represent its distances from perpendicular lines that intersect at a point called the origin.

Table 9.3	Terminologies of the Various Movements of the Body (11)
PLANES	**BODY MOVEMENT**
Sagittal	Flexion, extension, and hyperextension
Frontal	Abduction, adduction, lateral flexion, elevation and depression, deviation, eversion, and inversion
Transverse	Rotation, supination, pronation, abduction, and adduction
Other	Circumduction

center can be measured with respect to the two axes, described as (x, y), where x the number of horizontal units away from the y-axis and y is the number of verti cal units away from the x-axis. These units can be measured in both positive an negative directions as illustrated in Figure 9.8. When a body movement is thre dimensional, the analysis can be extended to the third dimension by adding a z-ax perpendicular to the x- and y-axes and measuring units away from the x, y plane i the z direction. In a two-dimensional coordinate system, the y axis is vertical an the x-axis is horizontal. In a three-dimensional coordinate system, the z-axis is ver tical with the x- and y-axes representing the two horizontal directions (11).

Qualitative Analysis of Human Movement

Often the analysis of human movement takes a **qualitative** form. The abilit of exercise science and allied healthcare professionals, as well as sport and ath letic coaches, to qualitatively assess human movement requires knowledge of th movement characteristics desired and the ability to observe and analyze whethe a given performance incorporates these characteristics (11,21). Visual observatio is the most commonly used approach for qualitatively analyzing the mechanics c human movement, although many exercise science and allied healthcare profes sionals are employing the use of video recordings (See Chapter 10) to assist in th process. Using information gained from watching an athlete perform a skill or patient's movement pattern, coaches and clinical allied healthcare professional make judgments and recommendations based on movement patterns. Qualita tive analyses must be carefully planned and conducted with the knowledge of th biomechanics of the movement or motor skill (11,21).

Knowledge for a Qualitative Analysis

The analysis of a movement skill is a vital component of study in biomechanic Two important factors to consider in the quantitative analysis of a movemer are the techniques exhibited by the performer and the performance outcome Effective skill analysis requires the person performing the analysis to understan the specific purpose or outcome of the motor skill being studied. For example, i the clinical environment, the successful performance outcome of rehabilitatio from anterior cruciate ligament surgery of the knee is to have a normal walkir

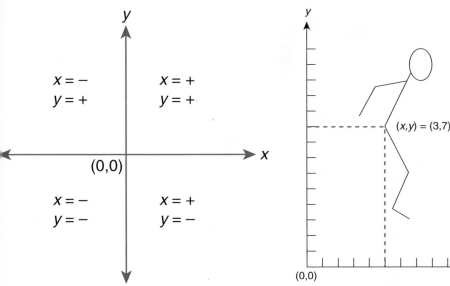

FIGURE 9.8 ▼ Positive and negative
positions in two-dimensional
Cartesian coordinate system.

ʒait that does not put excessive pressure on the joints of the lower extremity.
n a sport environment, the successful performance outcome of a placekicker in
American football is to kick the ball through the uprights to score points. A knowl-
ʒdge of this outcome is critical for understanding how to begin an examination of
he movements and forces required to perform the kicking skill (11). Knowledge
ɔf relevant biomechanical principles is important for identifying the factors that
ʒontribute to successful or unsuccessful performance. An analysis of a movement
kill requires several important planning steps including the following (11):

1. Identifying the major question or questions of interest.
2. Determining the optimal perspective(s) from which to view the movement.
3. Identifying the distance from which to view the movement.
4. Determining the number of trials of the movement needed to formulate an
   analysis.
5. Determining whether visual observation alone is acceptable or the movement should be recorded with a motion capture system.

A **qualitative analysis** requires the progressive identification of the aspects
ʒritical to the movement or motor skill. Movements affecting the outcome of the
ɱotor skill are identified through a systematic process that often requires the indi-
ʋidual performing the analysis   to view multiple trials of the motor skill from
ʒifferent viewpoints. For a physical therapist, observing an individual from all sides
ʒuring walking allows for the determination of whether a normal gait pattern has

Qualitative analysis Requires the progressive identification of the aspects critical to the movement through
a systematic process that often requires the analyst to view multiple trials from different viewpoints.

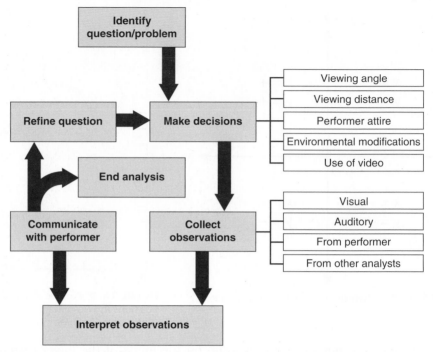

FIGURE 9.9 ▼ Cyclical process of an analysis of a movement skill (11).

been established during the rehabilitation program. For an athletic coach trying to improve the performance of the placekicker in football might observe the athlete from each side during the performance of several repetitions of a kick. This allows multiple viewpoints from which the coach might make corrections to the movement being performed and therefore improve the chances of success (i.e., kicking the ball through the goal posts). It is important to remember that the performance of a movement skill is affected by the physical, developmental, and psychological characteristics of the performer (11). The qualitative analysis of a movement skill can often result in the refinement of the movement and then possibly a new analysis of the revised skill. Figure 9.9 shows how a qualitative analysis of a movement skill can result in cyclical process to improve performance (11).

> ➤ *Thinking Critically*
> *What qualitative information about a sport technique would you need to help an athlete improve performance of a complex movement skill?*

BASIC CONCEPTS RELATED TO KINETICS

The term kinetics describes the effects of forces on the motion or movement of the body or body part. When sufficient external forces are produced by muscles, body movement and the manipulation of objects can occur. During the course of daily activities and participation in sports, the human body generates and responds to forces. For example, recovery from injury requires the systematic increase of forces by muscles and muscle groups during rehabilitation. During the early phase of rehabilitation, small forces are generated during muscular contraction so that the required body part is not damaged any further. As the rehabilitation program proceeds, there is a progressive increase in force production during muscular contraction. Often the decision for an individual to return to work or competition is based on how much force can be generated during an assessment of muscle and joint movement. Sport participation requires muscles to apply forces to a variety of objects including balls, bats, racquets, and clubs and also requires the absorption of forces from impacts with ball, the playing surface, and opponents in contact sports (11). Individuals studying and using biomechanics to improve human performance must understand the basic concepts related to kinetics that are displayed in Table 9.4 (11).

Mechanical Loads on the Human Body

External forces acting on an object impose a **mechanical load** on the object. Forces from gravity and muscles and forces external to the body all affect the

Table 9.4	Basic Concepts and Definitions Related to Kinetics (11)
BASIC CONCEPT	**DEFINITION**
Inertia	Tendency of a body to maintain its current state of motion, whether motionless or moving with a constant velocity.
Mass	Quantity of matter contained in an object.
Force	Something that causes a change in the motion of a body.
Center of gravity	Point around which the body's weight is equally balanced, no matter how the body is positioned.
Weight .	Force with which an object is attracted toward the center of the earth by gravity; weight depends on an object's mass and the strength of the gravitational pull.
Pressure	Force per unit area that one region of a gas, liquid, or solid exerts on another region.
Volume	Amount of space occupied by a three-dimensional object or region of space.
Density	Measure of the quantity of some physical property (usually mass) per unit length, area, or volume.
Torque	Tendency of a force applied to an object to make the object rotate about an axis.
Impulse	Change of momentum of a body or physical system over a time interval; equal to the force applied times the length of the time interval over which it is applied.

Mechanical loads Forces that act upon a body or object including those from gravity, the muscles, and external to the body.

Table 9.5	Basic Concepts and Definitions Related to Mechanical Loads (11)	
BASIC CONCEPT	**DEFINITION**
Compressive force (compression)	Force that tends to shorten or squeeze something, decreasing its volume.
Tensile force (tension)	A force which tends to stretch or elongate something.
Shear force	Force acting on a substance in a direction perpendicular to the extension of the substance.

human body differently. The effect of a given force or forces on the body or an object depends on the direction, duration, and magnitude of the force. The mechanical loads on the human body are defined in Table 9.5 (11,21). The action of forces on the human body can be affected by the way in which the force is distributed on the body. There are two terms that are key to understanding the action of forces on the body. Pressure represents the distribution of force that is applied externally to a body. Stress represents the resulting force distribution inside a body when an external force acts upon the body (11,21).

Tension and Combined Loads

Pure compression and tension are directed along the longitudinal axis of the body and are called axial forces. When an **eccentric** (called nonaxial) force is applied to a structure, the structure bends, creating compressive stress on one side and tensile stress on the opposite side. For example, when an athlete performs the pole vault the end of the pole is placed in the vaulting box. The forces exerted on the pole cause a compressive stress on one side of the pole and tensile stress on the other side of the pole (Figure 9.10). **Torsion** occurs when a structure is caused to twist around its longitudinal axis, typically when one end of the structure is fixed. For example, many movements in aerobic dance require the upper body to twist in one direction while the feet remain planted on the floor. In this instance, torsion is applied to the upper body. The most common type of loading on the body is combined loading, which is the presence of more than one form of force on the body (11).

Effects of Loading

There are two potential outcomes when a force acts on an object: acceleration and deformation. Acceleration is the rate of change in velocity of an object or the human body. When a baseball player throws a ball, the force imparted upon the ball causes the ball contained in the hand and travelling at a velocity of 0 m per second to leave the hand at an increased velocity and travel through space. Increased force production by the muscles of the body can increase the velocity of objects on which the body is acting (11). For example, professional baseball pitchers can generate enough force to throw a baseball over 100 mi per hour.

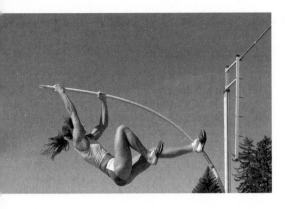

FIGURE 9.10 ▼ An example of compression and tension during a pole vault. (Photo by UpperCut Images/Pete Saloutos/Getty Images.)

Deformation occurs when the external force causes a change in the shape or structure of an object or body component. For example, forces applied by an individual running down the track and placing the pole into the vaulting box will cause the pole to deform or bend. The bending of the pole creates a force that can propel the individual upward and over the top of the bar. However, if too much force is applied to the pole during the jump, the physical structure of the pole would not be strong enough to withstand the forces and therefore the pole would break. When an external force is applied to the human body, the structures of the body must withstand the external force. If too much force is applied, there is the potential for injury to a body part. The magnitude and direction of the force and the area over which the force is distributed play important factors in determining the potential for tissue injury. The material properties of the loaded body tissues also factor into determining the risk for injury. If the amount of force applied to the body causes the deformation of the body tissues to exceed the point at which change to the structure occurs some amount of deformation becomes permanent. In the human body, deformations exceeding the crucial failure point produce mechanical failure of the structure (called an injury) resulting in a fracturing of bone or rupturing of soft tissues (11).

Acute versus Repetitive Loads

During participation in physical activity, exercise, sport and athletic competition, the body is subjected to single (also called acute) loads and repetitive (also called chronic) loads. The distinction between acute loading and repetitive loading is important for understanding the response of the body tissues to physical activity and exercise. Understanding these concepts helps define the potential for the body tissues to experience a positive adaptation and define the potential for injury risk. When external loads of appropriate magnitude are applied to the body during physical activity and exercise, positive adaptations occur to the

Eccentric A movement that results in a lengthening of the muscle.

Torsion The production of force at one end of a body that results in a twisting motion whereas the other end of the body remains fixed or moves in the opposite direction.

tissues and systems of the body. For example, during chronic resistance exercise training, performing several sets of bench press exercise can result in positive adaptations such as an increase in bone density and muscular strength. These adaptations are referred to as a training effect. When a single force large enough to cause an injury acts on body tissues, the injury is termed acute. The force causing the injury is termed macrotrauma. A physical injury can also result from the repeated action of relatively small forces acting on tissue. Repeated bouts of chronic loading over a period of time can also produce an injury. In this instance, the injury is called a chronic injury or a stress injury, and the causative mechanism is called microtrauma. For example, long distance runners may experience stress fractures to the lower leg as a result of repeated microtrauma to the tibia and fibula (11).

AREAS OF STUDY IN BIOMECHANICS

Biomechanics and its associated principles of study are used in a wide range of exercise science and allied healthcare professional activities. Working as a clinician in an allied health profession, ergonomist, personal trainer, or strength and conditioning coach require a sound knowledge of biomechanical principles. Biomechanics contributes to a better understanding of numerous issues related to the safe and successful performance of individuals in physical activity, exercise, sport, and athletic competition through a wide variety of areas. The areas discussed in the following sections provide a sampling of some of the primary interest areas in clinical and sport biomechanics. The information provided is not meant to be an exhaustive list of areas of study in biomechanics.

Clinical Biomechanics

Clinical biomechanics focuses on the mechanics of injury and the principles of prevention, evaluation, and treatment of musculoskeletal problems. Clinical biomechanics professionals rely heavily on the fundamental knowledge and principles of anatomy, mathematics, and physics. Examples of the primary areas of interest in clinical biomechanics include designing individualized rehabilitation techniques, wheelchair design, tissue repair, surgical techniques, and bone and tissue design. With advanced study and preparation, clinical biomechanists can design environments that allow disabled individuals to live a satisfying and safe lifestyle and participate in recreational and sporting activities (11,21).

It is important for clinical biomechanists to know how the body responds in normal healthy situations. This information is then used to set goals for recovery for injured and disabled individuals and help prevent injuries. Understanding normal patterns of movement and their variations for healthy individuals is critical so that the movement pattern of an injured or disabled individual can be adjusted toward a normal and efficient movement pattern with a low risk of injury. Individuals using the principles of clinical biomechanics must be able to evaluate movement patterns in an injured or disabled individual to determine if movement can return to normal. If normal movement patterns cannot be attained, then adjustments in movement patterns must be made toward the most efficient and safe pattern for that atient. Clinical biomechanists work with other healthcare providers, such as hysicians and physical and occupational therapists, to help individuals return normal function as quickly as possible (18). Examples of areas where clini- l biomechanists and the application of clinical biomechanical principles help nprove physical function include osteoarthritis, gait patterns (e.g., Parkinson isease), and rehabilitation from knee injuries.

steoarthritis

steoarthritis is a dynamic, progressive disease causing the loss of joint function and gnificant disability. In osteoarthritis, a wearing away of the cartilage that covers and cts as a cushion inside joints causes a low-grade inflammation, which ultimately sults in pain in the joints (9). In osteoarthritis of the knee, the bone surfaces become ss well protected by the cartilage, and the individual experiences pain in weight- earing activities, including walking and standing. Osteoarthritis of the knee is two to ree times more prevalent in females compared to males (4) and females also have vofold higher risk of developing bilateral knee osteoarthritis (19). Intrinsic differ- nces between males and females in muscle strength (7), quadriceps angle (13), joint xity (2), and muscle activation patterns (27) may cause biomechanical differences nd contribute to the differentiated risk for developing knee osteoarthritis.

For allied healthcare professionals, a key factor in understanding how to create ehabilitation programs for injured or disabled individuals is understanding the ormal movement patterns of healthy individuals. Nonosteoarthritic individuals isplay similar joint kinetics at the knee (14), and similar knee joint kinematics nd stride characteristics have been observed when comparing gait characteristics etween females and males (17). Healthy and osteoarthritic populations have dif- erent gait patterns (Figure 9.11). Both male and female patients with osteoarthritis valk with an increased knee adduction movement (14), decreased knee flexion ovement (16), decreased knee flexion angle (6), and at a slower velocity than ealthy individuals (16). Osteoarthritic females also display certain gait biomechan- s that do not occur in males (22). It remains to be determined if the differences in ait biomechanics between males and females are the result of having osteoarthritis r a contributing factor that causes females to have higher rates of osteoarthritis.

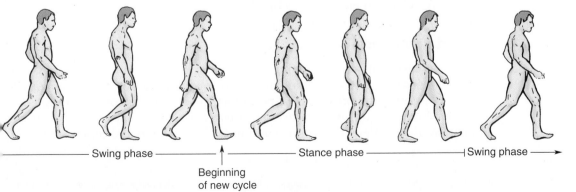

———— Swing phase ————↑———— Stance phase ————⊣Swing phase ——→

Beginning
of new cycle

IGURE 9.11 ▼ A normal gait cycle. (From Moore KL, Dalley AF II. *Clinical Oriented Anatomy.* th ed. Baltimore (MD): Lippincott Williams & Wilkins; 1999.)

Determining if differences exist in the biomechanics of gait movement i
males and females has significant implications for the treatment of osteoarthriti
Orthotic devices, knee braces, and total knee replacements are currently designe
to modify the biomechanical movement of the knee. Females with osteoarthrit
may walk differently than healthy females or males and as such treatment inte
ventions should be designed based on gender and the differences that are presen
between females and males. Gender-specific design of biomechanical interver
tions to slow the progression of osteoarthritis should be examined to determin
if these interventions significantly influence the disease condition (22).

Ergonomics

Ergonomics is the study of the interaction between humans, the objects they us
and the environments in which they function (25). Professional preparation i
ergonomics is similar to clinical biomechanics with ergonomists taking addition.
coursework in engineering. Ergonomists work to prevent workplace injuries an
improve the capacity for the individual to return to work after an injury has occurre
This includes the modification of the workplace environment and the working tech
niques employed by the individual worker (5). Ergonomists also design equipmer
and modify work and living conditions for special populations such as the elderl
and disabled. Ergonomists work to design and implement changes to improve env
ronments such as the home, recreational sites and facilities, motor vehicles, school
clinics, workplace, and other human-built environments (18,25).

Several physical factors can cause, maintain, or worsen musculoskeletal pai
and injury. Excessively forceful exertions, awkward postures, localized conta
loads, and repetitive motion may lead to musculo
skeletal disorders caused by **mechanical fatigue**
Ergonomists work to reduce the influence of thes
factors for causing pain and injury. Changing huma
movement patterns, redesigning work areas, an
developing protective equipment are examples o
how ergonomists might improve work performanc
and decrease the risk of pain and injury. Table 9.6 list
some of those factors that may increase the risk of pain and injury and therefor
be addressed by an ergonomist (18,25).

> ### ➤ *Thinking Critically*
> *What kinematic and kinetic informa-
> tion is helpful for an individual begin-
> ning a rehabilitation program to
> recover from an injury?*

Sport Biomechanics

Sport biomechanics includes the examination of factors of human movemen
associated with exercise training and sport for the purpose of improving perfor
mance. Information provided by sport biomechanics professionals through quan
titative investigations is often useful for coaches trying to provide a quantitativ
analysis of an athlete performing a motor skill or strength and conditioning coac

---

Mechanical fatigue When the expected force production of a muscle, tendon, ligament, cartilage, or bone
cannot be achieved or maintained.

Table 9.6	Factors Increasing the Risk of Injury and Pain (18,25)	
RISK FACTOR	**CONTRIBUTION TO INJURY AND PAIN**	
Forceful exertion	Used in activities that require a large magnitude of force to perform a task may easily lead to injury.	
Awkward postures	Using improper technique to perform a task can produce disabling injuries to active and supporting tissues and muscles.	
Localized constant loads	Occur between body tissues and objects in the environment and can cause increased compression and shearing on the tissues.	
Repetitious motions	Occur during repeated performance of tasks during the day and may cause injury through inflammation and repetitive stress	

teaching a movement pattern during training. Sport biomechanics combines the study of applied human anatomy with mechanical physics to describe how and why the human body moves the way it does and why individuals perform at varying levels of success in sports activities (15). Athletic coaches work with sport biomechanists to use neuromuscular and mechanical factors associated with human movement to describe the requirements necessary for an athlete to perform at an optimal level. Detailed biomechanical descriptions of movement performance help coaches and athletes to refine their knowledge and approaches to training, as well as consider new and innovative techniques for improving sport performance. This knowledge may also provide information into the mechanical causes of sport-related injuries, potentially leading to safer sport participation (11,21).

Technique Improvement

Improving an athlete's technique is one of the most common methods for bettering performance in sport and athletic competition (21). Using biomechanics to improve an athlete's technique can occur in two primary ways. First, coaches may use their knowledge of biomechanics to correct an athlete's technique to improve the execution of a movement skill. In this instance, coaches use qualitative biomechanical analysis methods to affect changes in the technique of the athlete. Second, research in biomechanics may discover a new and more effective technique for performing a sports skill. In this instance, a biomechanics researcher uses quantitative biomechanical analysis methods to discover new techniques, which will then be communicated to the coaches and athletes who will implement them (11,21).

Numerous examples exist for how sport biomechanics has helped improve athletic performance by changing techniques. Prior to the 1968 Olympics, most athletes performed the high jump by using techniques known as the Western roll, the straddle technique, or the scissors kick (Figure 9.12A). In the 1960s, Dick Fosbury developed a high-jump technique that allowed for increased height following the approach to the bar and takeoff from the ground. This technique, originally called the Fosbury Flop, allows the center of gravity to be lowered and a rotation of the body to occur immediately prior to the jump (Figure 9.12B).

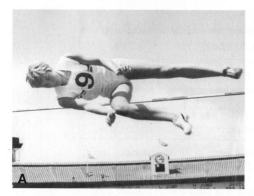 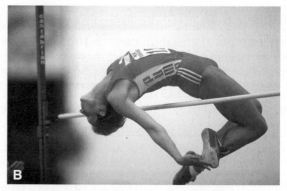

FIGURE 9.12 ▼ A: The Western roll high-jump technique (Photo by Hulton Archive/Evening Standard/Getty Images.). **B:** The Fosbury flop high-jump technique (Photo by Bob Thomas Sports Photography/Getty Images.).

As a result, there is more force being created to move the body up and over the bar. Another example of how a change in technique improves sport performance would be placekicking in American football. Prior to the late 1960s, all placekickers in professional football employed a straight-on (called conventional) approach to kicking the ball. In this technique, the leg served as a pendulum to impart force onto the ball and propel it toward the goal posts. Pete Gogolak was the first placekicker to approach the ball at an angle and kicked it with his instep. This style (called the soccer style) allows for greater forces to be impacted upon the ball. Virtually all American football kickers now use this soccer style approach. Table 9.7 provides brief examples of how biomechanics may be used to improve the performance of an athlete during sport or athletic competition (11,21).

Equipment Improvement

Biomechanics also contributes to performance enhancement by improving designs for the shoes, apparel, and equipment used in various sports (21). For example, significant changes in shoe design and construction since the 1980s (Figure 9.13A) have most likely contributed to improved performance by athletes in all types of sports. Athletes can now choose from a wide range of shoe options that are specific to the structural features of the foot and body, the playing surface, or the environmental conditions (Figure 9.13B). Alterations in clothing design have resulted in reduced friction through the air and water and improvements in body temperature regulation. For example, competitive swimmers can wear full body suits in an effort to reduce friction on the body when swimming in the water. Equipment worn by athletes may have an effect on performance, either directly or through injury prevention. Improvements in helmet design in football (Figures 9.14A and B), ice hockey, and lacrosse have reduced the force impact felt by athletes competing in contact sports (24). Lighter and better designed equipment have contributed to improved performances by competitive athletes and recreational participants as well. For example, professional and amateur baseball players often carve out the end of their bat in an effort to make the bat lighter and increase the movement velocity of the bat when swung at a pitch (21). Cyclists can benefit from using

Table 9.7	Examples of How Biomechanics May be Used to Improve the Technique and Performance of an Athlete (11,21)			
	PERFORMANCE TECHNIQUE	PERFORMANCE ANALYSIS	CHANGE IN TECHNIQUE	CHANGE IN PERFORMANCE
Coach improving performance	A baseball pitcher experiences a decrease in throwing velocity.	The coach observes the pitcher from different positions around the pitcher's mound.	The coach suggests opening up the front foot when stepping toward home plate during the pitch delivery.	This allows the pitcher's hips to open sooner creating more force with the body and greater throwing velocity.
Biomechanist improving performance	A swimmer has a slow start off the stand resulting in a poor entry into the water.	The biomechanist films a group of swimmers using different starting techniques and analyzes the video to determine which technique results in the fastest entry into the water.	The biomechanist recommends a change in foot placement on the starting block.	This allows the swimmers to generate more force during entry into the water resulting in a faster entry into the water.

ighter weight bicycles during training and competition, effectively reducing he amount of force required by the muscles to move the bicycle over the urface.

Training Improvement

The principles of biomechanics can be used to modify training and improve performance in many ways. A biomechanical analysis of skill performances may identify deficiencies in technique that can be improved by altering training. For example, if an athlete participating in the high jump is having difficulty in determining the correct distance to run during the approach to the bar he/she may spend more time in practice working on the approach to the bar. If an athlete is limited by the strength or endurance of certain muscle groups, a biomechanical analysis may be helpful in determining which muscle groups are limiting performance. The training program of the athlete may then be altered to focus on improving the strength of the muscle group, which in turn may then improve the performance technique (15,21). For example, if a biomechanical analysis reveals that poor jumping technique is the result of a weakness in the strength of the quadriceps muscles, then a training program can be devised to improve the strength of that muscle group.

Plyometric exercise training is an example of how muscle biomechanics can be used to enhance force and power production in the muscles. This type of

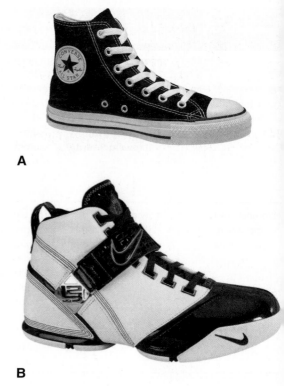

FIGURE 9.13 ▼ **A:** Original basketball sneakers (photo courtesy of Converse). **B:** Biomechanically improved basketball sneakers.

exercise training involves practicing motor movements to strengthen tissues and train nerve cells to stimulate a specific pattern of muscle contraction. The theoretical basis behind plyometric training is in creating a prestretch of the muscle so that it generates as much force as possible during the contraction. A plyometric contraction involves an initial rapid muscle lengthening movement, followed by a short resting phase, and then an explosive muscle contraction movement. The combination of these movements enables the muscles involved in the contraction to generate maximal force. Plyometric exercise training engages the myostatic-reflex, which is the automatic contraction of muscles when their muscle spindle receptors are stimulated. Plyometric exercises use explosive movements to generate a large amount of force quickly thereby improving muscle power. Plyometric exercise training acts on the nerves, muscles, and tendons of the body to increase an athlete's power output without necessarily increasing their maximum strength (3).

Injury Prevention

The use of biomechanical analyses helps athletic trainers and other sports medicine professionals identify factors that have caused an injury, how to prevent the injury from recurring (or occurring in the first place), and what activities and exercises may assist with rehabilitation from the injury. Biomechanics can also provide the basis for alterations in technique, equipment, or training to

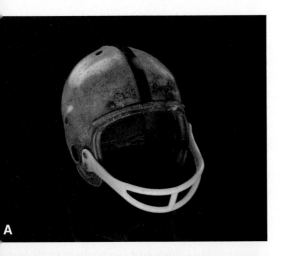

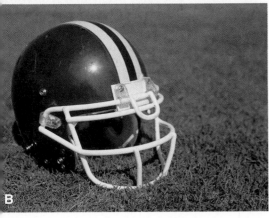

FIGURE 9.14 ▼ **A:** Old time American football helmet (Photo by Photodisc/ Alexander Nicholson/Getty Images.). **B:** Modern American football helmet (Photo by Stockbyte/Getty Images.).

prevent or rehabilitate injuries (15,21). For example, a kinematic analysis of an athlete running on a treadmill may reveal improper foot placement that is contributing to hip pain. Making adjustments in running mechanics may allow for a different foot placement that alleviates the pain in the hip caused by improper running mechanics.

> ➤ *Thinking Critically*
> *What kinematic and kinetic information is helpful for an athlete attempting to improve movement technique following the rehabilitation of a sport-related injury?*

ADVANCED BIOMECHANICAL CONCEPTS

Sport and athletic movement skills are very complex and often involve intricate coordination patterns among the nervous system and the musculoskeletal system. For example, throwing a baseball at maximum velocity to a specific location with great accuracy requires an athlete to generate force by the body and then transfer that force to the ball being thrown. Two advanced biomechanical concepts that can help exercise science professionals in the understanding of the principles involved include projectiles and kinetic link principles.

Projectiles

Many sport and athletic competitions involve the throwing or hitting an object through the air. Objects that fly through the air free of external forces (with the exceptions of gravity and air friction) are considered projectiles. Flying objects are undergoing displacement over time and are considered to be in a free-fall state, such that gravity and air friction are the only forces that affect the flight. The instant any other external force is applied to an object, the object is no longer considered a projectile because its free-fall state has been disrupted. If the external force is removed and the two objects separate, the original object will begin another free fall. The original object will, however, have different kinematic qualities than it had before the external force was applied. Projectiles moving in any direction can be defined using a three-axis Cartesian coordinate system. The prediction and quantification of numerous aspects of a projectile's flight can occur if the assumption is made that no air resistance affects the object while it is traveling through its arc. This does not occur in a real-world situation, but only in a vacuum. If one assumes no air resistance, then the only external force that must be accounted for is gravity. Gravity only affects the vertical motion. Numerous predictions regarding the flight of the object can be made if one assumes a parabolic flight and the symmetry of the resulting arc created during flight. Success in throwing, hitting, or catching projectiles ultimately depends on the projectile's release velocity, angle of projection, and the height of the release. Changes in throwing technique or force production by the muscles will alter the path of the projectile (15). The principles of biomechanics can be used to help an athlete improve the success when tracking a projectile. This is typically done by altering movement patterns and training programs of the athlete.

Kinetic Link Principle

Successful performance in sports and athletic competition depends on a coordination of muscle contraction for skilled movements. Highly skilled athletes often make very complex sports skills look simple and easy. Qualitative terms, such as good timing, smooth movement, effortless motion, and great skill, are used to indicate that the nervous system appropriately controls the musculature causing it to contract with the appropriate intensity or to relax at just the right time to produce the necessary movements for successful performance. Sport activities can be very challenging to perform because many requirements are necessary for success, including force production, velocity production, specific pattern of body motions and/or positions achieved, and conservation of energy while moving at a relatively fast velocity. Highly skilled athletes take advantage of the body's kinetic link system and create well-timed movements through coordinated muscle contractions. Two basic principles guide the body's kinetic link system: sequential movements and simultaneous movements of body segments (15).

The **sequential kinetic link principle** (also called sequential motion) means that segments of the body and joint rotations occur in a specific sequence. This coordinated movement typically leads to a high velocity of momentum enerated during the last segment of the performance. Sports skills that require he sequential kinetic link for success have the energy or momentum flowing rom one body segment to another. The creation of momentum in the big-er slower segments of the body leads to effective transferal of momentum o the smaller, faster moving segments (15). An example would be pitching baseball. To throw with maximum velocity, the pitcher must generate force y the body and then transfer that force to the ball. To successfully do this, a •itcher must generate force using the legs and hips, then transfer that force to he shoulder and elbow. This sequential motion process will lead to the force •eing imparted to the ball upon release from the throwing hand. This highly killed sequential motion must be performed with great accuracy when pitch-ng a baseball.

The **simultaneous kinetic link principle** means that major motor novements of the body occur at the same time (simultaneously) so that no •bservable difference in time exists between the contributions of the differ-nt body segments to the performance. Movements employing the simul-aneous kinetic link principle are engaged when the athlete is required to nove his or her body, an object, or another opponent, all of which offer ✓arying degrees of resistance. An example would be performing a supine •ench press. During the execution of the bench press, various muscle groups •ecome active during the lowering and raising the bar. Simultaneous con-raction of the pectoralis major muscles as well as other supporting muscles ncluding the anterior deltoids, serratus anterior, coracobrachialis, and the riceps occurs so that force can be generated by the muscles to move the veight. Many sports activities require both the sequential and simultane-»us kinetic link principles to occur during per-ormance of the movement. Additionally, some ictivities require both the production of great orce to move a massive object and the produc-ion of high velocity during the movement (15). ⁻or example, during the performance of a power •lean lift, the muscle of the body must generate ignificant force to lift the bar off of the floor and ιt the same time have the bar move at a fact veloc-ty so that the weight can be moved quickly to the finishing position. Only ∨hen the muscles involved in the movements contract simultaneously can he power clean lift be completed successfully.

> ➤ **Thinking Critically**
> *How might coursework in biomechan-ics and the associated disciplines pre-pare an individual for a career as a clinical biomechanist, physical thera-pist, or an athletic coach?*

Sequential kinetic link principle When segments of the body and joint rotations occur in a specific sequence or order.

Simultaneous kinetic link principle When major movements of the body occur at the same time.

INTERVIEW

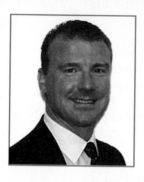

Mark A. Heidebrecht, MSE, CHFP, Managing Partner
of ErgoMethods

Brief Introduction

I graduated from the University of Kansas in 1992 with a bachelor of science degree in exercise science. Originally, I had planned to go into medicine or physical therapy and graduated with the prerequisites. After several internships and independent studies, I became interested in the field of ergonomics and decided to pursue a master's degree in exercise physiology and biomechanics, which I obtained in 1994. I have been working in the field of ergonomics and human factors since 1994 and started two companies ErgoMethods and Ergo-Online in 1998. As an ergonomic consultant I have to opportunity to work with such industries as apparel manufacturing, public accounting, card/paper manufacturing, shipping/cargo, meat and food processing, pharmaceuticals, automobile and truck manufacturing, aerospace, insurance, and private hospitals. In 2001, I was asked to develop and implement the Ergonomic Risk Reduction Process for the Customer Service Division of the United States Postal Service. When fully implemented, it will affect over 750,000 U.S. postal employees on a national level. In September of 2000, I was asked to present to the National Academy of Sciences in Washington DC regarding the effectiveness of ergonomic interventions and the early identification of musculoskeletal disorders.

➤ Why did you choose your professional career?

After completing several internships in the field of physical therapy, I decided rather than fixing the injuries I would rather prevent injuries from happening. Exercise physiology and biomechanics provided me with the knowledge base to get into the field of ergonomics. I utilize my knowledge of biomechanics to identify postures and forces that may be contributing to injuries or leading to an inefficient process. I utilize my knowledge of work physiology to identify contributing factors of fatigue and physical limits of human performance. This is becoming increasingly important as companies try to find ways to reduce the size of the workforce. In many instances, the machine capacity is optimized and the worker is asked to keep up. My background in work physiology allows me to design processes that are efficient but within the capabilities of the individual.

➤ Which individuals or experiences were most influential in your career development?

Dr Carol Zebas and Dr Jeffrey Potteiger were both very influential in providing the foundation for my success. I also took every opportunity to get involved in professional organizations and meet leaders in the field. Early in my career, I worked for a company that put on national conferences. This allowed me to meet and learn from individuals who were well respected in the field of ergonomics and occupational health and rehabilitation. Dr Don Bloswick, Anne Tramposh, and Regina Barker are individuals who I had the privilege to work with and contributed significantly to my success.

➤ What are your most significance professional accomplishments?

I consider being asked to present to the National Academy of Science and being listed as a "Contributor to the Report" published by the National Research Council as my most significant accomplishment to date in my professional career. Developing the ergonomic process for the customer service division of the United States Postal Service was a very challenging but rewarding process. There were many logistic factors, which had to be considered and overcome when developing a process that will be implemented in all 50 states, urban and rural environments and that will ultimately affect over 750,000 individuals.

(Continued)

> ➤ **What advice would you have for an undergraduate student beginning to explore a career in exercise science?**

Take advantage of internships and independent studies when in school. It is a great way to make contacts and learn about nontraditional fields that a background in exercise science can be very beneficial and rewarding. Find professionals who are established in the field and ask if they will mentor you. Look at others in the field as resources rather than competitors. Get a broad foundation and as much practical experience as possible.

I N T E R V I E W

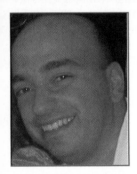

Daniel Pincivero, PhD, Professor, Department of
Kinesiology and Physical Education, Wilfrid Laurier University

Brief Introduction

I completed the Physical Education program at York University in Toronto, Canada with a career choice of Athletic Therapy, a Master of Education in Athletic Training at the University of Virginia, and a PhD in Exercise Physiology at the University of Pittsburgh. I began my professional career as an assistant professor in the Department of Physical Therapy at Eastern Washington University. In 2001, I moved to the Department of Kinesiology at The University of Toledo. While at the University of Toledo, I completed a BS in mechanical engineering.

> ➤ **Why did you choose to become a biomechanist?**

My first exposure to Biomechanics occurred during my undergraduate years at York University where I completed a three-semester sequence of courses. As I was developing an interest in athletic therapy as a career option, I was particularly intrigued by the fact that biomechanics provided me with a mechanical basis for understanding injury risk and occurrence. By developing my knowledge and expertise in the field of biomechanics, I felt I was able to gain a much deeper appreciation for the factors (i.e., forces) that drive human mechanical behavior that may eventually lead to musculoskeletal injury. I believed in the idea that to understand factors underlying human movement and function, one must appreciate anatomic details, physiologic mechanisms, and the biomechanics of the task. Today, my affinity to the field of biomechanics is held by the fact that the laws, principles, and analytic approaches of this discipline govern and describes all facets of biological systems.

> ➤ **Which individuals or experiences were most influential in your career development?**

My personal philosophy and approach as an educator and researcher is shaped by my continual interactions with students and colleagues on a daily basis. However, one of the most profound experiences that have shaped my career, to date, occurred early in my years in the Department of Physical Therapy at Eastern Washington University. As a new and young assistant professor ready to challenge the world, I was "blessed" with a $1,000 start-up budget and a storage room for my first research lab. I did the most basic thing I thought I had to do to get my research career on track: get into the laboratory and start collecting data! I credit the present state of my career to my initial experience of having to solve all problems myself; however, I would be remiss if I did not indicate that colleagues and students from the Department of Physical Education provided me with much needed assistance.

(Continued)

> ➤ **What are your most significant professional accomplishments?**

In regard to my career, I very much enjoy the work that I carry out every day. As a result of the career path that I have chosen and have come to embrace, I find it difficult to think that doing something that comes so naturally to me, as an accomplishment. I always gain a sense of personal excitement when we receive the latest copy of the journal that contains one of our research papers, or to see students that I have mentored explaining the results outlined in their poster at a national conference. However, I am at odds at considering such tasks as accomplishments, because I feel that this is "just what I do." I truly believe that any indication of accomplishment related to my professional activities must originate from others reviewing my work. In instances where I receive compliments from my peers, I do gain a sense of satisfaction for a job well done.

> ➤ **What advice would you have for an undergraduate student beginning to explore a career in athletic training?**

I believe that undergraduate students would be ill-advised to simply select a particular topic in exercise science that they develop interest, and to leave the remaining areas for others to worry about. Students' undergraduate years are, potentially, the most critical years of their lives, and decisions that they make will undoubtedly ripple for many years to come. As exercise science is the fundamental basis for many careers (i.e., physical therapy, occupational therapy, athletic training, coaching, and personal fitness, to name a few), I believe that undergraduate students must not dismiss any option until they have had an opportunity to experience it. In terms of curriculum, exercise science undergraduate students should also embrace coursework outside of the discipline that will only enhance their knowledge and competency. The principles and concepts in basic courses such as physics, chemistry, mathematics, and psychology all serve as the underpinning of the exercise science field, and will strengthen the students' academic abilities. Finally, my best advice to the undergraduate student intending to study exercise science, in addition to broadening their scope, is to feed off of their true interests and develop resolve in their studies. The field of exercise science can serve as a gateway to many interesting and promising careers that students should take full advantage of by immersing themselves in the complete undergraduate experience. In a nutshell, if a student can find herself/himself in a career they love, they will never have to work a day in their life!

SUMMARY

- Biomechanics is the study of the human body at rest and in motion using basic and advanced principles from the academic disciplines of mathematics, mechanics, physics, and engineering.

- The use of kinematics and kinetic techniques and principles provides insight into how the human body moves and responds to forces when healthy, injured, or performing a sport or movement activity.

- Biomechanics has important applications in the clinical environment for promoting recovery from injury and the industrial setting for improving work performance and reducing the risk of job-related injuries.

- Biomechanical principles are also used to enhance sport and athletic performance through improvements in technique, equipment, training methods, and injury prevention.

- Advanced biomechanical concepts are used to understand complex movements and sport skills to promote successful performance.

FOR REVIEW

1. Explain the difference between static and dynamic biomechanics.

2. What significant events happened during the Renaissance period that contributed to the development of biomechanics?

3. What are the two types of linear motion?

4. What is a biomechanical system of interest?

5. How are the three planes of the body (sagittal, frontal, or transverse) used to describe movements of the body?

6. How is a Cartesian coordinate system used in a biomechanical analysis of movement?

7. Describe the steps involved in a qualitative analysis of a soccer kick.

8. Define the three types of mechanical loads: compressive force, tensile force, and shear force.

9. How does mechanical loading cause the deformation of an object such as bone?

10. Why must a clinical biomechanist understand how the body responds to a normal situation or movement?

11. What is the difference between a clinical biomechanist and an ergonomist?

12. Describe how a biomechanist can improve performance by changing technique, equipment, or training techniques.

13. What is the difference between the sequential movements and simultaneous movements of body segments?

REFERENCES

1. Bates BT. The need for an interdisciplinary curriculum. In: *Third National Symposium on Teaching Kinesiology and Biomechanics in Sports Proceedings*; Ames, IA. 1991. p. 163–6.

2. Bridges AJ, Smith E, Reid J. Joint hypermobility in adults referred to rheumatology clinics. *Ann Rheum Dis.* 1992;51:793–6.

3. Brooks GA, Fahey TD, White TP, Baldwin KM. *Exercise Physiology:Human Bioenergetics and its Applications.* Mountain View (CA): Mayfield; 2000.

4. Buckwalter JA, Lappin DR. The disproportionate impact of chronic arthralgia and arthritis among women. *Clin Orthoped Relat Res.* 2000;458:159–68.

5. Chaffin DB, Andersson GB. *Occupational Biomechanics.* New York (NY): Wiley; 1991.

6. Childs JD, Sparto PJ, Fitzgerald GK, Bizzini M, Irrgang JJ. Alterations in lower extremity movement and muscle activation patterns in individuals with knee osteoarthritis. *Clin Biomech.* 2004;19:44–9.

7. Cureton KJ, Collins MA, Hill DW, McElhannon FM. Muscle hypertrophy in men and women. *Med Sci Sports Exerc.* 1988;20:338–44.

8. Fenn WO. Mechanical energy expenditure in sprint running as measured in moving pictures. *Am J Physiol.* 1929;90: 343–4.

9. Fisher NM. Osteoarthritis, rheumatiod arthritis, and fibromyalgia. In: Myers JN, Herbert WG, Humphrey R, editors. *ACSM's Resources for Clinical Exercise Physiology.* Philadelphia (PA): Lippincott, Williams & Wilkins; 2002. p. 111–24.

10. Haas RB. *Muybridge: Man in Motion.* Berkley (CA): University of California Press; 1976.

11. Hall SJ. *Basic Biomechanics.* Dubuque: McGraw-Hill; 2006.

12. Hay JG. *Biomechanics of Sports Techniques.* 1993.

13. Horton MG, Hall TL. Quadriceps femoris muscle angle: Normal values and relationships with

gender and selected skeletal measures. *Phys Ther.* 1989;69:897–901.

14. Hurwitz DE, Sumner DR, Andriacchi TP, Sugar DA. Dynamic knee loads during gait predict proximal tibial bone distribution. *J Biomech.* 1998;31: 423–30.

15. Johnson BF. Sports biomechanics. In: Brown SP, editor. *Introduction to Exercise Science.* Philadelphia (PA): Lippincott, Williams & Wilkins; 2001. p. 264–88.

16. Kaufman KR, Hughes C, Morrey BF, Morrey M, An K. Gait characteristics of patients with knee osteoarthritis. *J Biomech.* 2001;34:907–15.

17. Kerrigan DC, Todd MK, Della Croce U. Gender differences in joint biomechanics during walking. *Am J Phys Med Rehab.* 1998;77:2–7.

18. Leveau BF. Clinical biomechanics. In: Brown SP, editor. *Introduction to Exercise Science.* Philadelphia (PA): Lippincott, Williams & Wilkins; 2001. p. 236–63.

19. March LM, Bagga H. Epidemiology of osteoarthritis in Australia. *Med J Aust.* 2004;180:S6–10.

20. Martin, RB. A genealogy of biomechanics. Presidential Lecture at the 23rd Annual Conference of the American Society of Biomechanics. Pittsburgh (PA): American Society of Biomechanics; 1999.

21. McGinnis PM. *Biomechanics of Sport and Exercise.* Champaign (IL): Human Kinetics; 2005.

22. McKean KA, Landry SC, Hubley-Kozey CL, et al. Gender differences exist in osteoarthritic gait. *Clin Biomech.* 2007;22:400–9.

23. Nigg BM. Introduction. In: Nigg BM, Herzog W, editors. *Biomechanics of the Musculo-skeletal System.* Chichester England: John Wiley & Sons, Ltd.; 2007. p. 1–48.

24. Pellman EJ, Viano DC, Withnall C, et al. Concussion in professional football: Helmet testing to assess impact performance–part 11. *Neurosurgery.* 2006;58:78–96.

25. Pulat BM. *Fundamentals of Industrial Erogonomics.* Prospect Heights (IL): Waveland Press; 1997.

26. Stergiou N, Blanke DJ, Chen SJ, Siu KC. Biomechanics. In: Housh TJ, Housh DJ, Johnson GO, editors. *Introduction to Exercise Science.* San Francisco (CA): Pearson Education, Inc.; 2008. p. 207–31.

27. White KK, Lee SS, Cutuk A, Hargens AR, Pedowitz RA. EMG power spectra of intercollegiate athletes and anterior cruciate ligament injury risk in females. *Med Sci Sports Exerc.* 2003;35:371–6.

28. Wilkerson JD. Biomechanics. In: Massengale JD, Swanson RA, editors. *The History of Exercise and Sport Science.* Champaign (IL): Human Kinetics; 1997. p. 321–66.

10

Equipment and Assessment in Exercise Science

After completing this chapter you will be able to:

1. Describe the different types of equipment used in the assessment of cardiovascular and pulmonary function.

2. Describe the different types of equipment used in musculoskeletal assessments.

3. Explain the different types of equipment and instruments used in weight management and body composition assessments.

4. Describe the different types of equipment used in clinical rehabilitation.

5. Describe the different types of equipment used in motor performance assessment.

6. Explain the different types of instruments used in exercise behavior and sport psychology assessments.

The performance of individuals participating in physical activity, exercise, sport, and athletic competition can be affected by many factors including genetic endowment, health and injury status, physiologic status, psychological status, and biomechanical factors (13). Exercise science and allied healthcare professionals must accurately assess and evaluate those physical, physiologic, and psychological attributes that can provide insight into an individual's health status, the risk for certain diseases and illnesses, and the individual responses to training and rehabilitation programs. Furthermore, the assessment and evaluation of numerous factors related to success is important to athletes working to enhance performance in sport and athletic competition (14).

Evaluation and assessment procedures can be expensive and time consuming, so the most appropriate measurements using the best available equipment and instruments is critical to ensuring valid and reliable measures. Regardless of whether the assessments are made on an individual participating in a regular physical activity or exercise program or on a highly trained athlete the benefits derived from evaluation and assessment include (13,14)

- Identifying the individual's strengths and weaknesses from the measured variables
- Providing important feedback to the individual being tested, the exercise science or allied healthcare professional, or the coach on the assessment and evaluation results
- Identifying current health status, the risk for certain diseases, and the progress made on recovery from an injury or illness
- Providing educational information to the individual being tested on the assessment and evaluation process and the results of the testing

Much of the assessment and evaluation performed by exercise science professionals can be broadly categorized into **fitness and functional capacity testing** and **diagnostic testing**. Fitness and functional capacity testing is used to help assess the fitness and performance capabilities of an individual to do work- or job-related activity, physical activity, exercise, perform a sport, or participate in an athletic competition. Diagnostic testing is performed to help identify the presence of a disease condition, risk factors for a disease condition, or an existing injury within an individual. The type of assessments and evaluations performed will likely differ between a nonathlete and athlete as the purpose and use of the testing information is different for the two types of individuals. Whether performing fitness and functional capacity or diagnostic testing, there are certain guidelines and procedures that should be followed to ensure accurate and reliable results.

PRETESTING GUIDELINES AND PROCEDURES

To ensure that the most accurate and reliable information is obtained during assessments and evaluations, the exercise science and allied healthcare professional must establish and follow specific pretesting guidelines and procedures. Two of the most important issues to consider before testing include making sure that the assessments and evaluations that are selected are **valid** and **reliable** and that the data being collected are specific and relevant to the information that is required of the testing. An assessment or evaluation of a particular aspect of fitness or physical or psychological function is valid when it actually measures what it claims to measure and it is reliable when the results from the assessment or evaluation are consistent and reproducible. To ensure validity and reliability, the instruments used in testing must be calibrated according to the instructions of the manufacturer or according to established procedures. For example, the calibration of many metabolic gas and blood analyzers require the use of known reference standards in the calibration process. These standards are certified by the producers of the product to be of the exact value. When the known reference standards are used in the calibration of an instrument, the validity and reliability of the equipment are significantly enhanced (14).

When making an assessment or evaluation of a particular aspect of fitness or physical or psychological function, it is important to make sure that the measurement protocols, techniques, equipment, and instruments are specific to and designed for the item being measured. For the test results to have optimal significance, the testing must be specific to the desired question of interest. As testing procedures move further away from the actual physical or psychological function desired in the assessment and evaluation, the validity declines despite the fact that the results may be reliable. For example, if an exercise science professional wanted to know which muscles were being used during the performance of a job-related task, it would be best to perform the assessment in the work place environment. However, because specialized equipment is often needed to make this type of assessment, the measurements might have to be performed in a laboratory or clinical environment. This would necessitate constructing a test that would simulate the job-related task as closely as possible. If this is not possible, then the validity of the assessment might be compromised (14).

Upon identification of the specific assessments and evaluations to be made, it is important to closely control the test administration procedures to minimize the influence of extraneous factors of the results obtained (13,14). Important issues to consider and control during the assessment and evaluation process include the following:

- Ensure that standardized and clear instructions are given to subjects, patients, or clients
- Provide sufficient practice or warm-up procedures prior to testing
- Make certain that the order of the assessment and evaluation items does not influence the results
- Give sufficient recovery time between assessment and evaluation items
- Control the environmental conditions where the tests are being conducted

Fitness and functional capacity testing Used to provide an objective measure of an individual's safe functional abilities.

Diagnostic testing Used to determine a specific condition or possible illness.

Valid Providing an accurate measurement.

Reliable Providing a consistent measurement.

An inability to sufficiently account for or control these factors has the potential t significantly affect the results obtained during testing.

Individual Issues to Control

There are also numerous other issues to consider and possibly control for abou the subjects, patients, or clients so that accurate assessment and evaluation result are obtained (13,14). Some of these issues include

- Determine if and for how long an individual has been participating in a physical activity, exercise, or training program
- Consider whether the time of the most recent physical activity, exercise, or training session has any influence on the tests being conducted
- Consider if the time of day in which the assessments and evaluations are made have any relation to any previous assessments that have been conducted
- Evaluate the nutritional status of the individual to determine if this has an impact on the assessments being made
- Ensure that the amount of sleep or rest the individual has received is sufficien for testing
- Identify whether the individual has an injury or illness and decide if this will affect the assessments
- Ensure that the individual is properly hydrated
- Identify any drugs or medications used by the individual and consider whethe these will affect the testing results
- Identify the psychological status of the individual (i.e., anxious or nervous- ness) and consider the impact of the status on the testing results

Laboratory and Field Testing

Certain types of testing assessments and measurements must be made in a labora tory or clinical environment, whereas other tests can be made outside the laboratory and are usually called a field test. Laboratory tests and assessments are conducted in a controlled environment that uses protocols and equipment that simulate the physical activity, exercise, sport, or athletic performance. In general, a field test is a measurement procedure that is conducted while the individual is performing in a simulated physical activity or competitive situation. Results gained from field test are often not as reliable as those gained from laboratory tests, but can be more valid because of their greater specificity to the activity. Performance varies more in the field setting than in the laboratory environment because it is difficult to contro variables such as wind velocity, temperature, humidity, and other environmenta factors. Additionally, many of the "portable" data collection systems necessary fo field testing are generally not as accurate as those used in the laboratory; however recent advancements in technology have improved the validity and reliability o much of the equipment and instrumentation used in field testing (13,14).

The information received from fitness and functional capacity testing and diagnostic testing can be used to enhance health and improve physical perfor- mance. Many of the assessments of health and physical performance measures are performed by most all exercise science and allied healthcare professionals and are not limited to a particular field or discipline. Therefore, the information contained in this chapter will attempt to provide a description of the most commonly used equipment according to the following broad-based categories:

- Cardiovascular and pulmonary function
- Musculoskeletal function
- Energy balance assessment
- Body composition measurement
- Blood collection
- Injury rehabilitation
- Motor performance
- Behavioral and psychological function

CARDIOVASCULAR AND PULMONARY FUNCTION ASSESSMENT

The health and functional ability of the cardiovascular system and the pulmonary system play an important role in an individual's risk for developing cardiovascular and pulmonary diseases. Additionally, cardiovascular and pulmonary fitness can have considerable influence on the potential for successful performance in a variety of sports and athletic competitions that involve cycling, running, and swimming. The assessment of the cardiovascular and pulmonary functions can range from inexpensive field tests to very expensive time-consuming measurements performed in a controlled laboratory environment or clinical facility.

Treadmills and Ergometers

When assessing the health and functional capacity of the cardiovascular and pulmonary systems, the intensity and amount of exercise performed by the individual must be precisely controlled and accurately measured. Furthermore, the administration of safe and effective exercise and training prescriptions requires an accurate control of the exercise intensity. The motor-driven treadmill and cycle ergometer are the most commonly used pieces of equipment in both diagnostic and functional capacity exercise testing. The selection of equipment for testing should be based on the individual's primary mode of physical activity and exercise. The treadmill is the preferred equipment for individuals who participate in walking and running activities. Upright or **recombinant cycle ergometers** can be used for those individuals, such as the overweight/obese or disabled, who require support during exercise testing or whose primary physical activity and exercise activity are cycling (1).

During treadmill exercise, the intensity is controlled by manipulating the speed of the treadmill belt and the grade (i.e., slope) of the treadmill. This allows for a regulated and incremental increase in the workload administered to the individual

Recombinant cycle ergometers A cycle ergometer that allows the rider to be seated with the legs supine and the back supported.

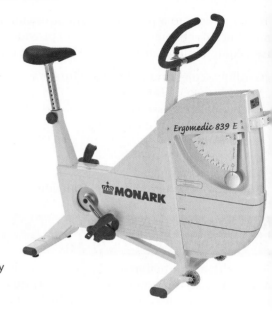

FIGURE 10.1 ▼ Laboratory cycle ergometer. (Photo courtesy of Monark.)

walking or running on the treadmill. The intensity of exercise is controlled on the cycle ergometer by increasing the resistance against which an individual must pedal when cycling. Many laboratory cycle ergometers administer resistance by the use of a friction belt against the rotating flywheel (Figure 10.1). In friction belt cycle ergometers, the individual pedaling rate will affect the workload and thus the intensity of the exercise. For example, if two individuals are pedaling against the same resistance, but one is pedaling at a faster rate, then that individual is doing more work at a higher exercise intensity. This limitation of the friction belt cycle ergometers can be overcome by using an electronically braked cycle ergometer that employs an electromagnet to impart resistance during exercise. An electronically braked cycle ergometer allows the intensity of exercise to be automatically adjusted without being affected by the pedaling rate. When using treadmill and cycle ergometers, it is important to allow the individual being tested to select the most comfortable walking, running, or cycling speed. During diagnostic and functional capacity testing of the cardiovascular and pulmonary systems, the exercise begins at a low intensity and increases until a predetermined workload or intensity is reached or until the subject reaches his/her maximal exercise capacity (1,14).

Other exercise equipment less commonly used in cardiovascular and pulmonary testing and exercise training includes arm cycle ergometers (Figure 10.2A) stairclimbers, elliptic machines, rowing machines (Figure 10.2B), simulated skiing machines (Figure 10.2C), and swimming flumes (Figure 10.2D). For example, arm ergometers can be used to test cardiovascular function in those individuals who cannot use their legs for physical activity or exercise. An arm cycle ergometer is similar to a cycle ergometer except arm pedals replace the foot pedals in this device (Figure 10.2A). Though stairclimbers and elliptic machines can be employed for exercise testing, their use is not widespread because many individuals do not commonly perform the movements required of those devices. Rowing machines, simulated skiing machines, and swimming flumes are frequently used

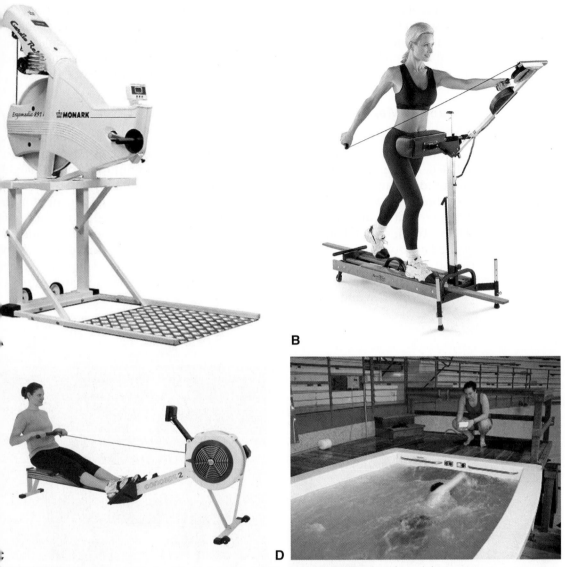

FIGURE 10.2 ▼ **A:** Arm ergometer (photo courtesy of Monark). **B:** Rowing machine (photo courtesy of Concept2, Inc). **C:** Simulated skiing machine (photo courtesy of Nordic Track). **D:** Swimming flume.

to test athletes in sport performance assessment settings. The use of this type of equipment allows an athlete to perform the activity he/she is engaged in during competition, resulting in a more accurate assessment of cardiovascular and pulmonary functions (14).

Though treadmills and ergometers are most commonly used in diagnostic and functional capacity testing of the cardiovascular and pulmonary systems, they can also be used for other purposes as well. For example, a biomechanical analysis of certain movement skills can be best performed in controlled conditions using treadmills, stationary cycle ergometers, simulated skiing machines, and swimming flumes.

Assessments of an individual's readiness to return to work, physical activity, c exercise can be more accurately made following the participation in a rehabilitatio program. Finally, measurements of energy expenditure for weight managemer can be best made during controlled exercise on a motor-driven treadmill or cyc ergometer where the exercise intensity can be accurately controlled.

Metabolic Measurement Equipment

The assessment of cardiovascular and pulmonary functions is commonly per formed while using equipment that measures the volumes of air inhaled an exhaled, the amount of oxygen consumed, and the amount of carbon dioxid produced during rest and exercise. This equipment, commonly referred to as **metabolic measurement cart**, includes highly sensitive instruments for th measurement of air volume and the oxygen and carbon dioxide concentration (Figure 10.3). A metabolic measurement cart collects and measures the volume c expired air from an individual's mouth, and then analyzes the air for oxygen an carbon dioxide concentrations to produce assessments of the amount of oxyge consumed and the type of fuel source (carbohydrates or fats) used to produc energy during rest and exercise.

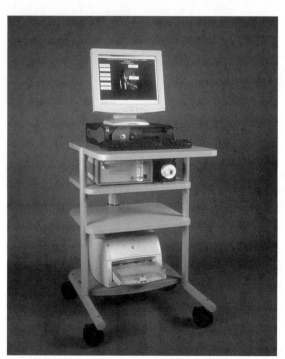

FIGURE 10.3 ▼ Metabolic measurement cart. (Photo courtesy of Parvo Medics.)

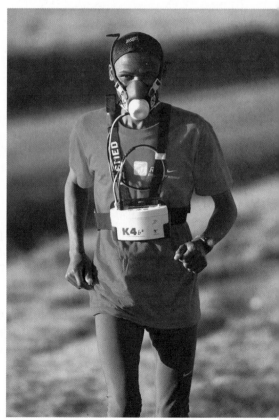

FIGURE 10.4 ▼ A portable metabolic measurement system. (Photo courtesy of Cosmed.)

During diagnostic and functional capacity testing, the levels of oxygen consumption attained at different workloads or at maximal effort exercise can be used to evaluate health and performance and develop individualized exercise prescriptions. The level of oxygen consumption at maximal effort exercise (VO_{2max}) is often called cardiorespiratory fitness and is a strong predictor of the risk for certain diseases (28) and performance during aerobic endurance sports and competitions (6). Most metabolic carts are large instruments designated for laboratory or clinical facility use. A portable metabolic cart has been developed that allows for the assessment of oxygen consumption and carbon dioxide production during activities outside a controlled laboratory testing facility (Figure 10.4). The freedom of movement allows for measurements during work, physical activity, or exercise.

The information collected by a metabolic measurement cart can also be used to determine the amount of energy expended during physical activity and exercise and the relative amounts of energy derived from carbohydrate and fat fuel sources. This information is often used during the development of individualized exercise prescriptions especially in weight management programs.

Pulmonary Function Equipment

Pulmonary function assessments include a broad range of tests that measure how well an individual inhales and exhales air from the lungs and how efficiently the lungs transfer oxygen into the blood and remove carbon dioxide from the blood. The measurement of the inhalation and exhalation rates and volumes, and the amount of oxygen that diffuses into the blood can assist in the diagnosis of restrictive and obstructive lung disease. **Restrictive lung disease** results when an individual cannot inhale a normal volume of air and may be caused by inflammation or scarring of the lung tissue or by abnormalities of the muscles or skeleton of the chest wall (2,12). Restrictive lung disease can be diagnosed by several lung volume measurements performed in one of two ways. The most accurate way is for an individual to sit inside a **whole body plethysmograph** (Figure 10.5). This instrument is a sealed, transparent box that resembles a telephone booth. When inside the whole body plethysmograph, the individual breathes normally into and out of a mouthpiece. Changes in pressure inside the plethysmograph allow for the determination of different lung volumes such as **residual lung volume** and **total lung capacity**. Lung volume can also be measured by having an individual breath nitrogen or helium gas through a tube for a specified period of time. The concentration of the gas in a sealed chamber attached to the tube is measured, allowing an estimation of the individual's lung volume (12).

Metabolic measurement cart An instrument that measures the volumes of oxygen consumed and carbon dioxide produced.
Restrictive lung disease Disease characterized by a reduced lung volume.
Whole body plethysmograph An instrument that allows for the measurement of lung volumes.
Residual lung volume The volume of air left in the lungs after a maximal exhalation.
Total lung capacity The volume of air in the lungs after a maximal inhalation.

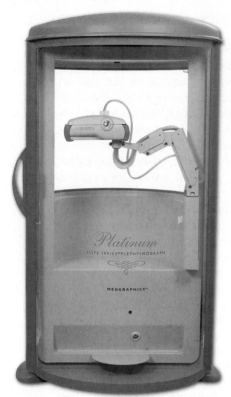

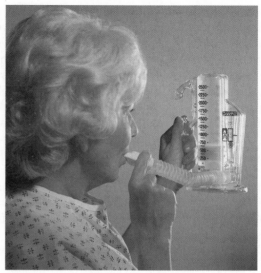

FIGURE 10.6 ▼ An incentive spirometer. (From Willis MC. *Medical Terminology: A Programmed Learning Approach to the Language of Health Care*. Baltimore (MD): Lippincott, Williams & Wilkins; 2002.)

FIGURE 10.5 ▼ A whole body plethysmograph. (Photo courtesy of Medical Graphics Corporation.)

The measurement of how well the lungs exhale air can be made through spirometer (Figure 10.6). The spirometer is a device that records the amount an the rate of air that is inhaled and exhaled over a specified time through the use c a pneumotach or turbine. The assessments are usually performed during norma quiet breathing, and during forced inhalation or exhalation after a deep breath The information gathered during this test is useful in diagnosing certain type of lung disorders, especially when making evaluations for **obstructive lun diseases** (e.g., asthma and chronic obstructive pulmonary disease) (12).

Testing the diffusion capacity of a gas permits an estimate of how efficientl the lungs transfer oxygen from the air into the bloodstream. The diffusion capac ity is measured when a person breathes carbon monoxide for a very short time often one breath. The concentration of carbon monoxide in exhaled air is the measured, often by a metabolic measurement cart. The difference in the amoun of carbon monoxide inhaled and the amount exhaled allows an estimation of hov quickly gas can travel from the lungs into the blood (12).

Obstructive lung disease A condition that results in the narrowing of the passageways of the lungs making the exhalation of air difficult.

Electrocardiograph Equipment

One of the primary instruments used during functional capacity and diagnostic testing of the cardiovascular and pulmonary systems is the electrocardiograph (ECG) machine (Figure 10.7). This instrument detects and records the electric impulses generated by the heart during and between contractions (Figure 10.8). When individuals are suspected of having heart disease or a cardiovascular

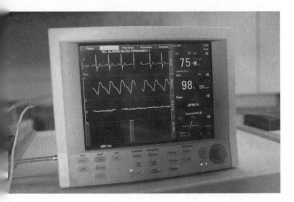

FIGURE 10.7 ▼ An ECG machine monitor.

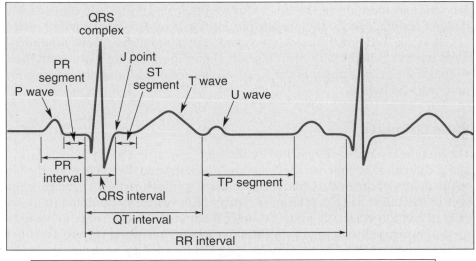

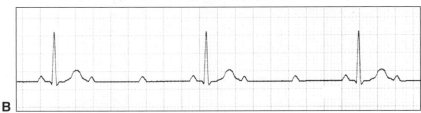

FIGURE 10.8 ▼ A normal ECG waveform **(A)**. Waveforms are shown on printouts from an ECG machine **(B)**. (**A**, from Ehrman JK, et al. (eds.). *ACSM's Resource Manual for Guidelines for Exercise Testing and Prescription.* 6th ed. Baltimore (MD): Lippincott, Williams & Wilkins; 2009. **B**, from Dunbar CC & Saul B. *ECG Interpretation for the Clinical Exercise Physiologist.* Baltimore (MD): Lippincott, Williams & Wilkins; 2009.)

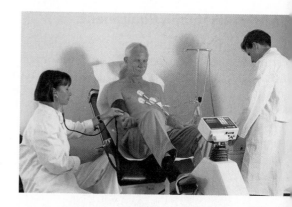

FIGURE 10.9 ▼ A graded exercise test using an ECG and metabolic measurement cart.

abnormality, an ECG test may also be included as part of a comprehensive physical examination (Figure 10.9). During functional capacity and diagnostic testing, the ECG is used to record the electric activity of the heart at rest and in response to graded or incremental exercise. An ECG uses 10 electrodes (also called leads) that are attached to an individual's chest. The electric activity of the heart is recorded from 12 different views, which the ECG displays as 12 separate readings. In addition to the standard recording of electric activity during rest and exercise, an ECG can assist in monitoring the heart during other diagnostic procedures such as thalium testing, and for therapeutic purposes in a cardiac rehabilitation program (1). Portable ECG instruments are called Halter monitors. These monitors are often used in patients with heart disease. Halter monitors are worn continuously so that the electric activity of the heart can be recorded for prolonged periods of time (e.g., 24 hours).

Pulse Oximeter

The pulmonary and cardiovascular systems are responsible for exchanging oxygen and carbon dioxide between the lungs and the blood and then delivering the blood to the tissues of the body. Often it is important to measure the oxygen concentration in the blood to help determine if any cardiovascular or pulmonary diseases exist in an individual. The pulse oximeter is a noninvasive instrument commonly used to measure the oxygen concentration in systemic blood (Figure 10.10). The pulse oximeter works using light-emitting diodes that can measure the amount of oxyhemoglobin and deoxyhemoglobin in blood passing through a translucent part of the body (e.g., fingertip or earlobe). The ratio of oxyhemoglobin to deoxyhemoglobin gives an indication of the individual's oxygen concentration in the blood.

Cardiac output The volume of blood pumped from the heart in a specified time, usually 1 minute.
Total vascular peripheral resistance The resistance to blood flow provided by the blood vessels of the body.

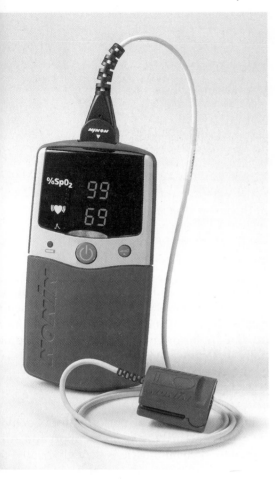

FIGURE 10.10 ▼ Pulse oximeter.
(Photo courtesy of Nonin Medical, Inc.)

Blood Pressure Assessment

The measurement of systolic and diastolic blood pressures is a commonly performed procedure that allows for the diagnosis of hypertension (e.g., high blood pressure) and provides an important assessment of the workload of the heart at rest and during physical activity or exercise. Blood pressure is the product of **cardiac output** and **total vascular peripheral resistance**, making the use of blood pressure measurements an indirect assessment of the health of the cardiovascular system. Hypertension is a common disease condition that can lead to other health problems if not diagnosed and properly treated. The assessment of blood pressure during a graded exercise test or during the performance of physical activity or exercise provides information about the health of the heart and cardiovascular system. Blood pressure can be measured using a sphygmomanometer, also known as a blood pressure cuff (Figure 10.11). The manual method of blood pressure assessment

> ➤ *Thinking Critically*
> *What types of measurements or assessments would you use to evaluate an individual's risk level for cardiovascular disease?*

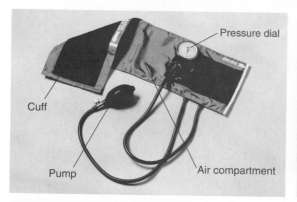
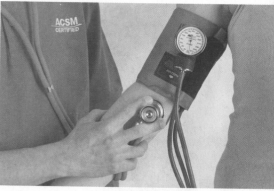

FIGURE 10.11 ▼ Blood pressure cuff and stethoscope. (From Thompson W, et al. (eds.). *ACSM's Resources for the Personal Trainer*. 3rd ed. Baltimore (MD): Lippincott, Williams & Wilkins; 2009.)

requires a trained individual to use a stethoscope and listen for sounds of blood flow after the blood pressure cuff has been inflated and the pressure is being released. Automated blood pressure cuffs (Figure 10.12) eliminate the need for a manual assessment of blood pressure and are becoming a more popular method of blood pressure assessment, especially in a clinical environment.

MUSCULOSKELETAL FUNCTION ASSESSMENT

The musculoskeletal system plays an important role in the performance of activities of daily living and in a wide range of physical activity, exercise, sport and athletic competition. The generation of force by skeletal muscle is strongly related to the successful performance of physically demanding movement and activities and most sports and athletic competitions (8). Additionally, the specific assessment of skeletal health and function can provide important information on the risk for developing bone disease such as osteoporosis.

Electromyography Equipment

Electromyography (EMG) is an assessment technique that allows for the measurement and recording of the electric activity of skeletal muscles at rest and during contraction. An electromyograph (Figure 10.13) is used to record the electric activity within the muscles when the muscles are stimulated by an internal signal from a nerve or by an external signal from an electric stimulation instrument. Muscles respond to both internal and external stimuli with the generation of electric signals in the individual muscle fibers, and the recording of this electric activity can occur through the use of an electromyograph. There are two forms of EMG: intramuscular and surface. Intramuscular EMG requires the insertion of a needle electrode containing a fine wire into an area, usually the belly of the muscle. The electric activity of the muscle at rest and during contraction is recorded and trained personnel can make evaluations about the condition and contractile properties of the muscle. Surface EMG can also be used to assess the condition of the muscle or

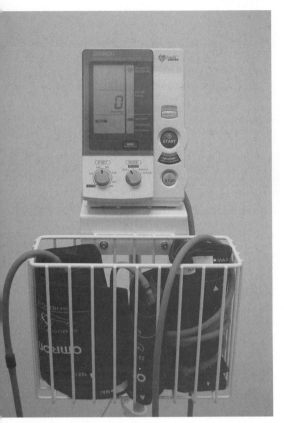

FIGURE 10.12 ▼ Automated blood pressure cuff.

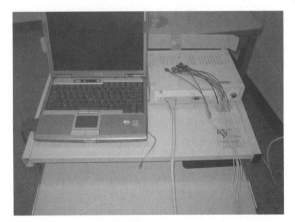

FIGURE 10.13 ▼ An EMG.

muscle groups. Surface EMG is typically used when an individual is performing a movement, when information about a large muscle or muscle groups action is needed, or when the insertion of a needle electrode is considered too invasive or unwarranted for the movement being studied (7).

Force Platforms

Force platforms are used to provide a measure of force production by a muscle or muscle group. A force platform provides voltage signals proportional to the forces exerted on the platform's surface in the vertical, horizontal, and lateral directions (Figure 10.14). The signals are recorded on a computer and analyses of pressure and muscle force and power output can be made. Force platforms are often used to analyze **ground reaction forces** during standing, walking, running, and jumping (8). This information can be used to make adjustments to motor movements

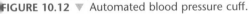

Ground reaction forces The force produced by a body part when in contact with the ground.

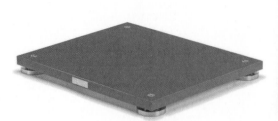

FIGURE 10.14 ▼ A Force platform. (Photo courtesy of Kistler Instrument Corporation.)

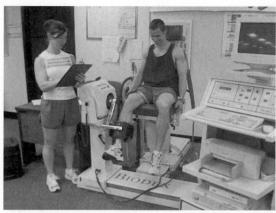

FIGURE 10.15 ▼ An isokinetic dynamometer.

or skill that will promote more efficient or more powerful movements. The results obtained from a force platform can also be used to assist in the correction of movements by injured or disabled individuals and for the creation of devices or instruments that may improve movement.

Pressure Sensitive Insoles

The measurement of pressure distribution in the foot and the vertical force generated during movement can be obtained using pressure sensitive insoles inserted into the footwear of the individual being assessed. Using principles similar in nature to the force platform, the pressure sensitive insoles allow for a more sophisticated and continuous measurement of pressure and force during ambulation, whether the movement is walking, running, or jumping. These measurements are important in the evaluation of abnormalities of walking and running for diagnostic and rehabilitation purposes and in the evaluation of sport and athletic performance.

Isokinetic Dynamometers

Isokinetic dynamometers are used to measure force during isometric and isokinetic movements of muscles and various body parts. When skeletal muscles contract force is generated, usually to an object external to the body. Isokinetic dynamometers measure muscular force (also called torque) at a constant velocity (Figure 10.15). Isokinetic dynamometers have computerized monitors that continuously alter the resistance of the dynamometer so that the movement velocity is held constant. Movement velocities can range from 0 to 450 degrees·s^{-1}. Typically, a joint is selected for assessment or evaluation and the maximum force or torque output is calculated for the movement by the muscles of the joint. Isokinetic dynamometers are used to measure static and dynamic muscle movements, perform muscle balance assessments, assist with pathology diagnosis, and in occupational and physical rehabilitation programs. Isokinetic dynamometers allow for assessments of force production from almost all of the muscles and joints

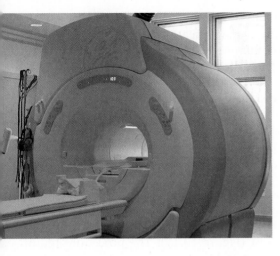

FIGURE 10.16 ▼ MRI instrument. (Photo courtesy of GE Healthcare.)

of the body as special attachments can be used to test numerous functional activities and movements (8).

Magnetic Resonance Imaging

Magnetic resonance imaging (MRI) is a radiology technique that uses application of a strong magnetic field, radio waves, and a computer to produce images of body structures. The MRI equipment includes a scanner tube surrounded by a giant circular magnet (Figure 10.16). During testing, the individual is placed on a moveable bed that is inserted into the magnet. The magnet creates a strong magnetic field that aligns the protons of hydrogen atoms within the tissues of the body. The atoms are then exposed to a beam of radio waves from a radiofrequency coil. This spins the various protons of the body, which produce a weak signal that is detected by the receiver component of the MRI scanner. The receiver information is processed by a computer, and a detailed digital image is created. The image and resolution produced by the MRI can allow for the detection of tiny changes of structures within the body. To increase the accuracy of the images, contrast agents can be used. An MRI scan can be used as an extremely accurate method of detecting abnormalities of the tissues of the body including glands, organs, joints, soft tissues, and bones (4).

Magnetic Resonance Spectroscopy

Magnetic resonance spectroscopy (MRS) can be used to measure the levels of different **metabolites** in body tissues. The principle of the MRS is similar to that of the MRI, only in the MRS technique the noninvasive measurement of tissue substrates and metabolites can occur. The principle of MRS is based on the spin of an atom. Any nucleus with an odd atomic number or an odd atomic weight will

Metabolite A substance produced during a chemical reaction.

produce a net spin like a spinning ball of energy. When a charged atom moves it creates a magnetic field. When the magnet creates a strong magnetic field and the atoms are exposed to a beam of radio waves they will create a magnetic field. Some biologically important nuclei that have spin include ^1H, ^{13}C, ^{17}O, ^{23}Na, and ^{31}P. Most MRS assessments of metabolites in body tissues use ^1H, ^{13}C, and ^{31}P. MRS can be used to assess disease status in various tissues including metabolic disorders, tumor growth, changes in tissue metabolism following exercise, and noninvasive identification of muscle fiber type (4).

Muscle Biopsy Equipment

Muscle biopsies can be used to assess the level of substrates and metabolites in skeletal muscle and determine the types of fibers in specific muscles. The muscle biopsy procedure requires the collection of a tissue sample, usually from the belly of the skeletal muscle of interest (Figure 10.17). The procedure requires a small incision on the surface of the skin and the insertion of a specialized needle through the muscle fascia into the largest area of the muscle. Upon removal of the needle (Figure 10.18), the tissue sample is immediately frozen (usually in isopentane cooled by liquid nitrogen). This snap freezing stops all metabolic processes from continuing to occur in the muscle sample. Various biochemical and analytic techniques can then be used to determine the concentrations of substrates such as glucose, glycogen, and fatty acids in the muscle sample and the concentrations of various enzymes that control the metabolic processes in the muscle cells. Muscle fiber type can also be determined using a muscle biopsy sample (15). Serial slices of tissue are made and then various analytic techniques are used to determine the fiber type within the tissue sample. The techniques used in fiber typing

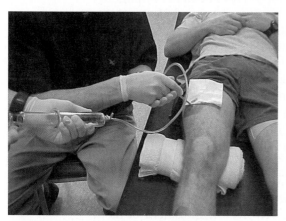

FIGURE 10.17 ▼ Muscle biopsy collection.

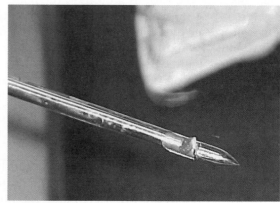

FIGURE 10.18 ▼ Muscle tissue sample.

Osteopenia A decrease in the density of bone.
Osteoporosis A disease that results in low bone mineral density and an increased risk of bone fractures.

include histochemical technique, gel electrophoresis, and immunohistochemical technique. Muscle biopsies are often collected in response to acute exercise and to examine the changes that occur following chronic training. Muscle biopsy samples may also be used to help predict the risk for certain metabolic and neuromuscular diseases.

Computed Tomography

Computed tomography (CT) is a diagnostic tool that provides scans or views of internal body structures using X-rays. The principle behind the CT scan involves the use of digital geometry to allow a computer to generate a three-dimensional image of an object from a series of two-dimensional images taken around a single axis of rotation. During a CT scan, the individual lies supine on a moveable bed that is inserted into the center of the scanner (Figure 10.19). The X-ray beam then rotates around the individual to collect the images. Precise locations of the body can be viewed as cross-sectional scans allowing for various densities of tissues to be easily distinguished. CT scans allow for the viewing of abnormal structures and organs, assessment of tumor growth in various areas of the body, strokes or lesions in the brain, and differentiation of tissue structure in the body. CT scans are commonly performed in a hospital or outpatient imaging center (21).

Dual Energy X-ray Absorptiometry

Dual energy X-ray absorptiometry (DXA or DEXA) is used to measure bone density, which is altered in diseases such as **osteopenia** and **osteoporosis**. Special equipment called a bone densitometer is used to measure the bone mineral content (Figure 10.20). Two X-ray beams with differing energy levels are used to scan the entire body or a specific body region. Different tissues of the body absorb and reflect the X-rays to varying degrees and using this principle

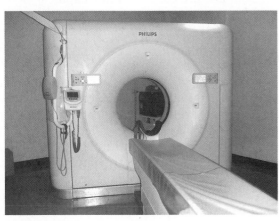

FIGURE 10.19 ▼ CT scanner.

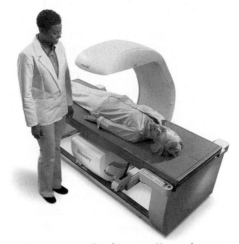

FIGURE 10.20 ▼ Dual energy X-ray absorptiometer. (Photo courtesy of Hologic Inc.)

➤ *Thinking Critically*
What assessments would you make and why would you make them, for an athlete attempting to improve performance in the sports of marathon running and Olympic weightlifting?

allows for the measurement of lean mass, fat mass and skeletal mass. When lean mass and fat mass are removed from the scan, the bone mineral density can be determined from the absorption of each beam by the bone. DXA is the most widely used technology to study bone mineral density and make a diagnosis of osteopenia and osteoporosis (21).

ENERGY BALANCE ASSESSMENT

The regulation of energy intake and energy expenditure is important for maintaining a healthy body weight and promoting weight loss or weight gain. Excess body weight and high levels of body fat increase the risk for developing cardiovascular disease, hypertension, diabetes mellitus, hyperlipidemia, and certain forms of cancer. Assessing energy balance and body composition can provide insight into the effectiveness of weight loss or weight gain intervention programs and the risk level for certain diseases.

Measuring Energy Intake

The assessment of energy intake can be valuable for determining the nutritional needs of individuals involved in weight management programs or for those individuals required to consume specialty diets (e.g., low sodium or low fat) for the purpose of disease risk reduction (e.g., hypertension) or personal choice (e.g., **vegetarian**). Individuals attempting to lose weight require the knowledge of dietary intake for the purpose of creating a negative energy balance for weight loss. For some individuals, weight gain or often more specifically the gain of lean muscle tissue is critical for enhancing performance in certain sports and athletic competitions. In this instance, the knowledge of total calorie intake and protein consumption is beneficial for creating a positive energy balance and creating an **anabolic state** of the body. The two most common methods for measuring nutritional intake are the dietary recall and dietary record (25). Descriptions of these two methods for measuring energy intake are contained in Chapter 6 "Exercise and Sport Nutrition."

Measuring Energy Expenditure

The assessment of energy expenditure during resting and nonresting conditions can be easily performed using a stationary or portable metabolic cart as described earlier in this chapter. The measurement of the carbon dioxide production and oxygen consumption provides a measure called the respiratory exchange ratio (RER). The RER is determined by the formula CO_2 production/ O_2 consumption. It is a valid measure of fat and carbohydrate oxidation rates during steady state metabolism. During rest or submaximal exercise, the RER is normally between 0.70 (100% of the energy expenditure from fat) and 1.0 (100% of the energy expenditure from carbohydrate). When the RER is used in conjunction with the volume of oxygen consumed, a measure of total energy

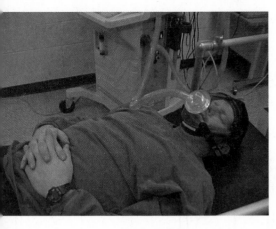

FIGURE 10.21 ▼ Resting energy expenditure.

expenditure can be determined. This is because fat and carbohydrate molecules require different amounts of oxygen to be completely metabolized to provide energy. Figure 10.21 shows the measurement of resting energy expenditure and **ubstrate** utilization. In addition to using metabolic measurement equipment, other methods and instruments can be used to measure the energy expenditure of the body during different metabolic conditions. The most technically advanced methods include the use of whole room calorimeters and doubly labeled water. Other methods include using pedometers, accelerometers, and physical activity questionnaires.

Whole Room Indirect Calorimeter

A whole room indirect calorimeter requires individuals to live in a small room (approximately 10' × 10') for a specific time period, usually 24–48 hours (Figure 10.22). Airflow into and out of the room is controlled allowing for the determination of oxygen consumption and carbon dioxide production by special gas analyzers. Food is delivered through a sealed passageway. Human waste is collected and analyzed for metabolic by-products. If needed, blood samples can be collected through a special portal. Over the designated time period, accurate assessments can be made for total energy expenditure, the relative energy production from carbohydrate, fat, and protein, and changes in various body metabolites. Whole room indirect calorimeters can also be used to determine the effects of different exercise regimens, nutritional programs, and pharmacologic interventions on whole body metabolism (16). Though the assessment of metabolism can be

---

Vegetarian The consumption of vegetables, fruits, grains, and nuts only in the diet.

Anabolic state The process where the body is building larger molecules or compounds from smaller molecules or compounds.

Substrate Substances in the body, which are acted upon by enzymes in a chemical reaction.

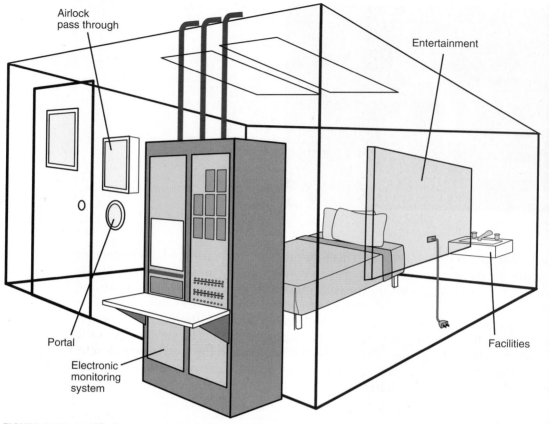

Airlock
pass through

Entertainment

Portal

Facilities

Electronic
monitoring
system

FIGURE 10.22 ▼ Whole room calorimeter.

accurately measured in a whole room indirect calorimeter, a limitation of this
technique is that it does not reflect a free-living environment.

Doubly Labeled Water

The use of the doubly labeled water technique allows for the assessment of energy
expenditure in a free-living situation unlike the whole room calorimeter, and
without the need to be connected to a portable metabolic measurement cart. The
doubly labeled water technique requires an individual to drink an **isotope**-based
solution of **enriched water**. The fundamental theory of the doubly labeled water
technique is that oxygen and hydrogen turnover in the body over time can provide a measure of oxygen consumption and carbon dioxide production. By collecting samples of body fluids (for example, saliva or urine) and then analyzing

Isotope One of the two or more atoms having the same atomic number but different mass numbers.
Enriched water Isotopic water that has the same atomic number as water but a different mass.
Accelerometers A device that measures and records the movement of the human body.

the fluids for the concentrations of oxygen and hydrogen, a measure of energy expenditure can be made. The more active an individual, the faster the turnover of enriched oxygen and hydrogen and the greater the measured energy expenditure. Measurement periods are usually 7 to 14 days in length (16). Although this technique provides an accurate measure of free-living energy expenditure, it is rather expensive to use and the analysis of the body fluids is very technical.

Other Assessment Instruments

Heart rate monitors, pedometers, accelerometers, and physical activity questionnaires are commonly used instruments for the determination of the volume of physical activity performed, which can then be converted to energy expenditure. Heart rate monitors are straps worn around the chest with a watchlike receiver worn around the wrist that can measure and record an individual's heart rate over a designated period of time (Figure 10.23). In advanced monitors, the heart rate information can then be downloaded to a computer and measures of energy expenditure can be made based on the measured relationship between heart rate and oxygen consumption during rest and exercise (14,16).

Pedometers measure the numbers of steps taken during a specific time period, usually a 24-hour period (Figure 10.24). These small instruments are worn on the waist and allow for free movement during physical activity or exercise. Pedometers, however, only measure movement when the foot strikes the ground at a sufficient force to create a recording of the movement. Pedometers do not make recordings of movement during other forms of activity such as cycling, swimming, or resistance exercise.

The use of accelerometers can increase the accuracy of physical activity and exercise measurement. **Accelerometers** can measure body movement in three planes allowing for the detection of movement during activities such as cycling, resistance exercise, machine stairclimbing, yoga, and pilates (Figure 10.25).

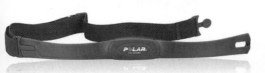

FIGURE 10.23 ▼ Heart rate monitor. (Photo courtesy of Polar Electro Inc.)

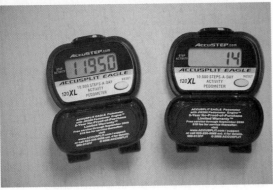

FIGURE 10.24 ▼ Pedometers.

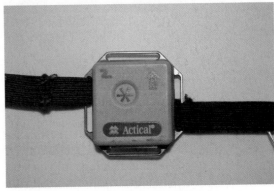

FIGURE 10.25 ▼ Accelerometer.

Accelerometers provide counts of movement that can be converted to energy expenditure (14,16).

Physical activity questionnaires are typically used when attempting to obtain information from large numbers of individuals. These instruments require individuals to answer questions about daily activities over a period of time, typically 7 days in duration. The physical activity questionnaires can provide information about total activity levels, but it is often very difficult to convert the information obtained to energy expenditure because of differences in body size among individuals and lack of precise information about the intensity of the activity (16).

MEASURING BODY COMPOSITION

An accurate assessment of body composition is necessary to correctly estimate an individual's risk for certain health conditions such as cardiovascular disease, hypertension, diabetes mellitus, hyperlipidemia, and certain forms of cancer. Additionally, the relative and sometimes total amounts of body fat mass and lean body mass can influence performance in certain types of sports and athletic competitions. Furthermore, the periodic measurement of body composition can be useful in determining the effectiveness of nutritional and exercise training interventions for both athletic and nonathletic individuals. There are several valid and reliable methods for assessing body composition to determine the amounts of fat mass, fat-free mass, and bone mass within an individual (26).

Densitometry

The assessment of body composition can be determined by **densitometry,** which is a process that provides a measure of body density. To calculate body density, a measurement of body mass and body volume is required. Body mass is easily determined from a calibrated scale. Body volume can be determined from hydrostatic weighing (Figure 10.26) or air displacement plethysmography (Figure 10.27).

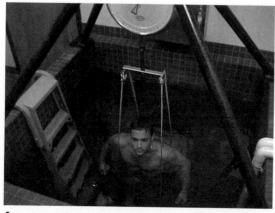
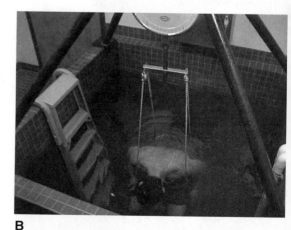

A   **B**

FIGURE 10.26 ▼ Hydrostatic weighing procedure. **A:** Initial body position. **B:** Body position when underwater weight is determined.

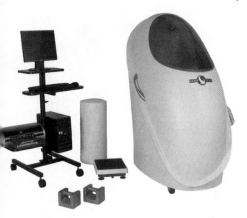

FIGURE 10.27 ▼ Air displacement plethysmography unit. (Bod Pod photo courtesy of Life Measurement, Inc.)

Hydrostatic weighing requires an individual to be weighed underwater when expiring all of the air from the lungs and achieving residual lung volume. The underwater weight is then used with the land weight (i.e., body mass) to calculate body density. **Air displacement plethysmography** requires an individual to sit inside a whole body plethysmograph while body volume is measured. The body volume is then used with the body mass value to calculate body density. In both hydrostatic weighing and air displacement plethysmography, the body density is then converted to a percentage body fat using mathematical regression equations (21).

Dual Energy X-ray Absorptiometry

In addition to measuring bone mineral density, DXA can also be used to measure body composition. As mentioned previously, the different tissues of the body absorb and reflect the X-rays from the DXA machine to varying degrees. When a complete body scan is performed, it is possible to determine the total amounts of lean mass and fat mass. The DXA can also partition the regional areas of lean mass and fat mass. These values, when combined with total body weight, can be used to determine the percentage of body fat within an individual (21).

Bioelectric Impedance

Bioelectric impedance analyzers can be used to measure body composition by sending a safe low voltage level electric current through the body (Figure 10.28). Electric currents travel faster in body tissues that have a higher water and electrolyte content than in those tissues with a lower water and electrolyte content. Lean body tissue, which has a high water content (approx. 50%–70%

Densitometry Process that determines the density of a body mass.

Air displacement plethysmography A process for measuring body composition that utilizes the inverse relationship between pressure and volume to measure body volume directly.

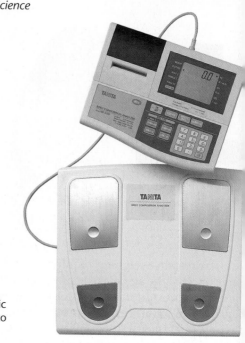

FIGURE 10.28 ▼ Bioelectric impedance analyzer. (Photo courtesy of Tanita Corp.)

water) allows the electric current to travel faster than in fat tissue, which has a low water content (approx. 15%–20%). The speed at which the current passes through the body can be used to determine the percentages of lean tissue and fat tissue in the body. By using an individual's height and weight, it is possible to calculate the percentage of body composition that is fat mass and fat-free mass (21).

Skinfold Assessments

The measurement of the skinfold thickness at various sites around the body can allow for the calculation of body density and the determination of body composition. The use of skinfold thickness measurements for determining body composition is based on the principle that a certain percentage of total body fat lies directly beneath the surface of the skin. Skinfold calipers are calibrated instruments that allow for the accurate determination of the thickness of fat immediately below the skin's surface (Figure 10.29). When predetermined sites are measured using standard measurement techniques, the resulting information can be used in a **regression equation** to calculate body density, which is then used to provide an estimate of body composition (21).

Regression equation A mathematical equation that measures the relationship between two different variables.

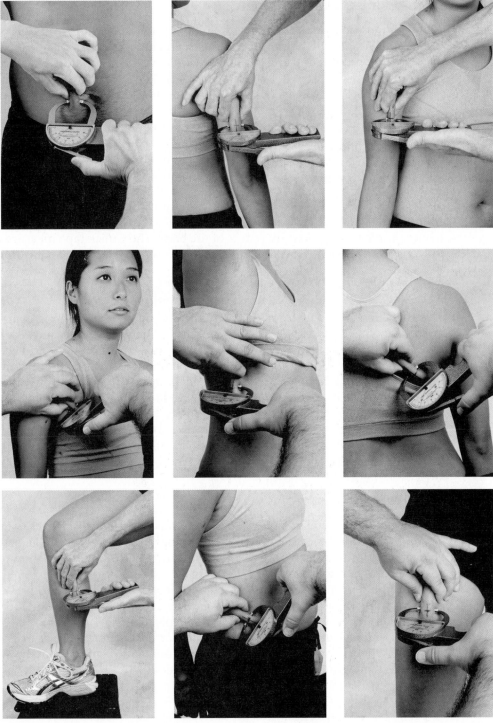

FIGURE 10.29 ▼ Assessment of body composition using skinfold calipers. (From Thompson W, et al. (eds.). *ACSM's Resources for the Personal Trainer*. 3rd ed. Baltimore (MD): Lippincott, Williams & Wilkins, 2009.)

Anthropometric Measurements

Body composition can be estimated simply by measuring the size and propor tion of the human body and its various segments. Measures of height using stadiometer and weight using a calibrated scale can be used to calculate the bod mass index (BMI). The BMI (Wt (kg)/Ht^2 (m)) can be used to provide an estimate of body fatness (5,17 and help determine the risk of certain disease condi tions and health outcomes (10). Circumference mea surements of various body segments can also be use to assess the risk for disease conditions and mortalit (20). In particular, a circumference measure of the waist at the level of the navel can be used to asses the level of risk for cardiovascular and other disease conditions (24). A spring loaded Gulick tape measure is the most commonly use device for measuring circumferences of the body. The Gulick tape measure allow for consistent tension to be applied to the tape when making the measurements

> **Thinking Critically**
>
> *What battery of assessments would you prescribe and why would you prescribe them for an individual attempting to achieve significant weight loss and maintain a healthy body weight?*

BLOOD COLLECTION AND ANALYSIS

The collection of blood from the body for the analysis of various compound and metabolites can provide insight into an individual's health and risk of dis ease conditions. The changes observed in these substances can also provide infor mation regarding the effectiveness of intervention or treatment programs an medications. For example, the blood lipid profile is frequently measured an typically consists of determining the total cholesterol, triglyceride, high-density lipoprotein (HDL), and low-density lipoprotein (LDL) concentrations. The bloo lipid profile is a strong predictor of cardiovascular disease risk (9). Various instru ments are needed for the safe and effective collection, storage, and analysis o blood and tissue samples.

General Equipment

The collection of blood samples is performed using needles, syringes, vacutain ers, and collection tubes (Figure 10.30). An analysis of blood in the laboratory i generally performed in two ways. Blood may first be collected and then permit ted to clot. When a clot forms, a liquid, called serum, escapes from the clotted cells and the serum is used in many tests. Anticoagulants are used to prevent the coagulation of the blood specimen. The anticoagulant used should not alter bloo components. The most commonly used anticoagulant in **hematology** is ethyl enediaminetetraacetic acid (EDTA). The proper anticoagulant must be used fo specific test procedures. Blood collected with one anticoagulant may be suitable for one test or a group of tests, but not for others.

Hematology The study of the nature, function, and diseases of the blood and of blood-forming organs.

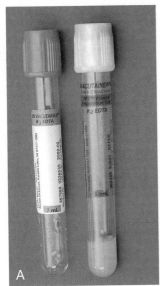
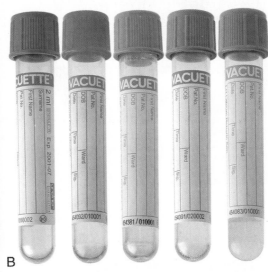
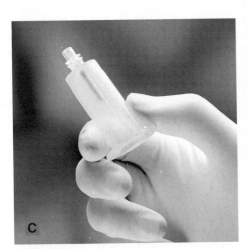
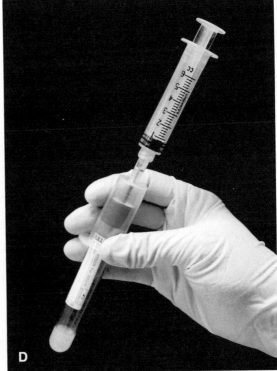

FIGURE 10.30 ▼ Blood collection equipment: evacuated tubes (Vacutainer Plus Plastic brand evacuated tubes **[A]** and Vacuette evacuated tubes **[B]**); syringe safety devices (a BD transfer device **[C]** and a Greiner transfer device attached to a syringe **[D]**); and examples of safety winged infusion sets (SAFETY-LOK **[E]**, Monoject Angel Wing **[F]**, and the Vacuette **[G]** safety butterfly blood collection systems). (From McCall RE, Tankersley CM. *Phlebotomy Essentials*. 4th ed. Baltimore (MD): Lippincott, Williams & Wilkins; 2008.)

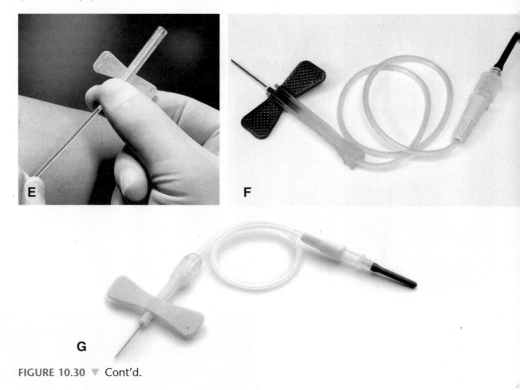

FIGURE 10.30 ▼ Cont'd.

Once the blood sample has been collected from the individual, the collection tube is placed into a centrifuge for the separation of serum, plasma, and blood cells. The serum or plasma sample can then be analyzed using special equipment or the sample can be stored in a deep freezer, usually at −80°C until analysis. The nature of the specific compound will determine the type of chemical analysis required. This, in turn, will dictate the specific equipment that will be used. Many times an automated analyzer will be used to determine the concentration of the compound in the collection sample. In other instances, specialized equipment will be used in the analysis. Examples of common equipment used by exercise science and allied healthcare professions include the **spectrophotometer**, the **fluorometer, high-pressure liquid chromatograph**, and a **gas chromatograph/mass spectrometer**.

Common Blood Measures

Some of the more common measures of blood and tissue samples in exercise science and related areas include hematocrit, glucose, lactic acid, and blood lipids. The hematocrit is an indirect measure of the red blood cell number. Red blood cells are responsible for carrying almost all of the oxygen in the blood to the tissues of the body. A reduction in the red blood cell number (anemia) may compromise oxygen delivery to the body. Increases in the red blood cell number often reflect in increased oxygen delivery to the tissues of the body. Glucose is the primary energy source for nervous tissues in the body and an important energy ource for skeletal muscles during exercise. An inability of the body to regulate blood glucose concentration may lead to insulin resistance and diabetes mellitus. Lactic acid is a metabolic by-product of carbohydrate metabolism in the body. Increased levels of lactic acid can contribute to muscular fatigue and a reduction in force production during muscular contraction. The primary blood lipids that increase the risk for cardiovascular disease include cholesterol, triglycerides, and LDL cholesterol. Conversely, HDLs reduce the risk of cardiovascular disease. Periodic monitoring of these blood lipids is important for reducing the risk of cardiovascular disease.

REHABILITATION ASSESSMENT AND EQUIPMENT

Various types of instrumentation and equipment are used to assist in the rehabilitation of an injured body part owing to participation in physical activity, exercise, sport, or athletic competition. This equipment is generally designed to enhance the recovery process and improve muscle and joint functions. Activities such as stretching and resistance exercise are commonly used to assist exercise science and allied healthcare professionals and sports medicine personnel during the rehabilitative process. Commonly used equipment in rehabilitation includes resistance bands, stability devices, resistance exercise equipment, devices for thermotherapy, and transcutaneous electric stimulation units.

Resistance Devices and Exercise Equipment

Various devices are used to overload the nervous system, skeletal muscle, and joints during rehabilitation assessment and exercise activities. Assessments of force production during rehabilitation and exercise training are important for initial assessments of muscle and joint performance and for determining the effectiveness of the intervention. A description of that equipment occurs earlier in this chapter. Elastic bands, medicine balls, stability devices, parachutes, weighted vests, and other types of equipment are used to increase the resistance against the muscles and joints involved during muscle contractions. By providing an overload on the muscle, improvements in force-generating capacity can be obtained. More traditional resistance exercise equipment includes free weights (dumbbells and barbells with weights) and resistance exercise machines. Resistance devices and exercise equipment are also used to promote muscular strength and endurance for improving health and fitness and for enhancing performance in sport and athletic competition (11,18).

Spectrophotometer An instrument used to determine the intensity of a variety of wavelengths in a spectrum of light.

Fluorometer An instrument used to measure the fluorescence being emitted from a substance.

High pressure liquid chromatograph An instrument used to separate, identify, and quantify compounds.

Gas chromatograph/mass spectrometer An instrument used to detect the presence of a substance in a test sample.

Thermotherapy

Thermotherapy is the use of cold or heat to assist in the rehabilitation and recovery from injury or surgery. **Cryotherapy** includes the use of ice massage, cold or ice water immersion, ice packs, and vapocoolant sprays. The purpose of cryotherapy is to reduce the temperature of the injured tissue. The reduction of temperature causes a decrease in tissue metabolism, inflammation, pain, muscle spasm, and blood flow. Heat therapy includes the use of a hot cloth, hot water, ultrasound, and heating pads. The purpose of heat therapy is to aid in recovery from injury by increasing blood flow to the injured area and decreasing muscle and joint stiffness and soreness (22).

Whirlpool Tubs

Whirlpool tubs are instruments used to circulate hot or cold water around an injured body part. The tubs are large enough to fit an entire person into the tub; however, there are smaller units that can be used for the limbs of the body. A small electronic motor is used to circulate water in the tub creating an enhanced thermal gradient between the water and the body part submerged in the water (Figure 10.31). The circulation of water assists with the rehabilitation and healing processes.

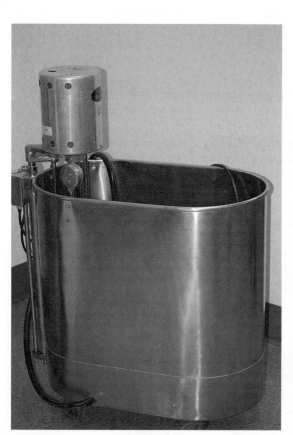

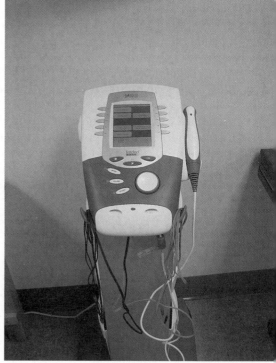

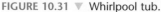

FIGURE 10.31 ▼ Whirlpool tub.   **FIGURE 10.32** ▼ A therapeutic ultrasound unit.

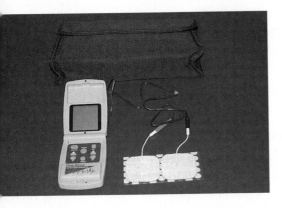

FIGURE 10.33 ▼ A TENS unit.

Therapeutic Ultrasound

Therapeutic ultrasound is a rehabilitation technique that uses high frequency sound waves to enhance the healing process of an injured joint or muscle. During therapeutic ultrasound, the body tissue at the site of application is heated creating an increase in blood flow, which assists with the healing process. At the same time, the therapeutic ultrasound unit creates cellular vibration of the tissues that may assist in the repair of damaged tissue (22). Figure 10.32 shows a therapeutic ultrasound unit.

Transcutaneous Electric Nerve Stimulation

A **transcutaneous electric nerve stimulator** (TENS) is a device that produces electric signals that stimulate nerves through the skin. A TENS unit consists of two or more electrodes that are placed over an area of the body that is designated to receive the stimulation. The frequency and intensity of the stimulation can be adjusted to assist with the alleviation of pain or to assist with muscular reeducation following an injury or surgery (22). Figure 10.33 shows a TENS unit.

> ➤ ***Thinking Critically***
> *What assessments and tests would you recommend and why would you recommend them for a recreational runner participating in a rehabilitation program for an injury to the lower leg?*

MOTOR PERFORMANCE

The assessment and evaluation of motor performance employs instruments and equipment that can be used to track movements and responses to stimuli. The knowledge gained is important for making corrections to motor movements to

Thermotherapy The use of heat or cold in rehabilitation therapy.

Cryotherapy The use of cold in rehabilitation therapy.

Therapeutic ultrasound An instrument that causes vibrations and a deep heating of the tissue it is used on.

Transcutaneous electric nerve stimulator An instrument that causes relief of pain or an enhanced healing of injured tissue.

enhance performance in daily activities, as well as improving performance i
sport and athletic competition. Movements of body parts can be directly mea
sured using a goniometer and potentiometer or through imaging techniques suc
as computerized cinematography. Other methods used to assess motor perfoi
mance include EMG, eye-tracking instruments, and equipment for measurin
brain activity.

Goniometers and Potentiometers

Goniometers are hinged devices that can be attached to a body part to recor
movement. Goniometers move with the body joint and provide informatio
about changes in the angle of movement (Figure 10.34). Many goniometer
are connected to a potentiometer that sends a voltage signal to a computer tha
accumulates and analyzes the information. **Potentiometers** can also be use
in conjunction with many other devices, including specialized equipment that i
physically moved by an individual and recorded by a computer (23).

Motion Capture Systems

The recording of physical movements is commonly used to assess motor per
formance. The digital recordings of body and limb movements can be analyze
using sophisticated computer software. During the assessment of a movemen
the individual being recorded usually wears reflective tape or fluorescent mark
ers that can easily be tracked during the analysis of the movement. Advance
computer software programs are now able to track body movements and make
very detailed analysis of motor performance (23). Figure 10.35 shows the use c
a high-speed motion capture system for recording body movement.

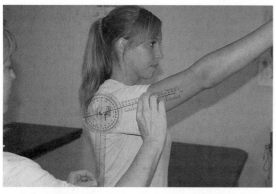

FIGURE 10.34 ▼ Goniometer for measurement of joint movement.

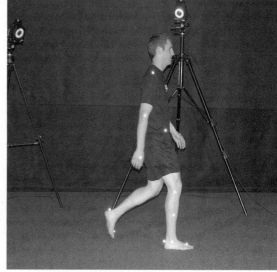

FIGURE 10.35 ▼ Motion capture system for recording body movements.

Electromyography

In addition to using EMG to evaluate musculoskeletal function, EMG recordings can be used to provide knowledge about the control of motor performance by the central nervous system. When combined with other **kinematic** information, the EMG activity obtained from skeletal muscle can provide additional insight into the execution of a motor skill (23).

Eye-tracking Instruments

The use of eye movement recording systems allows for the determination of what visual factors influence attention during motor tasks. Vision tracking is used to determine where the head and various other body parts are directed. Tracking eye movements requires the use of two video imaging techniques. One camera is mounted directly on the head or on a helmet that the individual is wearing. Information from this camera provides an image of the individual's line of vision. A second camera measures the movements of the eyes by means of corneal reflection. The combination of the two recording devices provides a measure of where the individual's eyes are directed during the performance of a motor task or movement (23).

Information Processing Measurement

The ability to identify a stimulus, select a response, and then program and initiate the response is very important for performing activities of daily living and responding to situations encountered during participation in exercise, sport, and athletic competition. An individual's response to a stimulus is referred to as reaction time. To accurately measure, reaction time devices that present a stimulus and then measure the time it takes an individual to respond to the stimulus are used (Figure 10.36). These reaction time devices have the ability to measure a

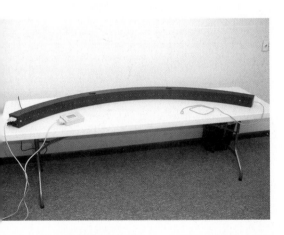

FIGURE 10.36 ▼ Reaction time measuring instrument. (Photo courtesy of Lafayette Instrument Co.)

Potentiometers An instrument that measures an unknown voltage to a standard known voltage.

Kinematic The study of motion of a body without consideration given to its mass or the forces acting upon the body.

response to a stimulus in hundredths and thousandths of a second. Changes i
reaction time are often measured in response to training programs or environ
mental distractions.

Measuring Brain Activity

The equipment and assessment techniques used to measure brain activity allow
for fast and flexible assessments of brain activity during motor performance
Electroencephalography (EEG) is the measurement of electric activity produce
by the brain and recorded by a computer through the use of electrodes placed o
the head. The primary advantage of using EEG is the almost instantaneous feedbac
that is provided during motor performance. Figure 10.37 shows the use of an EEG
Magnetoencephalography (MEG) is an imaging technique used to measure th
magnetic fields produced by the electric activity in the brain using extremely sensi
tive recording devices. These measurements are used to determine the function o
various parts of the brain. **Positron emission tomography** is a nuclear medicin
medical imaging technique, which can be used to produce a three-dimensiona

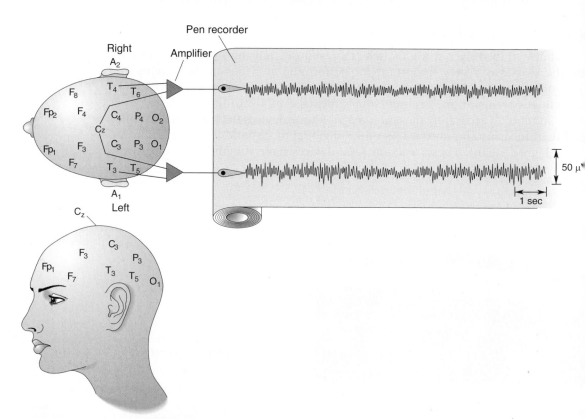

FIGURE 10.37 ▼ The standard placement positions of electroencephalograph electrodes. A, auri-
cle (or ear); C, central; Cz, vertex; F, frontal; Fp, frontal pole; O, occipital; P, parietal; T, temporal.
Wires from pairs of electrodes are fed to amplifiers, and these drive pen recorders. (From Bear MF,
Connors BW, Parasido, MA. *Neuroscience: Exploring the Brain.* 2nd ed. Philadelphia (PA):
Lippincott, Williams & Wilkins; 2001.)

age of brain structure and activity. A recently developed form of neuroimaging called **functional magnetic resonance imaging** allows for the measurement of blood flow related to neural activity in the brain or spinal cord (23). Each of the brain activity measurement techniques has advantages and disadvantages that must be considered when determining what equipment to use during testing (23).

BEHAVIORAL AND PSYCHOLOGICAL ASSESSMENTS

Assessments of behavioral and psychological issues associated with physical activity, exercise, sport, and athletic completion include the use of both quantitative and qualitative instruments. With appropriate training, an individual may use various quantitative instruments to assess variables of interest in exercise and sport psychology. These instruments are validated psychological tests or questionnaires. The use of a qualitative approach requires a more individualized approach to the assessment of variables of interest.

Quantitative Assessments

Assessing psychological phenomena in exercise and sport psychology requires a variety of analytic methods often not used in other areas of exercise science. The most common method has been to use a **constructionist approach** in which considerable consideration is given to the individual's subjective experience. The self-report, using standardized questionnaires or psychological inventories, is the predominant analytic strategy used in the constructionist approach. Some examples of commonly used questionnaires and inventories include (19)

Speilbergers State-Trait Anxiety Inventory
Profile of Mood States
Beck Depression Inventory
Sport Competition Anxiety Test
Competitive State Anxiety Inventory 2
Test of Attentional and Interpersonal Style

The use of these questionnaires and others can provide valuable information on an individual's psychological state in situations such as acute and chronic physical activity and exercise or in response to practice or game situations in sport or athletic competition (27).

Electroencephalography The measurement and recording of the electric activity of the brain.

Positron emission tomography A computer-generated image of metabolic or physiologic activity in the body generated through the detection of gamma rays.

Functional magnetic resonance imaging An imaging technique used to examine relationships between physical changes in the brain and mental functioning.

Constructionist approach A sociologic theory that considers how social phenomenon develops in a specific social context.

Table 10.1	The Most Commonly Used Types of Qualitative Research Techniques (3)
QUALITATIVE RESEARCH TECHNIQUE	**DESCRIPTION**
Grounded theory	Attempts to derive a theory from the views of the participants.
Life histories	Derives information about the lives of one or more individuals providing stories about their lives.
Case study	Provide an intensive, holistic, and in-depth understanding of a single event, activity, program, process, or individual.
Phenomenological	Identification of the core meaning of an experience.
Ethnographic	Provides a description and interpretation of a cultural or social group.
Basic and generic	Identifies recurrent patterns in the form of themes and categories and provides a descriptive understanding and exploratory interpretation.

Qualitative Assessments

The use of qualitative assessments for understanding the psychosocial phenomena in exercise and sport psychology helps understand the personal significance that individuals have constructed within their natural environment. Qualitative assessments have been used to develop deep understanding of the individual and personal factors that give meaning to why an individual believes and acts in a specific manner. There are numerous qualitative approaches used to help understand the meaning of what happens to an individual or group participating in an exercise or sport setting. Table 10.1 provides description of the most commonly used types of qualitative research techniques (3). A mixed methods approach, whereby both quantitative and qualitative assessment are used, can draw on the strengths of both types of assessment methods.

> ➤ *Thinking Critically*
> *How might a comprehensive testing program improve the health and physical performance of an athlete and nonathlete?*

SUMMARY

- Professionals from all areas of exercise science use the equipment and assessment methods for evaluating physical and psychological performances and functions.
- The assessment of physiologic, psychological, and biomechanical measures can provide useful information about an individual's risk for disease and illness.
- Periodical assessment of variables can provide insight into the acute responses to physical activity and exercise as well as practice and game situations in sport.
- The regular assessment of certain variables can provide information on the effectiveness of an individual exercise or team training program.

FOR REVIEW

1. Why should the type of ergometer (i.e., treadmill or cycle) used during testing be matched to the exercise mode of the individual being tested?

2. A metabolic measurement cart is used to make assessments of what physiologic measure?

3. The measurement of lung function provides an assessment of what two broad categories of pulmonary disease?

4. An ECG machine measures what aspect of cardiovascular function?

5. An EMG machine measures what aspect of muscular function?

6. An isokinetic dynamometer controls the speed of muscle contraction and makes a measurement of what muscle function?

7. Describe the basic scientific principle associated with the use of MRI and MRS.

8. Dual energy X-ray absorptiometry can be used to provide a quantitative assessment of what three body components?

9. What are the three most commonly used instruments for the determination of free-living physical activity and energy expenditure?

10. What is the conceptual basis for using bioelectric impedance analyzers to measure body composition?

11. The principle that a certain percentage of total body fat lies directly beneath the surface of the skin allows for the use of which technique for the assessment of body composition?

12. What are the two types of thermotherapy and how does each type work to enhance rehabilitation from injury.

13. High-speed motion capture systems are often used to assess what aspect of motor performance?

14. Electroencephalography (EEG) provides the assessment of what physiologic measure?

15. What is the difference between quantitative and qualitative instruments in the measurement of behavioral and psychological assessments of exercise and sport psychology?

REFERENCES

1. American College of Sports Medicine. *ACSM's Guidelines for Exercise Testing and Prescription*. Philadelphia (PA): Lippincott, Williams & Wilkins; 2006.
2. American College of Sports Medicine. *ACSM's Resource Manual for Guidelines for Exercise Testing and Prescription*. Philadelphia (PA): Lippincott, Williams & Wilkins; 2006.
3. Baumgartner TA, Hensley LD. *Conducting and Reading Research in Health and Human Performance*. New York (NY): McGraw-Hill Publishers; 2006.
4. Brooks GA, Fahey TD, White TP, Baldwin KM. *Exercise Physiology: Human Bioenergetics and its Applications*. Mountain View (CA): Mayfield; 2000.

5. Dietz WH, Bellizzi MC. Introduction: The use of body mass index to asses obesity in childlren. *Am J Clin Nutr*. 1999;70:123S–5S.

6. Hagberg JM, Moore GE, Ferrell RE. Specific genetic markers of endurance performance and VO_{2max}. *Exerc Sport Sci Rev*. 2001;29:15–9.

7. Hall SB. *Basic Biomechanics*. Dubuque (IA): McGraw-Hill;2006.

8. Harman EA. The measurement of human mechanical power. In: Maud PJ, Foster C, editors. *Physiological Assessment of Human Fitness*. Champaign (IL): Human Kinetics; 2006. p. 87–113.

9. Jeppesen J, Hein HO, Suadicani P, Gyntelberg F. Low triglycerides-high high-density lipoprotein cholesterol and risk of ischemic heart disease. *Arch Intern Med*. 2001;161:361–6.

10. Kirk S, Zeller M, Claytor R, Santangelo M, Khoury PR, Daniels SR. The relationship of health outcomes to improvement in BMI in children and adolescents. *Obes Res*. 2005;13:876–82.

11. Kohrt WM, Bloomfield SA, Little KD, Nelson ME, Yingling VR, American College of Sports Medicine. Physical activity and bone health. *Med Sci Sports Exerc*. 2004;36:1985–96.

12. Levitzky MG. *Pulmonary Physiology*. New York (NY): McGraw-Hill; 2007.

13. MacDougall JD, Wenger HA. The purpose of physiological testing. In: MacDougall JD, Wenger HA, Green HJ, editors. *Physiological Testing of the High-performance Athlete*. Champaign (IL): Human Kinetics; 1991. p. 1–6.

14. Maud PJ, Foster C. *Physiological Assessment of Human Fitness*. Champaign (IL): Human Kinetics; 2006.

15. McGuigan MRM, Sharman MJ. Skeletal muscle structure and function. In: Maud PJ, Foster C, editors. *Physiological Assessment of Human Fitness*. Champaign (IL): Human Kinetics; 2006.

16. Melby CL, Ho RC, Hill JO. Assessment of human energy expenditure. In: Bouchard C, editor. *Physical Activity and Obesity*. Champaign (IL): Human Kinetics; 2000. p. 103–31.

17. Morabia A, Ross A, Curtin F, Pichard C, Slosman DO. Relation of BMI to a dual-energy X-ray absorptiometry measure of fatness. *Br J Nutr*.1999;82:49–55.

18. Pearson D, Faigenbaum AD, Conley MS, Kraeme WJ. The National Strength and Conditioning Asso ciation's basic guidelines for the resistance training athletes. *Strength Cond J*. 2000;22:14–27.

19. Petruzzello SJ. Exercise and sports psycholog In: Brown SP, editor. *Introduction to Exercise Scienc* Philadelphia (PA): Lippincott, Williams & Wilkin 2001. p. 310–33.

20. Pischon T, Boeing H, Hoffmann K, et al. General ar abdominal adiposity and risk of death in Europ *N Engl J Med*. 2008;359:2105–20.

21. Pollock ML, Kanaley JA, Garzarella L, Graves J Anthropometry and body composition measuremen In: Maud PJ, Foster C, editors. *Physiological Assessmen of Human Fitness*. Champaign (IL): Human Kinetic 2006.

22. Prentice WE. *Arnheim's Principles of Athletic Training: Competency-based Approach*. New York (NY): McGraw Hill Companies; 2006.

23. Schmidt RA, Lee T. *Motor Control and Learning: A Beha ioral Emphasis*. Champaign (IL): Human Kinetic 2005.

24. Seidell JC, Perusse L, Despres JP, Bouchard C. Wai and hip circumferences have independent and opposi effects on cardiovascular disease risk factors: The Que bec Family Study. *Am J Clin Nutr*. 2001;74:315–21.

25. Thompson FE, Subar AF. Dietary assessment meth odology. In: Coulston AM, Rock CL, Monsen E editors. *Nutrition in the Prevention and Treatmen of Disease*. San Diego (CA): Academic Press; 200 p. 3–30.

26. Wagner DR, Heyward VH. Techniques of body con position assessment: A review of laboratory and fiel methods. *Res Q Exerc Sport*. 1999;70:135–49.

27. Weinberg RS, Gould D. *Foundations of Sport and Exe cise Psychology*. Champaign (IL): Human Kinetic 2007.

28. Wing RR, Jakicic JM, Neiberg R, et al. Fitnes fatness, and cardiovascular risk factors in Typ 2 diabetes: Look AHEAD study. *Med Sci Sports Exer* 2007;39:2107–16.

CHAPTER

11

Careers and Professional Issues in Exercise Science

After completing this chapter you will be able to:

. Describe the differences among the credentialing titles of certification, licensure, and registration.

. Identify various professional job opportunities available in exercise science and related areas.

. Identify the role and mission that professional organizations play in promoting the advancement of exercise science and related areas.

. Explain the role that governmental and international agencies and organizations play in advancing the professional growth of exercise science.

Graduates of programs in exercise science can gain professional employment and career development in a wide variety of job settings. Examples might include work as a personal trainer (Figure 11.1), health and wellness coordinator, or clinical exercise physiologist (Figure 11.2). In other instances, individuals will take advantage of opportunities in related professional fields where the knowledge base developed through a program of study in exercise science can be a valuable asset. This might include for example, a career in an allied healthcare field as a physical therapist, occupational therapist, or a physician assistant. In all of these professions, the knowledge, skills, and abilities developed as a student in an undergraduate program of study in exercise science will provide a solid foundation for a successful professional career.

Educational qualifications for professional employment can range from a bachelor's degree (e.g., BS) to an advanced professional degree (e.g., MD, DC, DD, DO, DPT) or educational degree (e.g., MS, EdD, PhD). It is also becoming increasingly common for employers to require potential employees to demonstrate achievement of certain skills and competencies prior to hiring. These may include successfully attaining **certification, licensure,** and **registration.**

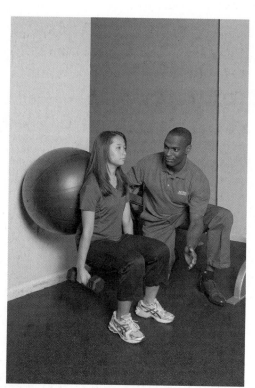

FIGURE 11.1 ▼ A personal trainer working with a client. (From Thompson W, ed. *ACSM's Resource for the Personal Trainer.* 3rd ed. Baltimore (MD): Lippincott, Williams & Wilkins; 2009.)

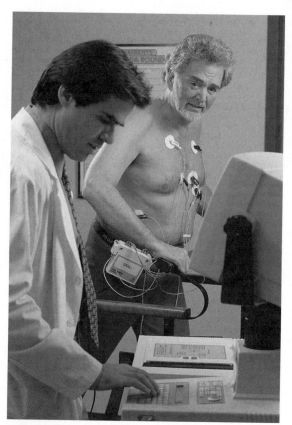

FIGURE 11.2 ▼ A clinical exercise physiologist working with a client. (Photo courtesy of Comstock Images/Getty Images.)

raduates of exercise science programs must pay close attention to the rofessional requirements for working with individuals in physical activity, xercise, sport, and athletic competition settings. Several professional organiza-ons have developed certification and registration programs to help individuals emonstrate knowledge and proficiency in content, skills, and abilities of the pecific areas for which they are intending to work. National organizations have lso worked with the state and federal governmental agencies to develop licen-ure programs for individuals in those professions that require a greater level f professional skills and competency when approving an individual for pro-essional practice. Professional organizations also provide membership benefits nd services to assist in the professional development for a career in an exer-ise science or allied health profession. Furthermore, numerous governmental nd private organizations promote and support initiatives and programs that are elated to the various areas of study in exercise science (23). This chapter pro-ides an overview of certification, licensure, and registration, and the role that rofessional and governmental organizations play in the credentialing processes. otential employment opportunities for graduates of exercise science programs re presented. Finally, information is provided about the various professional rganizations and governmental agencies that support exercise science and its elated areas of study.

CERTIFICATION, LICENSURE, AND REGISTRATION

Credentialing is defined as providing certified documents showing that an ndividual is entitled to recognition or has a right to perform certain functions or ctions. Credentialing is designed to ensure that, within a profession or service, tandards of a safe and ethical practice are being maintained (23). By achiev-ng a credential, an individual has demonstrated that he/she has achieved a et standard of knowledge, skills, and abilities as defined by the **credentialing organization** in a particular area of specialty. For many exercise science pro-essionals, the most common form of credentialing is certification. Professional ertification recognizes those individuals who possess the knowledge and com-etency to perform a variety of responsibilities in health, fitness, rehabilitative,

Certification A process whereby individuals demonstrate knowledge and proficiency in content, skills, and abilities of the specific areas for which they are intending to work.

Licensure Granting of permission by an official or legal authority (usually a government agency) to an individual or organization to engage in a practice or activity that would otherwise be illegal.

Registration Documentation of professional qualification information relevant to government licensing regulations.

Credentialing Providing certified documents showing that an individual is entitled to credit or has a right to perform certain functions or actions.

Credentialing organization A professional organization or governmental agency that oversees and administers examinations for certification, licensure, or registration of an individual or program.

and sports medicine programs (23). Obtaining certification from a credentialing organization

- Provides recognition of competency to work with healthy, injured, diseased or disabled populations
- Demonstrates commitment to the profession and the standards that have been established
- Assists with job employment and advancement in professional development

Licensure and registration are credentials that require a higher level of professional competency and are often required to gain employment and practice as an allied healthcare professional (23).

Definitions of Certification, Licensure, and Registration

Within exercise science, graduates of degree and professional preparation programs can attain credentials from several professional organizations. There are distinctions among certification, licensure, and registration that allow individuals who possess a credential to perform specific duties within a defined area of professional practice. Higher education programs that receive certification or accreditation have demonstrated the ability to deliver to students a program or curriculum that meets standards acceptable to the credentialing organization. In some instances (e.g., athletic training, dietetics), students must graduate from an accredited program of study to qualify to take a national certification (athletic training) or licensure (dietetics) examination (23).

Certification

The certification process requires individuals, educational programs, or institutions to be evaluated and recognized as meeting predetermined standards through successful completion of a valid and reliable examination (e.g., for individuals) and review (e.g., educational programs and institutions) (23). Professional organizations usually administer certification, licensure, and registration examinations and reviews to individuals and programs that meet a defined level of curricular expectations. Individuals and programs voluntarily participate in the credentialing process; however, as professional expectations among employers and government agencies increase, certification or licensure is often desired (e.g., registered clinical exercise physiologist, RCEP) and/or required (athletic trainer certified, ATC and registered dietician, RD) in many exercise science areas.

The process for individuals seeking certification or licensure typically includes the following steps (23):

- Achievement of a core of knowledge, skills, and abilities through formal educational and/or professional experience
- Submission of an application form and candidacy credentials
- Review of prerequisite knowledge and skills through the use of study guides, resource manuals, review courses, and/or workshops
- Taking and passing the certification or licensure examination

Certification examinations generally include both written and **interactive components**. The written component is primarily comprised of objective questions of content knowledge, skills, and abilities. The interactive component typically requires candidates to view a video excerpt and then provide an answer to questions about a specific task or activity in the video clip. An individual who achieves a passing score on both the written and interactive components is recognized by the credentialing organization as a certified member.

Certified individuals are usually required to obtain **continuing education units** (CEUs) to retain certification in the credentialing organization. This can usually be accomplished by attending professional meetings and conferences, taking additional study courses, participating in online professional development programs, and/or becoming involved in the certification organization. Certification costs vary widely depending on the level of certification obtained and the fee structure of the organization administering the examinations (23,24).

Certification can also be extended to include educational programs and facilities. In this type of certification, individual programs or facilities are required to meet specific criteria related to curriculum, staff, facilities, and environment. For instance, **program accreditation** is currently required for academic programs in athletic training and dietetics. Students in these areas of study must graduate with a degree from an accredited program before being allowed to take the examinations for certification (e.g., athletic training) or licensure/registration (e.g., dietetics). Programs of exercise science can also become accredited. For example, the **Commission on Accreditation of Allied Health Education Programs** (CAAHEP) oversees the **Committee on the Accreditation for the Exercise Science** (CoAES). The role of the CoAES is to establish standards and guidelines for academic programs that facilitate the preparation of students seeking employment in the health, fitness, and exercise industry. Programmatic accreditation through CAAHEP is specifically intended for exercise science programs or the academic departments in which the program is contained (e.g., Kinesiology, Exercise Science) (8). The American Association of Cardiovascular and Pulmonary Rehabilitation (AACVPR) confers program certification for those cardiovascular and pulmonary rehabilitation programs in hospitals, medical centers, and outpatient facilities that meet specific guidelines of professional practice. The goal of program certification in this instance is to assure that programs meet the essential standards of patient care (23,24).

Interactive component A part of an examination whereby the candidate taking the examination must respond to a visual situation.

Continuing education units Additional professional education that is required to maintain certification, licensure, or registration.

Program accreditation The granting of an academic program the standing of meeting acceptable criteria for the preparation of students enrolled in the program.

Commission on Accreditation of Allied Health Education Programs The largest organization for program accreditation in the health and exercise sciences field.

Committee on the Accreditation for the Exercise Science An organization designed to establish standards and guidelines for academic programs that facilitate the preparation of students seeking employment in the health, fitness, and exercise industry.

Licensure

Licensure is the granting of permission by an official or legal authority (usually a state government agency) to an individual or organization to engage in the legal practice of a professional activity that would otherwise be illegal. Licensure requirements and regulations vary among states, and it is important for the exercise science and allied healthcare professional to be aware of the state requirements for professional practice. Individuals such as physicians, nurses, physical and occupational therapists, and dietitians are required to attain licensure to practice as a professional. Licensure is obtained after completing an approved educational curriculum from an accredited program in a college or university and passing a licensure examination. Licensure is usually permanent, but periodic fees, competency examinations, and/or CEUs may be required to maintain active licensure. Individual states usually establish the requirements for licensure and this allows individuals to legally practice a regulated profession. Professional certification does not allow an individual to practice a regulated occupation unless the individual state recognizes the certification requirements as equivalent to the licensure requirements (23).

Registration

In certain areas of exercise science and allied health, registration is required to engage in professional practice. Registration is the documentation of professional qualification information relevant to government licensing requirements (23). Individuals who are registered with an organization or agency must also complete CEUs to maintain professional registration. For example, the American Dietetic Association, through the Commission on Dietetic Registration, confers the title of RD upon those individuals who complete academic training and pass the American Dietetic Association examination (4). Registration and licensure are similar in scope except that a licensed professional generally has a broader range of professional practice. An individual who is registered as a professional typically has his or her name listed in the organizations' registry. This practice provides information to the general public and potential employers about the qualifications of the individuals listed in the registry. For example, an organization may provide the

Table 11.1	A Description of Certification, Licensure, and Registration (23)	
CATEGORY	**DESCRIPTION**	
Certification	• individual, institution, or educational program is evaluated and recognized as meeting certain predetermined standards through successful completion of a valid and reliable examination	
Licensure	• granting of permission by a competent authority (usually a government agency) to an organization or individual to engage in a practice or activity that would otherwise be illegal	
Registration	• recording of professional qualification information relevant to government licensing regulations; similar to licensure, except that the scope of practice is usually more narrow than for a licensed professional	

Table 11.2	Professional Organizations in Exercise Science and Related Areas and the Credentialing Each Provide
PROFESSIONAL ORGANIZATION	**CREDENTIALING**
ACSM	Certification in two tracks: Health and fitness • Certified personal trainer • Health Fitness Instructor Clinical • Exercise Specialist • RCEP
NSCA	• CSCS • Certified Personal Trainer (NSCA-CPT)
ACE	• Personal trainer certification • Advanced Health & Fitness Specialist Certification • Group Fitness Instructor Certification • Lifestyle and Weight Management Consultant Certification
American Dietetic Association	• Licensure • Registration • Certificate of training in weight management
NATA	• Offers certification through the NATA Board of Certification
YMCA	• Personal Training Instructor
Cooper Institute for Aerobics Research	• Personal Trainer Certification

names of professionals within a particular geographic area who are ACSM RCEPs. Table 11.1 provides a summary explanation of certification, licensure, and registration. The selection of an appropriate credential should be based on the professional requirements and the intended range of professional practice. Several professional organizations offer certifications, licensure, and registrations that have relevance to exercise science professionals. Table 11.2 lists some of the professional organizations and the credentialing that each organization provides to the members.

> ➤ *Thinking Critically*
> *How do certification, licensure, and registration promote an increase in the confidence of the general public when working with exercise science and allied healthcare professionals?*

CAREER EMPLOYMENT AND PROFESSIONAL OPPORTUNITIES

One of the most frequently asked questions of exercise science faculty by undergraduate students is: "What type of job can I get with a degree in exercise science?" Well, the possibilities for professional employment are numerous and vary widely. It is important that every undergraduate student take some time seriously consider what he/she is willing to invest in professional education ar career development and what he/she really wants to do with the profession aspect of their life. Thoughtful reflection is critical because it is important to cor sider the many different components of your professional education and develop ment as you prepare yourself for your professional career. Listed below are son questions every student should consider when deciding on a professional care in exercise science or related area (19).

- Do you participate in and enjoy physical activity, exercise, and sports?
- Have you enjoyed coursework in biology, chemistry, math, nutrition, physiology, and physical fitness?
- Are you willing to commit to the necessary investment in education, academi training, and professional education that are required of working exercise science professionals?
- Have you spoken to individuals who currently work in your particular field o interest?
- In what type of professional employment setting do you wish to work (e.g., hospital, clinic, school, fitness facility, industrial setting, outpatient clinic, college, university)?
- Do you enjoy working with all types of people or are you only interested in certain populations (e.g., athletes, children, elderly, or patients with a chronic disease condition)?
- Do you want to work with people to prevent disease and injury or with patients desiring treatment and rehabilitation?

Starting salaries for individuals with an undergraduate degree and no experienc will vary widely. Factors such as work experience, geographic location, employ ment setting, and market demand combined with other factors such as whethe you hold professional licensure or certification will influence your beginning sa ary. Speaking to a professional who currently works in your field of interest i your geographic location is a good way to obtain an approximation of an expecte starting salary (19).

There are numerous reasons for the increased opportunities for professiona careers in exercise science. The greater interest in overall health by the genera public has resulted in an explosion of possible career opportunities in exercis science–related fields such as personal trainers, fitness directors, and exercis and sport nutritionists. The rise in lifestyle-related diseases has resulted in th need for more highly trained medical doctors, dieti cians, physical and occupational therapists, reha bilitation specialists, and researchers. Advances i sport technology and product development, alon with increases in participation in sport and athlet ics, have resulted in the need for more highly traine persons as athletic trainers, strength and conditionin coaches, sport biomechanists, and researchers. Th U.S. Department of Labor, Bureau of Labor Statistic (www.bls.gov/) periodically projects the employment opportunities in all sector of the economy and is a good place to identify employment trends in many c

> ➤ *Thinking Critically*
> *How does academic coursework and experiences in exercise science prepare future professionals for working in the allied healthcare and exercise science professions?*

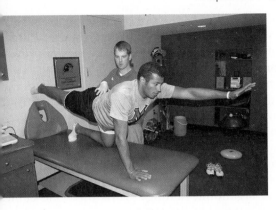

FIGURE 11.3 ▼ A clinical athletic trainer working with an athlete.

he professional jobs that exercise science graduates can expect to gain (18). The ollowing sections provide a short description of the major types of professional employment and career opportunities for graduates of exercise science programs. n some instances, an undergraduate degree is sufficient for employment, whereas n other professions an advanced or professional degree is required to work in a particular field. In almost every instance, obtaining a credential provides a benefit or gaining employment or is a required component of the job.

Athletic Trainer

An athletic trainer is a sports medicine professional, with a professional credential of athletic trainer certified (ATC), who is involved in the prevention, treatment, and rehabilitation of injuries to physically active individuals and athletes (see Chapter 5). Many people often view athletic trainers as only working with athletes in a sport setting; however, athletic trainers also work closely with other exercise science professionals, sports medicine physicians, and other allied health professionals o provide care to anyone who may have an injury caused by participation in physical activity, exercise, or sport (Figure 11.3). Only graduates of an athletic training program accredited by the **Commission on Accreditation of Athletic Training Education** may take the national Board of Certification examination and become a certified athletic trainer. In most states, athletic trainers must also become licensed by the state to practice athletic training. Athletic trainers are employed in a variety of work environments including secondary schools, colleges and universities, sports medicine clinics, professional sports programs, industrial and other occupational settings, as well as other allied healthcare employment settings (19,22).

Biomechanist

With proper academic training, an individual can work as a clinical or sport biomechanist and as an ergonomist. In general, an exercise science student will

Commission on Accreditation of Athletic Training Education The agency responsible for the accreditation of professional Athletic Training educational programs.

need additional undergraduate coursework in physics or engineering or possibly a graduate degree (MS or PhD) to work as a professional biomechanist. Clinical biomechanics focuses on the mechanics of injury and the principles of prevention, evaluation, and treatment of musculoskeletal problems. Sport biomechanic examines factors of human movement associated with exercise and training for the purpose of improving sport and athletic performance. Ergonomics is the study of the interaction between humans, the objects they use, and the environment in which they function and is similar to clinical biomechanics with ergonomist usually taking additional coursework in engineering (see Chapter 9). There is currently no credentialing available in the area of biomechanics. Employment opportunities include working in colleges and universities, performance enhancement centers, private business, industrial ergonomic settings sports medicine clinics hospitals, and other allied healthcare environments (19,22).

Clinical Exercise Physiologist

Clinical exercise physiologists work with healthy and diseased individuals in a variety of employment settings. Individuals who have chronic disease conditions including cardiovascular, respiratory, and metabolic diseases, can benefit from regular participation in physical activity and exercise. Clinical exercise physiologists are responsible for performing health and fitness assessments, developing and implementing exercise prescriptions, and monitoring the effectiveness of the interventions. Keeping appropriate records to determine the effectiveness of the physical activity or exercise intervention is often an important responsibility of the clinical exercise physiologist. Frequently advanced coursework in electrocardiography, pathophysiology, and specific populations (e.g., children or the elderly) is required. Certification and registration are becoming increasingly important and in many instances a requirement for employment as a clinical exercise physiologist. Employment opportunities exist primarily in hospitals outpatient and allied healthcare centers, cardiac rehabilitation centers, and within wellness and fitness programs (19,22).

Dietitian/Sport Dietician

A dietician is a licensed professional who assesses the nutritional needs of individuals, and then develops and assists with the implementation of nutritional programs for those individuals (Figure 11.4). Dieticians may also advise patients and clients on several health and disease-related conditions including weight loss, diabetes control, high blood pressure control, and cholesterol reduction. Only individuals who graduate from an American Dietetic Association accredited program, complete a 9-month, American Dietetic Association-approved internship, and pass the certification examination may become a licensed RD. RDs work in a variety of environments including private practice, long-term care facilities, medical institutions, health departments, social service agencies, residential care facilities, hospitals, primary and secondary school systems, colleges and universities, and other allied healthcare settings. RDs may also practice sports nutrition by working with individuals to develop nutritional programs that will serve to improve sport and athletic performance (19).

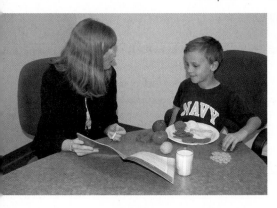

FIGURE 11.4 ▼ Dieticians perform counseling to healthy and diseased adults and children, as well as athletes.

Exercise and Sport Psychologist

Exercise and sport psychology professionals work with healthy and diseased individuals, as well as athletes of all performance and competition levels to enhance the psychological components related to successful performance. The principles of exercise and sport psychology are also used by other exercise science and allied healthcare professionals in a variety of employment settings, including the wellness and fitness industry, athletic training, coaching, and clinical exercise and rehabilitation settings. Individuals who are certified as consultants by the Association for the Advancement of Applied Sport Psychology (AAASP) can seek consultant positions with individual athletes and sport and athletic teams. Advanced academic coursework resulting in licensure as a clinical psychologist can also be valuable for developing a professional career in exercise or sport psychology. Attaining an advanced degree (PhD or EdD) can lead to employment as an instructor of exercise and sport psychology at a college or university (19,22).

Graduate School and Researcher

Individuals with an undergraduate degree in exercise science or related area who wish to pursue an advanced graduate degree in a particular area of exercise science or become actively involved in research have several opportunities to choose from. A masters degree (MS or MEd) generally requires 1 to 2 years of graduate coursework and experiences. The culminating experience may be a master's thesis, independent research project, or possibly an internship. The completion of a master's degree generally requires between 30 to 40 credit hours beyond the undergraduate degree. A doctoral degree (PhD or EdD) typically requires between 3 and 5 years of graduate coursework and research experiences. The traditional culminating experience is a doctoral dissertation demonstrating competency in conducting independent research. Table 11.3 provides some examples of areas of advanced study and research in exercise science. Advanced coursework and participation in research activities are the cornerstones of graduate school education. Additional coursework in research design and statistical analysis is critical for pursuing a career in research. Individuals with graduate degrees work in a variety of environments including

Table 11.3	Areas of Advanced Graduate Study in Exercise Science
Biomechanics	
Cardiac rehabilitation	
Environmental physiology	
Epidemiology	
Exercise and aging	
Exercise behavior and psychology	
Exercise biochemistry	
Exercise physiology	
Integrative physiology	
Motor behavior	
Motor control	
Motor development	
Neuroscience/Neurophysiology	
Occupational physiology	
Pediatric exercise physiology	
Sport psychology	
Therapeutic exercise	

pharmaceutical companies, colleges and universities, hospitals, medical school and institutions, governmental agencies including state and local health depart ments, and private research foundations (19).

Medical Doctor

A medical doctor is a licensed professional who is involved in the prevention treatment, and rehabilitation of illness and injuries to individuals. Medical doc tors can be educated to practice medicine in the following areas: allopathic chiropractic, osteopathic, podiatric, and ophthalmology. Each type of medica doctor has a defined scope of practice that can involve work with individual participating in physical activity, exercise, sport, and athletic competition. Man people often view medical doctors as only working with ill or sick individu als in a healthcare setting. Medical doctors, however, work closely with othe allied health professionals to provide preventive care to a wide range of health and diseased individuals. Individuals can also work as a sports medicine physi cian in private practice or with a local high school, college, or university sport teams. Only graduates of an accredited medical school may become a license medical doctor. Physicians also provide medical coverage at amateur, collegiate, and professional sport and athletic competitions. Certification as a sports medicine specialist is also becoming increasingly important if an individual has a desire to work with athletes. Medical doctors work in a variety of environments including private practice, long-term care facilities, medical institutions, health departments, residential care facilities, hospitals, colleges and universities, and other healthcare settings (19).

Occupational Therapist

Occupational therapists are licensed professionals who assist individuals with physically, mentally, emotionally, or developmentally crippling conditions to maintain or recover working skills and daily function. Often, occupational therapists teach individuals how to compensate for some temporary or permanent loss of motor function. Occupational therapists help individuals learn or regain the ability to perform activities of daily living, including dressing, preparing meals, and eating. To become a licensed occupational therapist, students must graduate from an occupational therapy program accredited by the Accreditation Council for Occupational Therapy Education, complete a fieldwork requirement, and pass a certification exam administered by the National Board for Certification in Occupational Therapy. Occupational therapists work in a variety of environments including private practice, long-term healthcare facilities, medical institutions, community health centers, residential care facilities, hospitals, school systems, adult daycare centers, and other healthcare settings (17,22).

Personal Trainer

Personal trainers work with individuals to assess functional capacity, and then develop and implement exercise programs for enhancing physical fitness and health. The exercise sessions are generally individual or small group (4–8 individuals) sessions and they typically occur in the client's home, the personal trainer's place of employment, or at a fitness facility. Personal trainers also conduct group exercise sessions in activities such as spinning, yoga, pilates, or aerobics. Personal trainers benefit from having a strong academic background in exercise physiology, biomechanics, fitness assessment, exercise prescription, exercise psychology, and nutrition as many aspects of this job involve the development of individualized muscular strength and endurance training programs and sound nutritional practices. In addition to obtaining an undergraduate degree in exercise science, gaining professional certification as a personal trainer or exercise leader from one of the organizations listed in Table 11.2 is essential (19).

Physical Therapist

Physical therapists are licensed professionals who help individuals recover from an injury or disabling physical condition (Figure 11.5). Physical therapists develop structured treatment and rehabilitation programs designed to improve mobility, reduce pain, and prevent or limit permanent disability. Physical therapists conduct evaluations of muscular fitness, range of motion, and muscle and joint functions

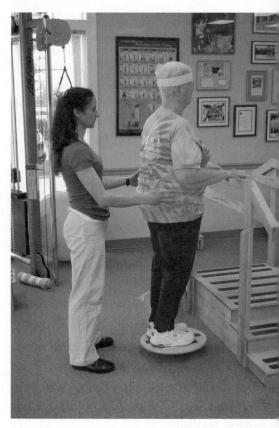

FIGURE 11.5 ▼ Physical therapist treating a patient.

and then use that information to develop and implement individualized treat
ment programs for patients. Only graduates of a physical therapy program accred
ited by the Commission on Accreditation in Physical Therapy Education ma
become a licensed physical therapist. The American Physical Therapy Associatio
now requires all graduates of accredited programs to have a Doctorate in Physica
Therapy (DPT) degree. Physical therapists work in a variety of employment envi
ronments including private practice, long-term care facilities, medical school an
institutions, community health centers, residential care facilities, hospitals, schoo
systems, adult daycare centers, and other allied healthcare (19).

Physician Assistant

A physician assistant is a licensed professional who works under the supervisio
of a medical doctor in the prevention, treatment, and rehabilitation of illness an
injuries to individuals (Figure 11.6). Physician assistants work closely with othe
allied health professionals to provide preventive care to a wide range of health
and diseased individuals. Physician assistants can benefit from undergraduat
coursework in fitness assessment, exercise physiology, biomechanics, nutritio
and exercise psychology. Only graduates of an accredited program may becom
a licensed physician assistant. Physician assistants work in a variety of environ
ments including private practice, long-term care facilities, medical institution

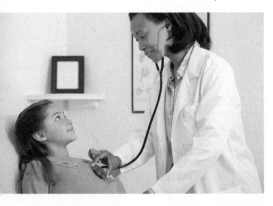

FIGURE 11.6 ▼ Physician assistant evaluating a patient. (Photo courtesy of Lifesize/Monica Rodriguez/Getty Images.)

ealth departments, residential care facilities, hospitals, colleges and universities, nd other allied healthcare settings.

ublic and Private School Teacher

eachers are licensed professionals who work to help children, adolescents, and oung adults develop motor skills, health, and physical fitness within a school tting. With proper academic training, an individual can pursue a career as a acher. Individuals interested in teaching health education and/or physical edu- ation must graduate from a National Council for the Accreditation of Teacher ducation–accredited program and pass a national licensing exam. This is typi- lly accomplished as an undergraduate teacher education major. However, many olleges and universities are offering graduate programs to prepare individuals to ecome licensed teachers. The cornerstone of teacher education programs is the racticum teaching experience, which must be completed before the licensure xamination. The majority of teachers work in public and private school systems aching kindergarten through grade 12. Coaching sport and athletic teams can ften be a part of the additional responsibilities of a health education or physical ducation teacher. Individuals can also pursue teaching careers at the college and niversity levels. Employment at this level does not require passing a licensure xamination but almost always requires a master's or doctoral degree, usually in ne of the areas of study listed previously in Table 11.3 (19).

trength and Conditioning Coach

trength and conditioning coaches are involved in the development and imple- entation of specialized training programs for athletes (Figure 11.7). Strength d conditioning coaches work with a variety of individual and team sport ath- tes to increase muscular strength and endurance, cardiovascular fitness, flexibil- y, and movement skills in an effort to improve performance. The evaluation and ssessment of physical performance and training improvements are important sponsibilities of the strength and conditioning coach. In addition to coursework an exercise science curriculum, individuals wishing to pursue this career option ould complete an internship or acquire volunteer training experience within established strength and conditioning program. Individuals should strongly nsider obtaining an appropriate certification credential and possibly a graduate

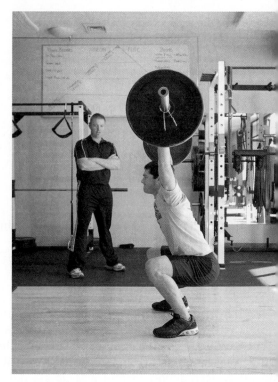

FIGURE 11.7 ▼ Strength and conditioning coaches work with athletes of all ages. (Photo courtesy of Stockbyte/DKP/ Getty Images.)

degree in an exercise science–related area of study. Strength and conditionin coaches work primarily in secondary schools, colleges and universities, profe sional sports programs, sports medicine clinics, and commercial sports develo ment businesses (19).

Wellness and Fitness Industry Professional

A wellness and **fitness industry** professional can expect to work with membe of the general public to develop and implement physical activity and exercis programs to improve health, wellness, and fitness. Exercise science graduates ca obtain employment in a variety of professional jobs within the wellness and fi ness industry. A broad knowledge of biomechanics, fitness assessment, exercis physiology, and exercise psychology is critical for an exercise science graduate t establish and develop a professional career in the wellness and fitness industr As more individuals use participation in physical activity and exercise as a mear to improve health, wellness, and fitness and reduce the risk of developing lifesty diseases there will be an increased need for professional employees in the wel ness and fitness industry (22). Table 11.4 provides examples of some employmer opportunities in the wellness and fitness industry. Within each of the work set tings, exercise science professionals have the opportunity to work as individua and group exercise leaders, fitness director, operations or facility manager, clu manager, or general manager. Each of these positions requires a specific conter knowledge base and in some instances years of experience (e.g., club manager c

Table 11.4	Employment Opportunities in the Wellness and Fitness Industry	
EMPLOYMENT OPPORTUNITY	**DESCRIPTION**	
Club fitness programs	For-profit business operating to provide a service to members who join the club	
Community programs	Operated by local communities and nonprofit organizations such as the YMCA and the YWCA	
Corporate wellness programs	Operated by large businesses and corporations as a means by which to provide employees with an opportunity to enhance health and wellness	
Spa fitness programs	For-profit business operating to provide a variety of traditional and nontraditional exercise, health, and relaxation programs to guests	

eneral manager). In many instances, professional certification is expected and ften required.

As a professional employed in one of the wellness and fitness industry set- ngs, you can expect to work with individuals across the lifespan from preschool ged children to the older adult. In many instances, the individuals will be healthy, ut physically **deconditioned**. There is the possibility of undiagnosed disease nd often individuals will want to begin an exercise rogram with risk factors for a variety of disease onditions. That makes it very important to follow ppropriate guidelines for exercise testing and exercise rescription (20). Participants in wellness and fitness rograms will also have a wide variety of knowledge, kills, and abilities related to physical activity and xercise. Within the wellness and fitness industry, xercise science professionals can be expected to be ivolved in health and fitness screening and assessment, fitness program develop- ent and implementation, and program evaluation and assessment (22).

> ➤ *Thinking Critically*
> *Why is it important to thoughtfully consider personal and professional goals when deciding on a career in an allied healthcare or exercise science profession?*

PROFESSIONAL ORGANIZATIONS N EXERCISE SCIENCE

he development of exercise science and the related areas of study have resulted 1 the establishment of several professional organizations that provide valuable ervices to professional members. Examples of these membership benefits and

---

Fitness industry A global term used to describe components related to improving health and fitness of indi- viduals through physical activity and exercise.

Deconditioned A state of being unfit to perform physical activity or exercise.

Table 11.5	The Missions of Various Exercise Science Professional Organizations
PROFESSIONAL ORGANIZATION	**MISSION**
AAHPERD	Promote and support leadership, research, education, and best practices in the professions that support creative, healthy, and active lifestyles.
AACVPR	To reduce morbidity, mortality, and disability from cardiovascular and pulmonary diseases through education, prevention, rehabilitation, research, and aggressive disease management.
ACE	A nonprofit organization committed to enriching the quality of life through safe and effective exercise and physical activity.
ACSM	Promotes and integrates scientific research, education, and practical applications of sports medicine and exercise science to maintain and enhance physical performance, fitness, health, and quality of life.
ASB	To encourage and foster the exchange of information and ideas among biomechanists working in different disciplines and fields of application, biologic sciences, exercise and sports science, health sciences, ergonomics and human factors, and engineering and applied science, and to facilitate the development of biomechanics as a basic and applied science.
ASEP	Represents and promotes the profession of exercise physiology, and is committed to the professional development of exercise physiology, its advancement, and the credibility of exercise physiologists.
AAASP	To provide leadership for the development of theory, research and applied practice in sport, exercise, and health psychology; to offer and deliver services to athletes, coaches, teams, parents and other groups involved in exercise, sport participation, and rehabilitation; to establish and maintain professional standards through the development of certification procedures, ethical guidelines, and the promotion of respect for and value of human diversity; to certify individuals who have met a minimal level of training and experience to provide professional services in applied sport and exercise psychology.
ISBS	Provide a forum for the exchange of ideas for sports biomechanics researchers, coaches and teachers; to bridge the gap between researchers and practitioners; to gather and disseminate information and materials on biomechanics in sports.
ISB	Promotes the study of the biomechanics of movement with a special emphasis on human beings; encouraging international contacts among scientists in this field, promoting knowledge of biomechanics on an international level, and cooperating with related organizations.
ISMC	To promote basic and applied research in the area of control of movements of biologic systems.
NASPSPA	To develop and advance the scientific study of human behavior when individuals are engaged in sport and physical activity; facilitate the dissemination of information; improve the quality of research and teaching in the psychology of sport, motor development, and motor learning and control.
NATA	To enhance the quality of healthcare provided by certified athletic trainers and to advance the athletic training profession.
NSCA	Supports and disseminates research-based knowledge and its practical application to improve athletic performance and fitness.

rvices range from the distribution of newsletters and professional journals to
ectronic employment bulletin boards. Many of these professional organizations
ffer discounted membership fees and reduced conference registration fees to
oth undergraduate and graduate students. The specific mission of an organiza-
on provides considerable insight into the scope of practice that the members
ho belong to the organization participate in as professionals. This can help guide
ou in the selection of an appropriate professional organization. Many individuals
elong to more than one organization in an effort to receive the valuable benefits
ffered by each organization. Table 11.5 provides the mission statements of the
rimary exercise science professional organizations. The following section pro-
ides a summary of the primary professional organizations in exercise science.

merican Council on Exercise

he American Council on Exercise (ACE) is a nonprofit organization commit-
:d to enriching quality of life through safe and effective exercise and physical
ctivity. Its purpose is to protect all segments of society against ineffective fitness
roducts, and promote programs and trends through its ongoing public education,
utreach, and research. ACE further protects the public by setting certification
nd continuing education standards for fitness professionals. ACE was founded
1 1985 and serves to provide fitness certification, education, and training to its
iembers. Membership benefits include career services, conferences, access to
eleconferences, and subscriptions to a variety of newsletters. Professional devel-
pment opportunities are available through numerous continuing education pro-
rams. Additional information can be obtained by visiting the ACE homepage at
ww.acefitness.org (23).

merican Alliance for Health, Physical Education,
ecreation and Dance

he American Alliance for Health, Physical Education, Recreation and Dance
AAHPERD) is the largest organization of professionals involved in physical edu-
ation, leisure, fitness, dance, health promotion, and education and all specialties
:lated to achieving a healthy lifestyle. Its purpose is to provide members with
vide-ranging and coordinated support, resources, and programs to help profes-
ionals improve their skills and abilities to help further enhance the health and
vell-being of the American public. Founded in 1885, AAHPERD is an alliance of
ve national associations and six district associations and serves more than 25,000
iembers. The national associations are

American Association of Health Education
National Dance Association
American Association for Physical Activity and Recreation
National Association for Girls and Women in Sport
National Association for Sport and Physical Education

here is also a Research Consortium for professional and student members of
AHPERD. Membership benefits include career services, discounts on confer-
nce registration fees, leadership conferences, interest group affiliations, and

subscription to journals such as *Research Quarterly for Exercise and Sport* and *Journa of Physical Education, Recreation, and Dance*. Professional development opportun ties are available through meetings and conferences. The AAHPERD also prc vides grants and scholarships to student members. Additional information can b obtained by visiting the AAHPERD homepage at www.aahperd.org (1).

American Association of Cardiovascular and Pulmonary Rehabilitation

Founded in 1985, the American Association of Cardiovascular and Pulmonar Rehabilitation (AACVPR) is the premier professional organization dedicated t the development of its members who are involved in the profession of cardic vascular and pulmonary rehabilitations. The AACVPR provides educational an networking opportunities that inform individuals of new advances, current legis lative and reimbursement initiatives, as well as member benefits to help improv the care and quality of life for patients with heart and lung diseases. The AACVP also provides certification for professional cardiac and pulmonary rehabilitatio programs. Membership benefits include career services, discounts on conferenc registration fees, access to teleconferences, and subscription to the *Journal of Ca diopulmonary Rehabilitation and Prevention*. Professional development opportunitie are available through meetings and conferences. Additional information can b obtained by visiting the AACVPR homepage at www.aacvrp.org (2).

American College of Sports Medicine

The American College of Sports Medicine (ACSM) was founded in 1954 for th purpose of bringing together individuals with an interest in exercise and health The ACSM has a diverse membership of professionals from all areas of exercis science. The ACSM is the largest exercise science and sports medicine organizatio in the world, with more than 20,000 international, national, and regional chapte members. ACSM offers individual certification programs in health and fitness an clinical tracks. Membership benefits include career services, interest group affili ations, discounts on conference registration fees, access to position stands, an subscription to the journals *Medicine and Science in Sports and Exercise* and *Exer cise and Sport Science Reviews*. Professional development opportunities are availabl through professional meetings and conferences. Continuing education credits an continuing medical education credits are available to members who participate i organizational activities. The ACSM also supports research activities through th ACSM Foundation and is active in advocacy for national and international issue related to exercise and health. Additional information can be obtained by visitin the ACSM homepage at www.acsm.org (3).

American Society of Biomechanics

The American Society of Biomechanics (ASB) was founded in 1977. The AS encourages and fosters the exchange of information and ideas among biomecha nists working in various disciplines and fields of application for the improvemen f health, well-being, and sport performance. Membership benefits include career ervices, interest group affiliations, and subscription to the *Journal of Biomechanics*. rofessional development opportunities are available through meetings and onferences. The ASB also provides awards and grants to professional and student nembers. Additional information can be obtained by visiting the ASB homepage t www.asbweb.org (5).

American Society of Exercise Physiologists

he American Society of Exercise Physiologists (ASEP) was founded in 1997 for he purpose of bringing together exercise physiology professionals. The ASEP is ommitted to the professional development of exercise physiology, its advance- nent, and the enhanced credibility of exercise physiologists. As part of its mission, ASEP offers an exercise physiology certified examination. Membership benefits nclude career services and subscription to the online *Journal of Exercise Physiology*. rofessional development opportunities are available through professional meet- ngs and conferences. Additional information can be obtained by visiting the ASEP omepage at www.asep.org (6).

Association for Applied Sport Psychology

ounded in 1986, the Association for Applied Sport Psychology (AASP) promotes he ethical practice, science, and advocacy of sport and exercise psychology. With bout 1,200 members, AASP is an international, multidisciplinary, professional rganization that is the largest applied sport and exercise psychology organiza- ion in the world. AASP incorporates information and expertise from exercise nd sport sciences and psychology into three interrelated focus areas: health and xercise psychology, performance enhancement/intervention, and social psychol- gy. The association offers an AASP Certified Consultants program to its mem- ers. Membership benefits include career services, interest group affiliations, and ubscription to the *Journal of Applied Sport Psychology*. Professional development pportunities are available through professional meetings and conferences and ontinuing education programs. AASP also provides an online resource center for rofessionals and the general public. Additional information can be obtained by isiting the AASP homepage at www.appliedsportpsych.org (7).

International Society of Biomechanics

he International Society of Biomechanics (ISB) was founded in 1973 to pro- note the study of all areas of biomechanics, although special emphasis is given to he biomechanics of human movement. The ISB promotes international contacts mongst scientists, promotes the dissemination of knowledge, and forms liaisons vith national organizations. Membership in the ISB includes individuals from the lisciplines of anatomy, physiology, engineering (mechanical, industrial, aerospace), rthopedics, rehabilitation medicine, sport science and medicine, ergonomics, lectrophysiologic kinesiology, and others. The ISB promotes the organization of biennial international congresses, publication of congress proceedings and biomechanics monograph series, distribution of a quarterly newsletter, sponsorship of scientific meetings related to biomechanics and affiliations with the *Journal of Biomechanics*, the *Journal of Applied Biomechanics, Clinical Biomechanics*, the *Journal of Electromyography and Kinesiology*, and *Gait and Posture*. Additional information can be obtained by visiting the ISB homepage at www.isbweb.org (10).

International Society of Biomechanics in Sport

Established in 1982, the International Society of Biomechanics in Sport (ISBS) provides a forum for the exchange of ideas for sport biomechanics researchers, coaches, and teachers. The ISBS also works to bridge the gap between researchers and practitioners and gather and disseminate information and materials on biomechanics in sports. The ISBS offers annual symposia, a regular newsletter, and additional resources for members. Membership in the ISBS also includes a subscription to the journal *Sport Biomechanics*. Additional information can be obtained by visiting the ISBS homepage at www.csuchico.edu/isbs (9).

International Society of Motor Control

Founded in 2002, the International Society of Motor Control (ISMC) is dedicated to the development of its members who are interested in basic and applied research in the area of control of movements in biologic systems. The ISMC provides educational and networking opportunities that inform individuals of current activities in motor control. The ISMC membership benefits include career services and subscription to the journal *Motor Control*. Professional development opportunities are available through professional meetings and conferences. Additional information can be obtained by visiting the ISMC homepage at www.i-s-m-c.org (11).

National Athletic Trainers' Association

The National Athletic Trainers' Association (NATA) was founded in 1950 and currently serves almost 30,000 national and international members. The NATA develops and presents the most advanced information regarding injury prevention and rehabilitation. Athletic training is practiced by certified athletic trainers who are healthcare professionals who collaborate with physicians to optimize the activity and participation of patients and clients. Athletic training encompasses the prevention, diagnosis, and intervention of emergency, acute, and chronic medical conditions involving impairment, functional limitations, and disabilities. The NATA offers the certification of athletic trainers through the Commission on Accreditation for Athletic Training Education. Membership benefits include discounts on conference registration fees, career services, interest group affiliations, a membership directory, and subscription to the *Journal of Athletic Training*. Professional development opportunities are available through national, regional, and state meetings, and conferences and continuing education programs. The NATA also provides grants and scholarships to student members through the NATA Research & Education Foundation. Additional information can be obtained by visiting the NATA homepage at www.nata.org (12).

National Strength and Conditioning Association

The National Strength and Conditioning Association (NSCA) was founded by strength and conditioning professionals in 1978. The NSCA serves nearly 30,000 members throughout the world. The NSCA develops and makes available the most advanced information regarding strength training and conditioning practices, performance enhancement, injury prevention, and research findings. The NSCA is comprised of a diverse group of professionals from the sport science, athletic, allied health, and fitness industries working together to bridge the gap between the scientist in the laboratory and the practitioner in the field. The NSCA offers the Certified Strength and Conditioning Specialist (CSCS) and the NSCS-Certified Personal Trainer credentialing programs. Membership benefits include career services, interest group affiliations, and subscription to the *Journal of Strength and Conditioning Research* and the *Strength and Conditioning Journal*. Professional development opportunities are available through professional meetings and conferences, and videos and electronic downloads. The NSCA also grants student scholarships through the National Strength and Conditioning Foundation. Additional information can be obtained by visiting the NSCA homepage at www.nsca-lift.org (13).

North American Society for the Psychology of Sport and Physical Activity

The North American Society for the Psychology of Sport and Physical Activity (NASPSPA) was founded in 1967. NASPSPA is a multidisciplinary association of scholars from the behavioral sciences and related professions that work together to disseminate information about the psychology of physical activity, exercise, and sport. NASPSPA promotes the development and advanced study of human behavior when individuals are engaged in physical activity, exercise, and sport. NASPSPA is also interested in improving the quality of research and teaching in sport psychology and motor behavior. Membership benefits include career services and subscription to a newsletter as well as access to abstracts in the *Journal of Sport and Exercise Psychology* and *Motor Control*. Professional development opportunities are available through national and regional meetings and conferences. Additional information can be obtained by visiting the NASPSPA homepage at www.naspspa.org (14).

Sports, Cardiovascular, and Wellness Nutrition Dietetics Practice Group

The Sports, Cardiovascular, and Wellness Nutrition Dietetics Practice Group (SCAN) was established in 1981 and is one of the largest dietetic practice groups of the American Dietetic Association. SCAN works to promote healthy active lifestyles through practice in sports, cardiovascular, and wellness nutrition and the prevention and treatment of disordered eating. RDs may become certified as a Specialist in Sports

> ➤ *Thinking Critically*
> *How do professional organizations within exercise science work to fulfill their organizational mission and meet the needs of their members and the general public?*

Dietetics by the Commission on Dietetic Registration. SCAN offers professional development opportunities through professional meetings, electronic newsletters, podcasts, and conferences. Additional information can be obtained by visiting the SCAN homepage at www.scandpg.org/ (16).

PROFESSIONAL ORGANIZATIONS RELATED TO EXERCISE SCIENCE

There are several other professional organizations that have an interest in exercise science–related activities. Each of these organizations has a specific mission of which some aspect of physical activity or exercise may be a component. It is also common for exercise science professionals to be members of one or more of these professional organizations if membership provides a benefit in the professional

Table 11.6	Primary Mission of Professional Organizations with an Interest in Exercise science
PROFESSIONAL ORGANIZATION	**MISSION**
American Cancer Society	Dedicated to eliminating cancer as a major health problem by preventing cancer, saving lives, and diminishing suffering from cancer through research, education, advocacy, and service.
American College of Epidemiology	Advocating for policies and actions that enhance the science and practice of epidemiology; promoting the professional development of epidemiologists through educational initiatives; recognizing excellence in epidemiology; developing and maintaining an active membership base of both fellows and members representing all aspects of epidemiology.
American Diabetes Association	To prevent and cure diabetes and to improve the lives of all people affected by diabetes.
American Dietetic Association	To lead the future of dietetics.
American Heart Association	To build healthier lives, free of cardiovascular diseases and stroke.
American Medical Association	To promote the art and science of medicine and the betterment of public health.
American Nurses Association	To advance the nursing profession by fostering high standards of nursing practice, promoting the rights of nurses in the workplace, projecting a positive and realistic view of nursing, and by lobbying the Congress and regulatory agencies on healthcare issues affecting nurses and the public.
American Physical Therapy Association	To further the profession's role in the prevention, diagnosis, and treatment of movement dysfunctions and the enhancement of the physical health and functional abilities of members of the public
American Physiological Society	To foster education, scientific research, and dissemination of information in the physiologic sciences.
American Psychological Association	To advance psychology as a science and profession and as a means of promoting health, education, and human welfare.

evelopment and employment of the individual. Table 11.6 provides the primary
ission of those professional organizations with a secondary interest in exercise
cience.

US GOVERNMENT AGENCIES WITH AN INTEREST IN EXERCISE SCIENCE

articipation in regular physical activity and exercise is recognized as a major
actor in improving health and reducing the risk for disease. As a result, major
nitiatives by agencies of the federal government address various aspects of health,
isease prevention and treatment, physical activity, and exercise. For example,
gencies and offices of the federal government were responsible for developing
nd promoting the Healthy People 2010 initiative (25) and using the 1996 Sur-
eon General's report (29) to guide decision making and policy development for
nhancing the quality and years of healthy life and the elimination of health dis-
arities. Healthy People 2020 will be the next guiding document for assessing the
najor risks to health and wellness, changing public health priorities, and address-
ng the emerging issues related to our nation's health preparedness and preven-
ion (26). There are several U.S. Government agencies that play an important role
n advancing the public health agenda of our nation through the promotion of
hysical activity and proper nutrition.

U.S. Department of Health and Human Services

he Department of Health and Human Services (DHHS) is the federal government's principal agency for protecting the health of all Americans and providing
ssential human services especially for those who are least able to help them-
elves. The DHHS's mission is to enhance the health and well-being of Ameri-
ans by providing for effective health and human services and fostering strong,
ustained advances in the sciences underlying medicine, public health, and social
ervices. The DHHS provides administrative oversight through the Office of the
ecretary of Health and Human Services. Figure 11.8 provides the current organi-
ational chart of the U.S. DHHS (28).

Furthermore, the DHHS provides resource support for over 300 programs
overing a wide range of activities (28). Table 11.7 provides some examples of
ctivities administered by the DHHS. The DHHS programs are administered by
1 operating divisions, including 8 agencies in the U.S. Public Health Service and
human services agencies. In addition to the services they deliver, the DHHS pro-
rams provide for equitable treatment of beneficiaries nationwide, and they enable
he collection of national health and disease data. The DHHS has established four
oals each having four objectives that support and carry out its mission (28):

- *Goal 1*—Healthcare: Improve the safety, quality, affordability, and accessibility
  of healthcare, including behavioral healthcare and long-term care.
- *Goal 2*—Public Health Promotion and Protection, Disease Prevention, and Emergency Preparedness: Prevent and control disease, injury, illness, and disability
  across the lifespan, and protect the public from infectious, occupational,
  environmental, and terrorist threats.

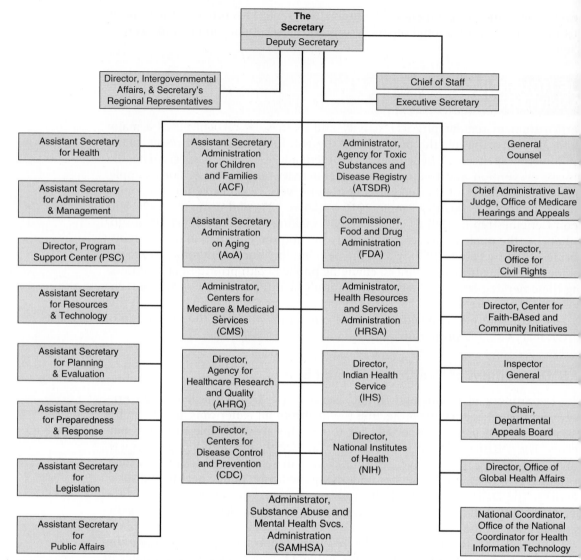

FIGURE 11.8 ▼ Organizational chart of the U.S. DHHS (28). (Available from http://www.hhs.gov/about/orgchart/index.html.)

- *Goal 3*—Human Services: Promote the economic and social well-being of individuals, families, and communities.
- *Goal 4*—Scientific Research and Development: Advance scientific and biomedical research and development related to health and human services.

The DHHS had identified four strategic objectives by which to accomplish each goal. Although all of the agencies of the DHHS are involved in the healthcare of the nation's population, some are especially important to exercise science and its related areas. For example, the Healthy People program (e.g., Healthy People 2010 and Healthy People 2020) is an initiative established by the DHHS that represents

Table 11.7	Examples of Activities Administered by the U.S. DHHS
Assuring food and drug safety	
Comprehensive health services for Native Americans	
Faith-based and community initiatives	
Financial assistance and services for low income families	
Head start preschool education and services	
Health Information technology	
Improving maternal and infant health	
Medical and social science research	
Medical preparedness for emergencies, including potential terrorism.	
Medicaid—health insurance for low income Americans	
Medicare—health insurance for the elderly and disabled Americans	
Preventing child abuse and domestic violence	
Preventing disease, including immunization services	
Services for older Americans including home-delivered meals	
Substance abuse prevention and treatment	

he nation's disease prevention agenda. Healthy People 2010 has two primary goals (25):

1. Increase quality and years of healthy life
2. Eliminate health disparities

t is the responsibility of the DHHS to work with other federal, state, and local government agencies, as well as additional public and private organizations to enhance the health and well-being of the nation's people.

National Institutes of Health

The National Institutes of Health (NIH) is the medical research branch of the DHHS. The NIH is the world's premier medical research organization, supporting over 38,000 research projects nationwide in diseases including cancer, Alzheimer's, diabetes, arthritis, heart ailments, and AIDS. Within the organizational structure of the NIH, there are 27 separate health institutes and centers (Table 11.8) (27). The budget of NIH, established by congress and the President of the United States, is used to support the mission of NIH, which is to promote science in pursuit of fundamental knowledge about the nature and behavior of living systems and the application of that knowledge to extend healthy life and reduce the burdens of illness and disability. The NIH uses much of its budget to fund grants and contracts

Table 11.8	Health Institutes and Centers of the NIH

National Cancer Institute—Est. 1937

National Eye Institute—Est. 1968

National Heart, Lung, and Blood Institute—Est. 1948

National Human Genome Research Institute—Est. 1989

National Institute on Aging—Est. 1974

National Institute on Alcohol Abuse and Alcoholism—Est. 1970

National Institute of Allergy and Infectious Diseases—Est. 1948

National Institute of Arthritis and Musculoskeletal and Skin Diseases—Est. 1986

National Institute of Biomedical Imaging and Bioengineering—Est. 2000

National Institute of Child Health and Human Development—Est. 1962

National Institute on Deafness and Other Communication Disorders—Est. 1988

National Institute of Dental and Craniofacial Research—Est. 1948

National Institute of Diabetes and Digestive and Kidney Diseases—Est. 1948

National Institute on Drug Abuse—Est. 1973

National Institute of Environmental Health Sciences—Est. 1969

National Institute of General Medical Sciences—Est. 1962

National Institute of Mental Health—Est. 1949

National Institute of Neurological Disorders and Stroke—Est. 1950

National Institute of Nursing Research—Est. 1986

National Library of Medicine—Est. 1956

Center for Information Technology (CIT formerly DCRT, OIRM, TCB)—Est. in 1964

Center for Scientific Review—Est. in 1946

John E. Fogarty International Center for Advanced Study in the Health
   Sciences—Est. in 1968

National Center for Complementary and Alternative Medicine—Est. in 1999

National Center on Minority Health and Health Disparities—Est. in 1993

National Center for Research Resources—Est. in 1962

NIH Clinical Center—Est. in 1953

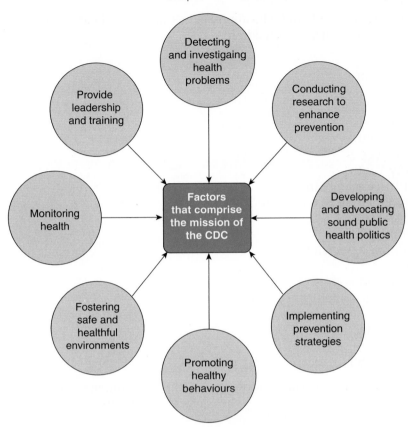

FIGURE 11.9 ▼ Mission of the CDC.

upporting research and training throughout the United States and abroad. Many f the grants and contracts funded by NIH are connected to research in various reas of exercise science.

Centers for Disease Control and Prevention

The Centers for Disease Control and Prevention (CDC) are under the administrative oversight of the DHHS. The mission of the CDC is to promote the health and quality of life by preventing and controlling disease, injury, and disability. Figure 11.9 illustrates the factors that constitute the mission of the CDC (21). Of the CDC's six Coordinating Centers, the Center for Health Promotion has the closest link to exercise science. Within the Center for Health Promotion is the National Center for Chronic Disease Prevention and Health Promotion. The mission of the National Center for Chronic Disease Prevention and Health Promotion is to provide national leadership in areas of health promotion and chronic disease prevention by conducting public health surveillance, epidemiologic studies, and behavioral interventions; by disseminating guidelines and recommendations; and by assisting state health and education agencies to increase their capacity to prevent chronic diseases and promote healthful behaviors. These programs provide national leadership by offering guidelines and recommendations and

by helping state health and education agencies promote healthy behaviors (21
These major programs are listed here:

- Arthritis
- Cancer Control
- Diabetes
- Epilepsy
- Genomics
- Global Health
- Healthy Aging
- Healthy Youth
- Heart Disease and Stroke
- Nutrition, Physical Activity and Obesity
- Oral Health
- PHHS Block Grant
- Prevention Research Centers
- REACH
- Safe Motherhood
- Steps to a Healthier United States
- Tobacco
- WISEWOMAN

Office of Public Health and Science

The Office of Public Health and Science (OPHS) is under the direction of th
Assistant Secretary for Health, who serves as the DHHS Secretary's senio

Table 11.9	Missions of Offices Located within the OPHS that are Related to Health and Exercise Science
OFFICE	**MISSION**
Office of Disease Prevention and Health Promotion	To provide leadership, coordination and policy development for public health and prevention activities with OPHS.
Office of the Surgeon General	To protect and advance the health of the nation.
President's Council on Physical Fitness and Sports	An advisory committee of volunteer citizens who advise the president through the secretary of Health and Human Services about physical activity, fitness, and sports in America.
Office for Human Research Protections	Supports, strengthens, and provides leadership to the nation's system for protecting volunteers in research that is conducted or supported by the DHHS.
Office of Research Integrity	Promotes the integrity in research programs of the OPHS, both intramural and extramural, including responding to allegations of research misconduct.
Office on Women's Health	Strives to improve the health of American women by advancing and coordinating a comprehensive women's health agenda throughout the DHHS.

viser for public health and science. The OPHS
ovides leadership and coordination across the
HHS in public health and science, provides direc-
on to program offices within the OPHS, and pro-
des advice and counsel on public health and sci-
ce issues to the DHHS secretary. The OPHS is
mprised of 12 core public health offices and the
ommissioned Corps, a uniformed service of more
an 6,000 health professionals who serve at DHHS and other federal agen-
es (15). Many of the offices within the OPHS address issues directly related
 health, wellness, and exercise science. Those offices and their respective
issions are listed in Table 11.9.

> ➤ *Thinking Critically*
>
> *In what ways do governmental agencies work to accomplish their individual missions and provide for the improved public health of the nation?*

ADDITIONAL ORGANIZATIONS AND AGENCIES N EXERCISE SCIENCE

umerous other organizations and agencies are involved in a variety of activities
at are related to the various areas of study in exercise science. Some of these
rganizations contribute to enhancing the educational development of exercise
ience professionals and the general public, whereas other organizations attempt
 provide guidance and support for addressing public health issues. Table 11.10
cludes some of those organizations that are involved in exercise science–related
ctivities.

Table 11.10	Additional Organizations that are Involved in Various Aspects of Exercise Science and Related Areas
ORGANIZATION	**RELATIONSHIP TO EXERCISE SCIENCE**
World Health Organization	Supports projects, initiatives, activities, information products, and contacts for various health and development topics including disease conditions such as cancer, diabetes mellitus, obesity, and poor nutrition.
Board of Certification in Professional Ergonomics	The certifying body for individuals whose education and experience indicate broad expertise in the practice of human factors/ergonomics.
Aerobics and Fitness Association of America	World's largest fitness educator delivering comprehensive cognitive and practical education for fitness professionals; grounded in industry research, using both traditional and innovative modalities.
The Cooper Institute	Conducts research in epidemiology, exercise physiology, behavior change, hypertension, children's health issues, obesity, nutrition, aging, and other health issues. It also provides training and certification programs for fitness leaders and health professionals.

SUMMARY

- Credentialing is an important aspect of professional development that demonstrates individual competency in knowledge, skills, and abilities.
- Professional careers in exercise science and allied healthcare require a core base of knowledge and additional preparation in specialty areas.
- Professional organizations strive to enhance the development of their profession, their members, and their mission by providing member benefits and services.
- Departments and agencies within the Federal Government and other professional organizations work to enhance the health and wellness of Americans through policy initiatives and program development.

FOR REVIEW

1. Describe the differences among the following credentials:
   a. certification
   b. licensure
   c. registration

2. What are the primary benefits of certification?

3. What are the principal certifications offered by the primary exercise science professional organizations?

4. What are the primary employment opportunities in the fitness industry?

5. What is the difference between an occupational and a physical therapist?

6. In what ways do physician and a physician's assistant work together to promote health and reduce disease risk?

7. Why are professional certifications important for athletic trainers and clinical exercise physiologists?

8. Describe the mission of the following professional organizations:
   a. American College of Sports Medicine
   b. National Athletic Trainers Association
   c. American Alliance for Health, Physical Education, Recreation and Dance
   d. American Association of Cardiovascular and Pulmonary Rehabilitation
   e. North American Society for the Psychology of Sport and Physical Activity
   f. American Society of Exercise Physiologists
   g. International Society for Motor Control
   h. International Society of Biomechanics

9. What branches of the federal government are charged with enhancing the health and reducing the disease risk of the American public?

REFERENCES

1. American Alliance for Health, Physical Education, Recreation, and Dance Web Site [Internet]. Available from: http://www aahperd org. 2008.
2. American Association of Cardiovascular and Pulmonary Rehabilitation Web Site [Internet]. Available from: http://www aacvpr org/. 2008.
3. American College of Sports Medicine Web site [Internet]. Available from: www acsm org. 2008.
4. American Dietetic Association Web site [Internet]. Available from: www eatright org. 2008.
5. American Society of Biomechanics Web Site [Internet]. Available from: http://www asbweb org/. 2008.
6. American Society of Exercise Physiologists Web Site [Internet]. Available from: http://www asep org/. 2008.
7. Association for Applied Sport Psychology Web Site [Internet]. Available from: http://appliedsportpsych org. 2008.
8. Commission on Accreditation of Allied Health Education Programs Web site [Internet]. Available from: www caahep org/. 2008.
9. International Society of Biomechanics in Sport Web Site [Internet]. Available from: http://www csuchico edu/isbs/. 2008.
10. International Society of Biomechanics Web Site [Internet]. Available from: http://isbweb org/. 2008.
11. International Society of Motor Control Web Site [Internet]. Available from: http://www i-s-m-c org/. 2008.
12. National Athletic Trainers Association Web Site [Internet]. Available from: http://www nata org/. 2008.
13. National Strength and Conditioning Association Web Site [Internet]. Available from: http://www nsca-lift org/. 2008.
14. North American Society for the Psychology of Sport and Physical Activity Web Site [Internet]. Available from: http://www naspspa org/. 2008.
15. Office of Public Health and Science. Available from: http://www hhs gov/ophs/. 2008.
16. Sports, Cardiovascular, and Wellness Nutrition Dietetics Practice Group Web site [Internet]. Available from: www scandpg org/. 2008.
17. The American Occupational Therapy Association. Available from: www aota org. 2008.
18. U.S. Department of Labor, Bureau of Labor Statistics [Internet]. Available from: www bls gov. 2008.
19. American College of Sports Medicine. Careers in sports medicine and exercise science. *American College of Sports Medicine Webpage*. 2003.
20. American College of Sports Medicine. *ACSM's Guidelines for Exercise Testing and Prescription*. Philadelphia (PA): Lippincott, Williams & Wilkins; 2006.
21. Centers for Disease Control and Prevention. Centers for Disease Control and Prevention Internet Source. *Center for Disease Control and Prevention*. 2008.
22. Kravitz L. Job activities and employment. In: Brown SP. *Introduction to Exercise Science*. Philadelphia (PA): Lippincott, Williams, & Wilkins; 2001. p. 82–96.
23. Kreider RB, Cahill KM. Exercise science and fitness certifications. In: Brown SP. *Introduction to Exercise Science*. Philadelphia (PA): Lippincott, Williams & Wilkins; 2001. p. 67–81.
24. Thompson WR, Brown SP. Professional issues. In: Brown SP. *Introduction to Exercise Science*. Philadelphia (PA): Lippincott, WIlliams & Wilkins; 2001. p. 117–29.
25. U.S. Department of Health and Human Services. Healthy People 2010. *Healthy People 2010 Website*. 2008.
26. U.S. Department of Health and Human Services. *2008 Healthy People 2010 Web site* [Internet] [Online]. 2008.
27. U.S. Department of Health and Human Services. National Institutes of Health. *National Institutes of Health Webpage*. 2008.
28. U.S. Department of Health and Human Services. U.S. Department of Health and Human Services. *U S Department of Health and Human Services Webpage*. 2008.
29. U.S. Department of Health and Human Services, Centers for Disease Control and Prevention, National Center for Chronic Disease Prevention and Health Promotion, and The President's Council on Physical Fitness and Sports. Physical Activity and Health: A Report of the Surgeon General. 1995.

Exercise Science in the Twenty-First Century

After completing this chapter you will be able to:

1. Describe how past research by exercise science professionals has influenced future trends in health promotion and disease prevention.

2. Identify major public and private initiatives for enhancing health promotion and disease prevention that include areas of study from exercise science.

3. Describe the impact of exercise science on sport and athletic performance enhancement.

4. Identify some future trends for exercise science in the area of sport and athletic performance enhancement.

rying to predict what will happen in the future is obviously a very difficult ask. This is especially true for the areas of study that comprise exercise science where numerous factors can have a significant influence on the direction any particular exercise science profession or related allied healthcare field may move. One only needs to examine the historic developments of exercise science to construct a vision of how the profession has been influenced by individuals, discovery, societal change, and visions for the future. Although one could probably construct a reasonably accurate vision of the future for each area of study or discipline within exercise science, it is probably more realistic to take a larger view of the direction that exercise science and related areas of study and professions will take. It is however, fairly safe to assume that many of the challenges facing exercise science and allied healthcare professionals and the opportunities derived from those challenges will be in the areas of health promotion, disease prevention and disease risk reduction, and rehabilitation from injury or illness. For a variety of reasons, each of these has become major areas of focus for state and federal governments, politicians, scholars, and professionals. In addition, because so many individuals of all ages participate in sport and athletic competition exercise science professionals will continue to play important roles in the development of new training and nutritional strategies for enhancing performance, better equipment for greater safety protection and improved performance, and more effective diagnostic, surgical, and rehabilitative programs for injured athletes.

EXERCISE SCIENCE AND HEALTH

Over the last 50 years, there has been considerable research conducted that strengthens the belief that physical activity, exercise, and physical fitness can reduce the risk of morbidity and early mortality from lifestyle-related diseases. Much support for this belief comes from research obtained from **epidemiologic studies** and long-term **clinical trials**. For example, considerable evidence about the role of physical activity and exercise in decreasing the risk for cardiovascular disease (CVD) and the identification of factors that increase the risk for heart disease comes from data collected in research projects such as the Framingham Heart Study (8), the Harvard alumni study (25,33), and the Aerobics Center Longitudinal Study (11). CVD has been the leading cause of death in the United States for the past 50 years and much of the research in this disease area has been directed toward gaining a greater understanding of the factors that contribute to the development of CVD and what lifestyle changes and behavioral interventions can reduce the risk of disease development. Table 12.1 illustrates many of those risk factors for CVD that cannot be altered and those which can be affected by intervention strategies (3).

Epidemiologic studies Research investigations conducted to identify factors that affect the health and disease of populations.
Clinical trials Comparison test of a medical intervention versus a control condition, placebo condition, or the standard medical treatment for a patient's condition.

Table 12.1	Risk Factors for CVD
Risk Factors that cannot be changed	• Increasing age • Male sex • Heredity, including race
Risk factors that can be changed or modified	• Tobacco smoke • High blood cholesterol • High blood pressure • Physical inactivity • Obesity and overweight • Diabetes mellitus

One very important risk factor that has been studied extensively by exercise science professionals is physical activity/inactivity. As a result of much research, physical inactivity is now considered a primary risk factor for coronary heart disease, similar to smoking, high blood pressure, and high serum cholesterol level (24,25,29,34). Physical inactivity is also a risk factor for several disease conditions including hypertension, diabetes mellitus, obesity, and certain forms of cancer. Conversely, higher levels of physical activity and regular exercise are beneficial for helping to maintain a healthy body weight, and strengthening muscles, bones, and joints. Figure 12.1 shows the levels of physical activity in 2003 for each state and territory in the United States. Physical activity and exercise can also enhance mental health and reduce the risk of falls in older adults (35).

Much of what we know about physical inactivity and disease risk and the role of physical activity and exercise in minimizing disease risk comes from epidemiologic studies. Information derived from these longitudinal research studies is used to guide future **health promotion** and disease prevention strategies by public and private organizations (Figure 12.2). Though not a foolproof method for predicting the future of exercise science, an examination of some of these studies can give an indication as to the continued future direction of exercise science in promoting good health and reducing the risk of disease among individuals of all ages.

> ➤ *Thinking Critically*
> *Why is research an integral component of the future of those areas that comprise exercise science?*

EPIDEMIOLOGY AND HEALTH PROMOTION

Epidemiology is the study of the causes, distribution, and control of disease in specifically defined populations. Epidemiology serves as the foundation of support for interventions made for the improvement of public health and the promotion of better health and medical care. It is a fundamental methodology of public health.

Health promotion The process of enabling people to increase their control over and improvements in their health.

Epidemiology The study of factors affecting the health and illness of populations.

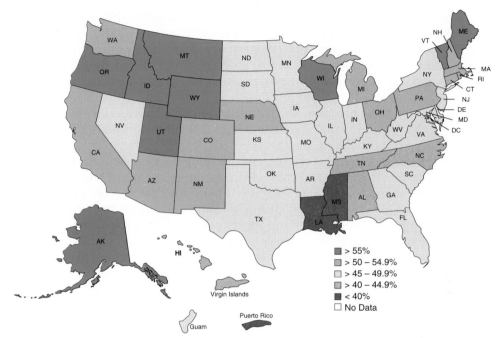

FIGURE 12.1 ▼ Physical activity levels in the United States 2003. (From Centers for Disease Control and Prevention.)

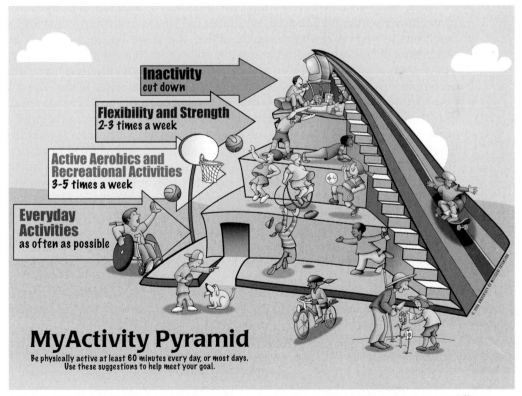

FIGURE 12.2 ▼ MyActivity pyramid for children. (From University of Missouri Extension Office.)

research, and is highly regarded in **evidence-based medicine** for identifying ris
factors for disease and determining optimal treatment approaches for use in clinic
practice. Epidemiologic research is essential for examining the efficacy of treatmen
and preventive measures, and to elucidate their relationships among the variou
factors that affect the disease condition. Information about the frequency an
prevalence of disease and health threats is essential for the development of effe
tive prevention programs and treatment interventions for disease, and for elucida
ing the environmental, behavioral, and biologic factors associated with good an
poor health conditions. Information derived from epidemiologic research is used t
inform and advance future research, develop public policy, and support initiative
designed to improve the health of large groups of people. Though there have bee
countless epidemiologic investigations performed on all types of health issues an
problems, several have provided significant information about public health that
relevant to exercise science and allied health professionals. Examples of some of th
more noteworthy epidemiologic studies include the Framingham Heart Study, th
Heritage Family Study, and the National Health and Nutrition Examination Surve
(NHANES). It is the use of information from these types of studies that helps ider
tify the future direction of healthcare and indirectly the future of many of thos
areas comprising exercise science and the allied health professions.

Framingham Heart Study

CVD is the leading cause of death and serious illness in the United States. In 1948
the Framingham Heart Study, under the direction of the National Heart Institut
(now known as the National Heart, Lung, and Blood Institute), embarked on a
ambitious project in health research. When the study began, little was know
about the general causes of heart disease and stroke, but the death rates for CVI
had been increasing steadily since the beginning of the twentieth century and ha
become an epidemic in the United States. The primary objective of the Framinghar
Heart Study was to identify the common factors or characteristics that contribut
to CVD by following its development over a long period of time in a large grou
of participants who had not yet developed overt symptoms of CVD or suffered
heart attack or stroke. The investigators recruited 5,209 men and women betwee
30 and 62 years of age from the town of Framingham, Massachusetts, and bega
the first round of extensive physical examinations and lifestyle interviews tha
would later be analyzed for common patterns related to CVD development (2
For additional detailed information about the Framingham Heart Study, pleas
see the Web page at http://www.framingham.com/heart/.

Since its inception the Framingham Heart Study has produced man
major discoveries that have helped scientists, physicians, and allied healthcar

---

Evidence-based medicine A process whereby the quality of evidence relative to the risks and benefits of treatment is determined.

Genotype Genetic makeup of an organism is distinguished from its physical characteristics.

Genetic epidemiology The study of the role of genetic factors in determining health and disease in families and in populations.

Phenotype The physical appearance of an organism as distinguished from its genetic makeup and the interaction with the environment.

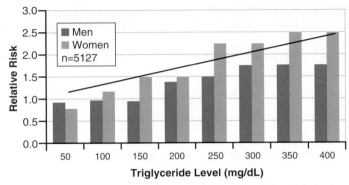

FIGURE 12.3 ▼ Relative risk of heart disease by triglyceride levels in those individuals participating in the Framingham Heart Study. (From The American Board of Family Practice. 2004;17:424–437.)

rofessionals understand the development and progression of CVD and its risk actors (2). For example, Figure 12.3 illustrates the relative risk of heart disease y increasing triglyceride levels. Some of the important milestones are included in able 12.2. The information and knowledge gained have helped generate new esearch questions for additional study; promoted drug development for the treatment of CVD; and facilitated behavioral, nutritional, and physical activity interventions for the reduction of disease risk and the promotion of recovery from CVD.

ERITAGE Family Study

he HERITAGE Family Study began in 1992 under the coordinated efforts of Claude Bouchard and other well-known scholars such as James K. Skinner, rthur S. Leon, Jack H. Wilmore, and D. C. Rao. The justification for conducting he study included the following components:

Regular aerobic exercise has favorable effects on the risk profile for CVD and type 2 diabetes.
There are considerable individual differences in the response to regular exercise.
Genes are thought to play an important role in determining the general benefits derived from participating in regular physical activity.

The primary objectives of the Heritage Family Study was to examine the role f the human **genotype** in the cardiovascular and metabolic responses to aerobic xercise training and the changes brought about by regular exercise for several CVD and diabetes risk factors (14). There have been three phases to the study. hase I involved the testing and exercise training of 742 subjects. Responses of ardiovascular and metabolic variables to submaximal and maximal exercise were nade prior to and following exercise training. Phase 2 included an investigation f **genetic epidemiology** issues pertaining to exercise **phenotypes** and CVD nd type 2 diabetes. Phase 3 included the expansion and further refinement of he search for genes and mutations affecting cardiorespiratory endurance and CVD and type 2 diabetes risk factors as well as their response to regular exercise 6). For further information about The HERITAGE Family Study, please see the Web page at http://www.pbrc.edu/heritage/Home.htm.

Table 12.2	Milestones in the Framingham Heart Study (2)
YEAR	SIGNIFICANT MILESTONE
1948	Start of the Framingham Heart Study
1960	Cigarette smoking found to increase the risk of heart disease
1961	Cholesterol level, blood pressure, and electrocardiogram abnormalities found to increase the risk of heart disease
1967	Physical activity found to reduce the risk of heart disease and obesity found to increase the risk of heart disease
1970	High blood pressure found to increase the risk of stroke
1971	Framingham Offspring Study initiated to assess the familial and genetic factors as determinants of coronary heart disease
1974	Overview of diabetes, its complications, and association to the development of CVD described
1976	Meno pause found to increase the risk of heart disease
1978	Psychosocial factors found to affect heart disease
1981	Major report issued on the relationship of diet and heart disease
1987	High blood cholesterol levels found to correlate directly with the risk of death in young men; Fibrinogen found to increase the risk of heart disease; Estrogen replacement therapy found to reduce the risk of hip fractures in postmenopausal women
1988	High levels of HDL cholesterol found to reduce risk of death; Association of type "A" behavior with heart disease reported; Isolated systolic hypertension found to increase the risk of heart disease; Cigarette smoking found to increase risk of stroke
1990	Homocysteine (an amino acid) found to be a possible risk factor for heart disease
1994	Lipoprotein (a) found as a possible risk factor for heart disease; Apolipoprotein E found to be possible risk factor for heart disease
1995	OMNI Study of Minorities starts.
1997	Cumulative effects of smoking and high cholesterol on the risk for atherosclerosis reported
1998	Work identifying a gene (angiotensin-converting enzyme deletion/insertion polymorphism) associated with hypertension in Framingham men published
2002	Excess body weight/obesity linked with an increased risk of heart failure; BMI (Body mass index) to be an independent risk factor
2002	Third Generation Study enrolls 3,900 grandchildren of the Framingham Heart Study's original enrollees; Key goals are to identify new risk factors for heart, lung, and blood diseases; identify genes that contribute to good health and to the development of heart, lung, and blood disease; and to develop new imaging tests that can detect very early stages of coronary atherosclerosis in otherwise healthy adults.
2003	Likelihood of heart attack three times greater in individuals with common genetic variation in an estrogen receptor.
2004	Having a parent with a CVD history doubles the personal risk of the disease.
2005	An increase of up to 45% for risk of heart attack, stroke, or arterial disease may occur in middle-aged people with a sibling who suffered a similar cardiovascular event.

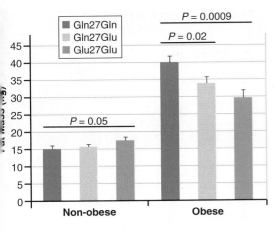

FIGURE 12.4 ▼ Association between the gene polymorphism and the total fat mass in nonobese and obese white men in the Heritage Family Study. (With permission from Garenc C, Pe'russe L, Chagnon YC, et al. Effects of 2-adrenergic receptor gene variants on adiposity: The HERITAGE family study. *Obes Res.* 2003;11:612–8.)

To date, the results from the study have yielded some significant findings about the relationships between genetic factors, cardiorespiratory endurance, risk factors for CVD, and type 2 diabetes. For example, genetic factors explain about 40% of the individual variations in cardiorespiratory fitness (13). There was however, large variation in the response to exercise training. For example, there was about 2.5 times more variance between families than within families for the improvement observed in cardiorespiratory fitness (13). Furthermore, it appears that one set of genes influenced the initial level of cardiorespiratory fitness and another set of genes influenced the response to exercise training (30). Also, it appears that familial/genetic factors are more important in determining the amount and distribution of subcutaneous body fat than in the response to exercise training (27). Figure 12.4 shows the association between the gene polymorphism and the total fat mass in nonobese and obese white men in the Heritage Family Study. The information gained from this study has led to countless other investigations of the role of genetics in health and disease risk reduction.

National Health and Nutrition Examination Survey

The goal of NHANES is to assess the health and nutritional status of adults and children in the United States. To achieve this goal, a complex series of statistical techniques are used to obtain a nationwide sample of the population. The country is divided into geographic areas, called primary sampling units, which are then combined to form strata, and each strata is then divided into a series of neighborhoods. From these neighborhoods, households are chosen at random, and inhabitants of the households are interviewed to determine eligibility for participation in the survey. Theoretically, each selected survey participant represents approximately 50,000 other U.S. residents (1).

Once a household has been identified through the sampling procedure, an interviewer conducts an initial in-house interview to determine study eligibility. Eligible participants are scheduled for an in-person appointment at a mobile examination center. Figure 12.5 shows a mobile examination center used in the NHANES. The mobile examination center consists of four large trailers that contain all of the equipment and personnel necessary to perform the following evaluations: (a) A physical examination; (b) Dental examination; (c) Blood and urine specimen collection; and (d) Personal interviews to collect information about nutrition, alcohol and tobacco

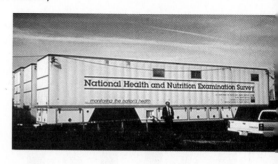

FIGURE 12.5 ▼ A mobile examination center used in the NHANES.

use, sexual experience, mental illness, and assessments of cognitive development and learning achievement (1). For further information about NHANES, please see the Web page at http://www.cdc.gov/nchs/nhanes.htm.

Since its inception, NHANES has produced a wealth of valuable information that has helped improve the health and healthcare of the United States population. Results of NHANES benefit the people of the United States in many ways. Facts about the distribution of health problems and risk factors in the population give researchers important clues to the causes of disease. Information collected from the current survey is compared with information from previous surveys. This allows health planners to detect the extent various health problems and risk factors have changed in the United States population over time. By identifying the healthcare needs of the population, government agencies and private organizations can establish policies and plan research, education, and health promotion programs that help improve present health status and will prevent future health problems (1). Examples of some of the important accomplishments derived from NHANES are listed below:

> ➤ **Thinking Critically**
>
> *In what ways will some of the more significant longitudinal epidemiologic research studies contribute to identifying the future trends in exercise science?*

- Past surveys have provided data to create the growth charts used nationally by pediatricians to evaluate children's growth.
- Blood data were instrumental in developing policy to eliminate lead from gasoline and food and soft drink cans.
- Overweight prevalence figures have led to the proliferation of programs emphasizing healthy weight management, stimulated additional research, and provided a means to track trends in obesity.
- Data have continued to indicate that undiagnosed diabetes is a significant problem in the United States.

The continuation of NHANES contributes to our knowledge about health and provides for new initiatives including (1):

- Determining if there is a need to change vitamin and mineral fortification regulations for the Nation's food supply.
- National programs to reduce hypertension and cholesterol continue to depend on NHANES data to steer education and prevention programs toward those at risk and to measure success in curtailing risk factors associated with heart disease.
- New measures of lung function will further the understanding of respiratory disease and better describe the burden of asthma in the United States.

USING PAST INFORMATION TO IMPROVE FUTURE HEALTH

Information that is collected from epidemiologic research studies can be used to support subsequent research, develop healthcare plans and policies to guide future decision making, and allow for recommendations of programs to enhance the health and wellness of individuals. For example, the endorsement of the health benefits obtained from physical activity and exercise by the U.S. Surgeon General in 1995 was a significant milestone in the promotion of physical activity and exercise for enhancing health and reducing diseased risk within individuals. The Surgeon General serves as the chief health educator for the United States by providing Americans with the best scientific information available on how to improve their health and reduce the risk of illness and injury. Using a structured process, a panel of experts and scholars reviewed past research in physical activity and health and developed a set of conclusions based on that information. In 1995, the Surgeon General's Office issued a report that highlighted the positive effects of physical activity on the health of the musculoskeletal, cardiovascular, respiratory, and endocrine systems including a reduced risk of premature mortality and reduced risks of coronary heart disease, hypertension, colon cancer, and diabetes mellitus. The report also suggested that regular participation in physical activity appears to reduce depression and anxiety, improve mood, and enhance the ability to perform daily tasks throughout the life span. Recommendations for the appropriate amount of physical activity and exercise helped establish the standards for using exercise to assist in the treatment of diseased individuals (26). The publication of this landmark report is an example of how past research can be used to assist in making new policy recommendations and decisions.

Another example of using research to support health promotion initiatives is the Federal Government's **Healthy People Program**. The Healthy People Program (Figure 12.6) has been in existence since the latter part of the twentieth century. The Healthy People 2020 initiative consists of a set of health objectives for the United States to achieve during the second decade of the twenty-first century. It is intended to be used by individuals, states, communities, professional organizations, and others to help them develop programs to improve health. Healthy People 2020 builds on the public health initiatives pursued over the previous three decades. The 1979 Surgeon General's Report, *Healthy People* (36), and *Healthy People 2000: National Health Promotion and Disease Prevention Objectives* (23) established national health objectives and served as the basis for the development of the state and local community plans. Like its predecessors, *Healthy People 2010* (http://www.healthypeople.gov/) was developed through a broad consultation process, built on the best scientific knowledge, and designed to measure goals and outcomes over time (5). The next set of health promotion initiatives including goals, objectives, and action plan for *Healthy People 2020*, can be found at http://www.healthypeople.gov/.

Healthy People Program A program administered by the United States Department of Health and Human Services to improve the health of the nation's population.

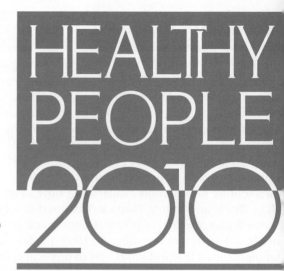

FIGURE 12.6 ▼ Healthy People 2010 and 2020 programs are designed to enhance the health of our nation's population.

WHAT WILL THE FUTURE BRING?

The health of the people of the United States is a critically important issue. It is clear that physical activity and exercise play an important role in promoting good overall individual health. It is important however, to not forget about the broader impact of health and disease conditions. Individuals who are not healthy have an increased risk of premature morbidity and mortality, poor quality of life, increased medical and healthcare expenses, and lost time from work. As a society, the poor health of many Americans is creating an economic burden, not only on the individual citizens of the United States, but also on businesses to provide health insurance, and on the healthcare systems of the state and federal governments to provide quality healthcare to everyone. For example, in 2005 the total national healthcare expenditures rose two times the rate of inflation (15) and was 16% of the **gross domestic product**. These rising costs are creating considerable economic burden on our nation's healthcare system. Healthcare expenditures are expected to rise to 20% of the gross domestic product by 2015 (12). Continued cost increases of this magnitude cannot be endured by individuals, business, and federal and state governments. It is clear that a cooperative effort must be made among all stakeholders to address the health issues of our nation. It is without question, that exercise science and allied health professionals can and must play an important role in this effort to solve these problems. Past and current information must be used to guide future research programs, program development and policy initiatives and advocacy. The scope of importance ranges from developing and implementing the most effective physical activity programs for individuals across the lifespan to being an integral part of the comprehensive healthcare team for treating and rehabilitating individuals from disease and illness.

Gross domestic product The total market value of all the goods and services produced within the borders of the United States during a specified period, usually one calendar year.

uture Research

ederal and state governments and private organizations and foundations play a vital le in supporting future research on health and healthcare issues. Exercise science rofessionals will continue to play an active role in research as greater insight into ow improvements in individual health, the overall health of Americans, and effective healthcare is delivered. Research into broad program initiatives will be central enhancing the understanding of how to develop the most cost effective and efficacious treatments. Additional research will need to continue to occur at the cellular nd molecular levels as we attempt to further understand the role of genetics and nolecular responses to physical activity and exercise in both healthy and disease onditions. A better understanding of what genes are affected by lifestyle behaviors uch as nutritional intake, physical activity, and exercise will provide key knowledge or the development of safe and effective prevention and treatment programs. arge-scale clinical trials and smaller efficacy studies will be essential for creating knowledge base for advancing both the individual and public health efforts of ublic and private organizations. Some prospective areas of principal future research re highlighted in Table 12.3. Each of these areas will require a coordinated effort mong exercise science and allied health professionals to develop sound research udies that answer our most important questions about the health and healthcare.

Table 12.3	Future Research in Health and Disease Risk Reduction
EXERCISE SCIENCE AREA	**POTENTIAL RESEARCH AREAS**
Exercise physiology	• Genetic influence on disease risk and health • Mechanisms involved with improvements in physiologic function
Clinical exercise physiology	• Role of exercise and reduction of disease risk including CVD, cancer, diabetes, hypertension, obesity, and metabolic syndrome • Promotion of effective rehabilitation programs for diseased individuals
Athletic training and sports medicine	• Development of effective treatment and rehabilitation strategies for individuals injured during participation in physical activity and exercise • Further development of medical interventions that enhance physical activity in health and disease conditions
Exercise and sport nutrition	• Role of nutrition in health promotion • Efficacy of specialty diets in weight management programs
Exercise and sport psychology	• Development of effective strategies for promoting behavioral change and enhancing exercise adherence • Role of behavior in promoting physical activity and exercise
Motor behavior	• Understanding how individuals with differing levels of ability or development can effectively participate in exercise • How does neurophysiologic functioning affect health and/or prevent disease
Clinical and sport biomechanics	• Developing effective movement patterns for individuals with biomechanic limitations • Prevention of injuries and rehabilitation

Program Development

As exercise science and allied health professionals work to enhance the health and reduce the disease risk of the clients and patients they work with, it will be important to expand effective programs and develop new and innovative intervention programs and examine the efficacy of those interventions. Exercise science professionals must and will play a major role in the implementation and advancement of programs. Effective program development and execution must occur at both the national and local levels. As a result, exercise science professionals will be at the forefront of program delivery working with clients and patients of all ages in diverse healthcare settings including private practice, hospitals, fitness centers, outpatient clinics, and residential care facilities. Numerous private and public organizations and businesses will continue to develop and implement programs at the local level for enhancing health and promoting disease risk reduction. For example, employee health and well-being programs are being effectively used to improve the health of working individuals and reducing healthcare costs for both individuals and business (Figure 12.7). Governmental agencies such as the Centers for Disease Control and Prevention and the President's Council on Physical Fitness and Sports, as well as state and local health departments will continue to work with organizations such as the American Heart Association and the American College of Sports Medicine to develop and implement programs to improve the health of individuals. For example, Exercise is Medicine is a national health promotion program that is a combined initiative of the American Medical Association and the American College of Sports Medicine. This overarching vision of this program is to make physical

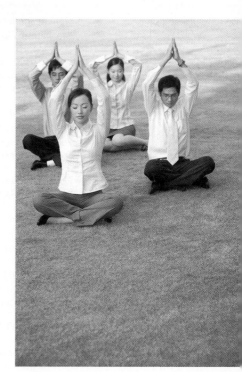

FIGURE 12.7 ▼ Employee fitness programs can be used to reduce healthcare costs. (Photo courtesy of IMAGEMORE Co, Ltd./Getty Images.)

:tivity and exercise a standard part of a disease prevention and medical treatment aradigm in the United States (4). As a primary goal, Exercise is Medicine desires 1at "physical activity be considered by all healthcare providers as a vital sign in very patient visit, and that patients are effectively counseled and referred as to 1eir physical activity and health needs, thus leading to overall improvement in the ublic's health and long-term reduction in healthcare cost" (4). Exercise is Medi- 1e provides physicians, the public, health and fitness professionals, and the media 'ith important and useful knowledge and information about the role of physical :tivity and exercise in the promotion of good health. Some examples of other 1rrent programs for the promotion of good health and disease risk reduction are sted in Table 12.4. For additional information about program initiatives, you are 1couraged to visit the Web sites of the various governmental, private, and profes- onal organizations that have as a mission the goal to promote good health. This 'ill be a good way to gauge some of the future directions of exercise science.

olicy Initiatives and Advocacy

ederal and state governments and private organizations promote and support olicy initiatives designed to enhance health and reduce disease risk. The evelopment of sound policies includes having an infrastructure that provides

Table 12.4	Programs Designed to Enhance Health and Reduce Disease Risk
AGENCY/ORGANIZATION	**PROGRAM INITIATIVE**
Centers for Disease Control and Prevention	• Coordinated School Health Program • School Health Index • CDC's State-based Nutrition and Physical Activity Program to Prevent Obesity and Other Chronic Diseases
American Heart Association	• Choose to move program • The Heart of Diabetes • Power to end stroke • Cholesterol low down
American College of Sports Medicine	• Exercise is Medicine
Robert Wood Johnson Foundation	• Healthy Schools Program • Active Living Research • Healthy Eating by Design
Directors of Health Promotion and Education	• School Employee Wellness: A Guide for Protecting the Assets of our Nations Schools
American Alliance for Health, Physical Education, Recreation and Dance	• Physical Best Program • Backyards and Beyond
American Diabetes Association	• Education Recognition Program
American Dietetic Association	• National Nutrition Month

Table 12.5	Policy Initiatives and Advocacy Efforts in Exercise Science
AGENCY/ORGANIZATION	**POLICY/ADVOCACY INITIATIVE**
American Heart Association	• Heart disease and stroke: you are the cure
American College of Sports Medicine	• Science Partner of the President's Council on Physical Fitness and Sport
National Association of State Boards of Education	• Fit, Healthy, and Ready to Learn: A School Health Policy Guide
American Dietetic Association	• Policy Initiatives and Advocacy Report – On the Pulse
American Diabetes Association	• Diabetes Advocacy Action Center
United States Department of Agriculture Food and Nutrition Division	• National School Lunch Program
Institute of Medicine	• Nutrition Standards for Food in Schools
The Obesity Society	• Weight Bias Task Force Policy Statement

➤ *Thinking Critically*

How will increased knowledge about the human genome and molecular biology contribute to developing new and effective strategies for treating lifestyle-related diseases?

sophisticated data collection and analysis, professional guidance, funding for the initiation of the policies, and an evaluation to assess the effectiveness of the policies. Professional and private organizations also use advocacy efforts to support the policy initiatives. Examples of some policy initiatives and advocacy efforts in exercise science are contained in Table 12.5.

EXERCISE SCIENCE AND SPORT AND ATHLETIC COMPETITION

Performance enhancement is critical for helping individuals participating in sport and athletic competition reach their highest potential. Individuals from beginner to professional athletes are continuously looking for ways to improve practice and competition and game performance. Performance enhancement can take the form of improving individual and team strategy and movement skills, as well as conducting a comprehensive assessment of physical and psychological abilities and developing an individualized training prescription and nutritional program. Performance enhancement also includes aspects of mental preparation and training, the reduction of injury risk, and the recovery from illness and injury.

Exercise science professionals have long played an important role in improving sport and athletic performance. From the early work of Coleman R. Griffith (1893–1966), who in 1925 established the first Athletic Research Laboratory at the University of Illinois (37) to the recent work of Edward F. Coyle with seven-time Tour de France Champion Lance Armstrong (17) exercise science rofessionals have been working to enhance individual and team sport and hletic performance. Professional organizations such as the American College of ports Medicine, the National Athletic Trainers Association, the National Strength nd Conditioning Association, and the Association r Applied Sport Psychology have been instrumen- l in advancing the knowledge base of physiologic, sychological, nutritional, and rehabilitative aspects f performance enhancement. Though it is difficult to redict where the future of exercise science will move sport and athletic performance enhancement, it is fe to say that exercise science professionals will play important role in that future.

> ➤ *Thinking Critically*
>
> *Why should athletes and coaches rely on the knowledge of exercise science professionals for enhancing individual and team sport and athletic performance?*

WHAT WILL THE FUTURE BRING?

Many of the areas of study comprising exercise science have a component focused n improving performance in sport and athletic competition. It is without ques- on that the exercise science professionals working in exercise physiology, ath- tic training and sports medicine, sport nutrition, sport psychology, and motor ehavior and biomechanics will use the knowledge gained from prior research formulate future trends of study. Sporting events and athletic competition quire athletes of all ages to perform activities that last from a few seconds to veral hours and sometimes days. From a single weightlifting event (Figure 12.8) the one-hundred-meter sprint (Figure 12.9) to the Iron Man Triathlon igure 12.10), athletes are required to coordinate the various systems and compo- ents of the mind and body into a coordinated effort that results in their best indi- dual performance. Whether it is playing competitive tennis (Figure 12.11), driving race car (Figure 12.12), or climbing a mountain (Figure 12.13), the psychologi- l and physiologic components of the body must optimally function together so at individual performance is maximized. Team sports (Figure 12.14) must have ch individual athlete performing at his or her physical and psychological best

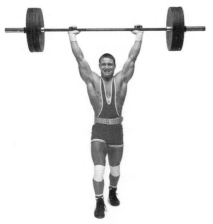

FIGURE 12.8 ▼ Weightlifting. (Photo courtesy of Photodisc/Jack Mann/Getty Images.)

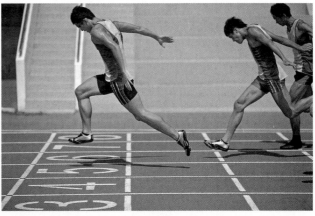

FIGURE 12.9 ▼ One-hundred-meter sprint. (Photo courtesy of IMAGEMORE Co, Ltd./Getty Images.)

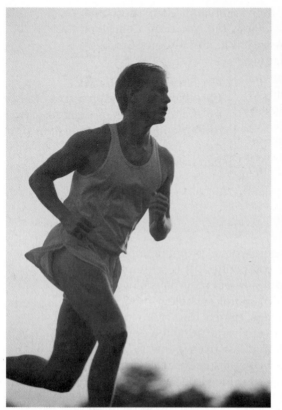

FIGURE 12.10 ▼ Iron Man Triathlon. (Photo courtesy of Comstock Images/Getty Images.)

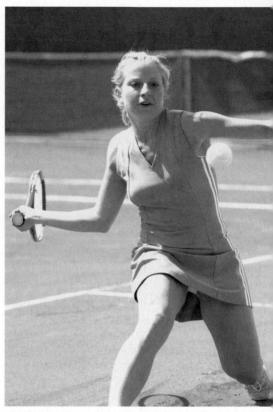

FIGURE 12.11 ▼ Competitive tennis. (Photo courtesy of Score by Aflo/Getty Images.)

to have a successful performance. However, to examine performance during th
sporting event or competition only provides part of the picture. Athletes partic
pate in regular training and practice for numerous hours each week often for yea
at a time to maximize their performance during a competition that sometim
lasts only a few seconds. During training, athletes refine their movements throug
repetitive practice and adjustments to their biomechanical movement patterns. T
be best prepared for rigorous practice and difficult competition it is imperative th
athletes have optimal nutritional intake. Appropriate macronutrient and micr
nutrient consumption allows athletes to meet the energy demands of training, a
well as enhance the function of the various systems of the body that are importar
for successful performance in sport and athletic competition. When injured, atl
letes rely on athletic trainers and sports medicine personnel to make an accura
diagnosis, develop an effective medical intervention, and implement an effectiv
rehabilitation strategy so that they may return to competition quickly.

Plyometric training A type of exercise training designed to produce fast, powerful movements, and improve the functions of the neuromuscular system for the purposes of improving sport performance.

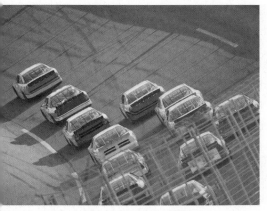

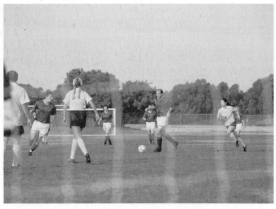

FIGURE 12.12 ▼ Race car driving. (Photo courtesy of Digital Vision/David Madison/Getty Images.)

FIGURE 12.14 ▼ Team sport performance. (Photo courtesy of Photodisc/Ryan McVay/Getty Images.)

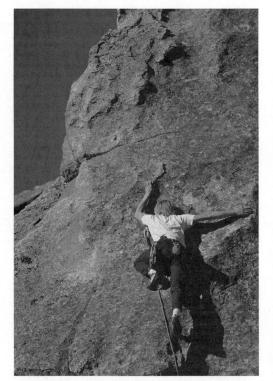

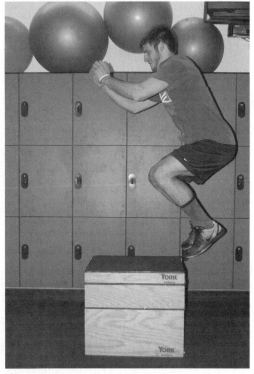

FIGURE 12.13 ▼ Mountain climbing. (Photo courtesy of Photodisc/Karl Weatherly/Getty Images.)

FIGURE 12.15 ▼ Plyometric training.

As long as individuals are participating in sport and athletic events, exercise science professionals will play an important role in assisting athlete's in maximizing their performance. Over the years the various disciplines of exercise science have been instrumental in advancing our understanding of performance and developing new strategies for training, enhancing equipment for competition, and providing insights into the best nutritional intake for optimal performance. For example, recent advances in exercise science have led to the use of **plyometric training**

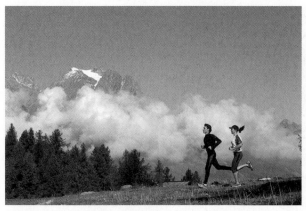

FIGURE 12.16 ▼ High-altitude training. (Photo courtesy of Digital Vision/AGENCE ZOOM/Getty Images.)

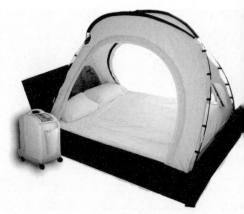

FIGURE 12.17 ▼ Simulated high altitude tent. (Photo courtesy of Hypoxico, Inc.)

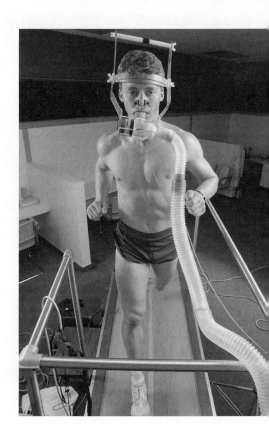

FIGURE 12.18 ▼ Genetics plays an important role in successful sports performance. (Photo courtesy of Stockbyte/Getty Images.)

Female athlete triad A combination of three different disorders that affect female athletes: osteoporosis, eating disorders, and amenorrhea.

High-altitude training The practice of athletes living and performing exercise at high altitudes with the expectation of an improved sport performance at lower altitudes.

Figure 12.15) for improving muscle power output (28), a greater understanding of issues surrounding the **female athlete triad** (7). Recently there has been considerable interest in **high altitude training** for enhancing endurance performance (10). This has led to conducting training programs at high altitude (Figure 12.16) and the development of a simulated altitude tent (Figure 12.17) for those individuals who do not live at a geographically high elevation.

Exercise science professionals have been instrumental in enhancing sport and athletic performance through the development and evaluation of equipment (18,22) and strategies for training (31) and competition (16), nutritional supplements (32), pharmacologic agents (39), psychological strategies (9), and the evaluation (19,20) and rehabilitation of injured athletes (21). Recently, exercise science professionals have become more interested in the role that molecular biology can play in identifying the different genes that are responsible for predicting athletic performance (Figure 12.18) (38). Table 12.6 provides examples of possible future trends in exercise science that are centered on the enhancement of sport and athletic performance.

> ➤ *Thinking Critically*
> *How can exercise science professionals continue to contribute to enhancing individual and team performance in sport and athletic competition?*

Table 12.6	Potential Trends of Future Sport and Athletic Performance Enhancement in Exercise Science
EXERCISE SCIENCE AREA	**FUTURE TRENDS**
Exercise physiology	• Identifying the mechanisms of legal and illegal human growth–promoting agents • Further refinement of optimal training programs for individuals of different genetic profiles, different sports, and different ages
Athletic training and sports medicine	• Identification of techniques and signals to improve the detection of injuries and the prevention of potential injuries • Improvement of treatment modalities including enhanced medical and surgical techniques that will improve individual outcomes following an injury
Exercise and sport nutrition	• Refinement of appropriate macronutrient and micronutrient intakes for performance enhancement of different sports and different age groups • Clarification of the role of nutritional supplements in performance enhancement
Exercise and sport psychology	• Identification of effective performance enhancement techniques for individuals of various ages and their coaches • Increased utilization by athletes of all ages
Motor behavior	• Further refinement of effective motor learning and control strategies • Continued clarification of optimal practice strategies
Clinical and sport biomechanics	• Improvement of movement patterns for sport techniques • Development of equipment that will enhance performance

SUMMARY

- Much of the information used to predict future health promotion and disease risk reduction trends in exercise science comes from longitudinal epidemiologic research.
- Future trends in health promotion and disease risk reduction will be in the areas of research, program development, and policy initiatives.
- The enhancement of sport and athletic performance requires all areas of exercise science to provide an integrated and coordinated effort to improve the psychological and physiologic components that affect performance.
- Future trends in sport and athletic competition will most certainly be centered on the molecular and genetic factors that influence performance.

FOR REVIEW

1. Define the following terms:
   a. Epidemiological
   b. Longitudinal
   c. Clinical trial

2. What was the primary purpose of the Framingham Heart Study?

3. List five important outcomes of the Framingham Heart Study that help guide the current recommendations for reducing disease risk.

4. What is the primary purpose of the continuous NHANES?

5. What was the primary rationale for conducting the Heritage Family Study?

6. Describe the primary conclusion of the 1995 United States Surgeon General's report on Health Promotion and Disease Prevention.

7. What is the primary purpose of the Healthy People 2010 and 2020 programs?

8. Describe the relationships among research, program development, and policy initiatives as they relate to the future of exercise science.

9. How might each of the following exercise science areas contribute to enhancing individual sport and athletic performance:
   a. Exercise physiology
   b. Athletic training and sports medicine
   c. Sport nutrition
   d. Sport psychology
   e. Motor behavior
   f. Sport biomechanics

REFERENCES

1. Centers for Disease Control and Prevention National Center for Health Statistics Website [Internet]. Available from: http://www cdc gov/nchs/ 2007.

2. Framingham Heart Study Website [Internet]. Available from: http://www framinghamheartstudy org/ 2007.

3. American Heart Association Diseases and Conditions Web Site [Internet]. Available from: http://www americanheart org 2008.

4. Exercise is Medicine Website [Internet]. Available from: http://www exerciseismedicine org/ 2008.

5. Healthy People 2010 Website [Internet]. Available from: http://www healthypeople gov/ 2008.

6. The HERITAGE Family Study Website [Internet]. Available from: http://www pbrc edu/Heritage/ 2008.

7. American College of Sports Medicine. The female athlete triad. *Med Sci Sports Exerc*. 2007;29:i–x.

8. Ashley FW, Kannel WB. Relation of weight change to changes in atherogenic traits: The Framingham Study. *J Chronic Dis*. 1974;27:103–14.

9. Barwood MJ, Thelwell RC, Tipton MJ. Psychological skills training improves exercise performance in the heat. *Med Sci Sports Exerc*. 2008;40:387–96.

10. Beidleman BA, Muza SR, Fulco CS, et al. Seven intermittent exposures to altitude improves exercise performance at 4300 m. *Med Sci Sports Exerc*. 2008;40:141–8.

11. Blair SN, Kohl HW, Paffenbarger RS, Clark DG, Cooper KH, Gibbons LW. Physical fitness and all-cause mortality. *JAMA*. 1989;262:2395–401.

12. Borger C, Smith S, Truffer C, et al. Health spending projections through 2015: Changes on the horizon. *Health Aff*. 2006;25:w61–w73.

13. Bouchard C, An P, Rice T, et al. Familial aggregation of VO_{2max} response to exercise training: results from the HERITAGE Family Study. *J Appl Physiol*. 1999;87:1003–8.

14. Bouchard C, Leon AS, Rao DC, Skinner JS, Wilmore JH, Gagnon J. The HERITAGE family study. Aims, design, and measurement protocol. *Med Sci Sports Exerc*. 1995;27:721–9.

15. Catlin A, Cowan C, Heffler S, Washington B. National Health Spending in 2005. *Health Aff*. 2006;26:142–53.

16. Chatard JC, Wilson B. Effect of fastskin suits on performance, drag, and energy cost of swimming. *Med Sci Sports Exerc*. 2008;40:1149–54.

17. Coyle EF. Improved muscular efficiency displayed as Tour de France champion matures. *J Appl Physiol*. 2005;98:2191–6.

18. Curtis CK, Laudner KG, McLoda TA, McCaw ST. The role of shoe design in ankle sprain rates among collegiate basketball players. *J Athl Train*. 2008;43:230–3.

19. Gluck GS, Bendo JA, Spivak JM. The lumbar spine and low back pain in golf: A literature review of swing biomechanics and injury prevention. *Spine J*. 2008;8:778–88.

20. Guskiewicz KM, Marshall SW, Bailes J, et al. Association between recurrent concussion and late-life cognitive impairment in retired professional football players. *Neurosurgery*. 2005;57:719–26.

21. Kuster MS, Spalinger E, Blanksby BA, Gachter A. Endurance sports after total knee replacement: A biomechanical investigation. *Med Sci Sports Exerc*. 2000;32:721–4.

22. Luttrell MD, Potteiger JA. Effects of powercranks training on cardiovascular fitness and cycling efficiency. *J Strength Cond Res*. 2003;17:785–91.

23. National Center for Health Statistics. *Healthy People 2000 Final Review*. 76–641469. Hyattsville (MD): Public Health Service; 2001.

24. Paffenbarger RS, Hale WE. Work activity and coronary heart mortality. *N Engl J Med*. 1975;292:545–50.

25. Paffenbarger RS, Hyde RT, Wing AL, Hsieh CC. Physical activity, all-cause mortality, and longevity of college alumni. *N Engl J Med*. 1986;314:605–13.

26. Pate RR, Pratt M, Blair SN, et al. A recommendation from the Centers for Disease Control and Prevention and the American College of Sports Medicine. *JAMA*. 1995;273:402–7.

27. Perusse L, Rice T, Province ME, et al. Familial aggregation of amount and distribution of subcutaneous fat and their responses to exercise training in the HERITAGE Family Study. *Obes Res*. 2000; 8:140–50.

28. Potteiger JA, Lockwood RH, Haub MD, et al. Muscle power and fiber characteristics following 8 weeks of plyometric training. *J Strength Cond Res*. 1999;13:275–9.

29. Powell KE, Thompson PD, Caspersen CJ, Kendrick JS. Physical activity and the incidence of coronary heart disease. *Annu Rev Public Health*. 1987;8:253–87.

30. Rankinen T, Perusse L, Borecki IB, et al. The Na + -K + -ATPase alpha 2 gene and trainability of cardiorespiratory endurance: The HERITAGE Family Study. *J Appl Physiol*. 2000;88:346–51.

31. Rodriguez FA, Truijens MJ, Townsend NE, Stray-Gundersen J, Gore CJ, Levine BD. Performance of runners and swimmers after four weeks of intermittent hypobaric hypoxic exposure plus sea level training. *J Appl Physiol*. 2007;103:1523–35.

32. Schroeder CA, Potteiger JA, Randall J, et al. The effects of creatine dietary supplementation on anterior compartment pressure in the lower leg during rest and following exercise. *Clin J Sports Med*. 2001;11:87–95.

33. Sesso HD, Paffenbarger RS, Lee IM. Physical activity and coronary heart disease in men: The Harvard Alumni Health Study. *Circulation*. 2000;102: 975–80.

34. Siscovick DS, Weiss NS, Fletcher RH, Schoenbach VJ, Wagner EH. Habitual vigorous exercise and primary cardiac arrest: Effect of other risk factors on the relationship. *J Chronic Dis*. 1984;37:625–31.

35. U.S. Department of Health and Human Services, Centers for Disease Control and Prevention, National Center for Chronic Disease Prevention and Health Promotion, and The President's Council on Physical Fitness and Sports. Physical Activity and Health: A Report of the SurgeonGeneral. 1995.

36. U.S. Department of Health, Education and Welfare. Healthy People: The Surgeon General's Report on Health Promotion and Disease Prevention. 79–55071. Public Health Service, Office of the Assistant Secretary for Health and the Surgeon General. 1979.

37. Vealey RS. Smocks and jocks outside the box: The paradigmatic evolution of sport and exercise psychology. *Quest.* 2006;58:128–59.

38. Yang N, MacArthur DG, Gulbin JP, et al. ACTN genotype of associated with human elite athletic performance. *Am J Hum Genet.* 2003;73:627–31.

39. Yesalis CE. *Anabolic Steroids in Sport and Exercise.* Champaign (IL): Human Kinetics; 2000.

Index

Page numbers in *italics* denote figures; those followed by a 't' denote tables.

413

RRS0911